Praise for *Healthy Herbs*

"*An extensive collection of concise, practical applications of herbal medicine that is useful to anyone. Both practitioners and the general public will love this book.*"

~Michael T. Murray, N.D., one of the leading researchers
in natural health, faculty member of Bastyr University and author of
over twenty books, including *Encyclopedia of Nutritional Supplements.*

"*It is good to see a new herb book on the Canadian market that is both credible and user friendly. Linda Woolven and Ted Snider have been able to walk the fine balance of giving enough new information to make this new volume truly useful for the general public, but not so technical that it is hard to read. I highly recommend this book as a good addition for anybody's bookshelf, no matter if herbal medicine is a casual affair or a serious pastime. This book can replace many hours of research for herbal enthusiasts.*"

~ Terry Willard ClH Ph.D., author of several books on herbs,
including *Encyclopedia of Herbs* and *Textbook of Advanced Herbology*. He
is also president of the Canadian Association of Herbal Practitioners
and director of Wild Rose College of Natural Healing.

"*This is a wonderful little herb book! The authors have taken the wisdom of herbal lore, blended it with clinical trials and scientific studies, and presented it all in simple, easy-to-read language. There's just enough information about each plant to be informative but not overwhelming. Rather like a well laid out herb garden, it's richly abundant with what's essential about herbalism.*"

~ Rosemary Gladstar, herbalist and author of
Herbal Healing for Women and the *Gladstar's Family Herbal.*

"*This is one of the most thorough and easy-to-use guides to herbal supplements available today. It provides clear and reliable information on safe and effective use of common herbs, including potential drug interactions.*"

~ Donald Brown, N.D., is a leading authority on evidence-based
herbalism, author of *Herbal Prescriptions for Health and Healing* and
coauthor of *The Natural Pharmacy*, 2nd edition, and *The A-Z Guide to
Drug-Herb-Vitamin Intractions.*

Healthy Herbs

Your Everyday Guide to Medicinal Herbs and Their Use

Linda Woolven, M.H., C.Ac. and Ted Snider

Fitzhenry & Whiteside

Healthy Herbs
Copyright © 2006 Linda Woolven and Ted Snider
First published in the United States 2007

Fitzhenry and Whiteside Limited
195 Allstate Parkway, Markham, Ontario L3R 4T8

In the United States:
311 Washington Street, Brighton, Massachusetts 02135

www.fitzhenry.ca godwit@fitzhenry.ca

Fitzhenry & Whiteside acknowledges with thanks the Canada Council for the Arts, and the Ontario Arts Council for their support of our publishing program. We acknowledge the financial support of the Government of Canada through the Book Publishing Industry Development Program (BPIDP) for our publishing activities.

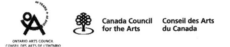

Library and Archives Canada Cataloguing in Publication
Woolven, Linda
Healthy herbs : your everyday guide to medicinal herbs
and their use / Linda Woolven & Ted Snider.
Includes bibliographical references and index.
ISBN-13: 978-1-55041-329-8
ISBN-10: 1-55041-329-5
1. Herbs—Therapeutic aspects. I. Snider, Ted II. Title.
RM666.H33W665 2006   615'.321   C2006-904454-6

United States Cataloguing-in-Publication Data
Woolven, Linda.
Healthy herbs : your everyday guide to medicinal herbs and their use /
Linda Woolven and Ted Snider.
[240] p. : cm.
Includes index.
ISBN-10: 1-55041-329-5 (pbk.)
ISBN-13: 978-155041-329-8 (pbk.)
1. Herbs – Therapeutic use. I. Snider, Ted. II. Title.
615.321 dc22   RM666.H33.W66 2006

Cover and interior design:
Karen Thomas, Intuitive Design International Ltd.
Cover photo: Firstlight.ca

Printed and bound in Canada

1 3 5 7 9 10 8 6 4 2

CONTENTS

INTRODUCTION TO HERBS AND HERBAL PROPERTIES

For thousands of years, herbs have been used all over the world to both prevent and treat a wide variety of common and not so common ailments. They can be used for everything from colds and flus to cancer and everything in between. And, most importantly, herbs can be used safely and easily, as very few of them have any serious cautions or side effects. They can be used on the very old and the very young, and many herbs can even be used by pregnant and breast-feeding women. They are affordable and growable – so everyone can have access to them – and herbs have a history of use that proves they are both effective and safe. In the last several decades, many of them have also been very well studied. Because herbs have been used by cultures all over the world, we are left with a great deal of written and recorded material to add to the growing body of scientific literature. We also have the wisdom of unwritten herbal lore from virtually every country and culture around the word. What does all this mean? That herbs have a lot to offer the modern world to help promote good health and vitality no matter where we live or who we are.

In this book, we have tried to take the wisdom of the old herbal lore as well as clinical experience, and add to it (in easy-to-read language) any relevant studies, clinical trials or other scientific information that is available. But the world of herbs is an ever growing one that constantly reveals new possible uses of herbs and new proofs of their effectiveness. We hope you will enjoy the information presented here, learn from it, use it, and continue to pursue this fascinating world of ancient knowledge.

Many countries and cultures are represented in this book, among them South America (cat's claw, pau d'arco, passion flower, muira puama), North American Aboriginal culture (echinacea, goldenseal, black cohosh, devil's club), Africa (devil's claw, pygeum, rooibos), China (ginseng, dong quai, licorice, astragalus, ho shou wu, shiitake and reishi mushrooms), India (Indian myrrh, turmeric, ashwagandha, andrographis) and many more. It combines the east and the west, the north and the south, the old and the new.

Teas: Infusions and Decoctions

Traditionally, herbs were used as whole, unaltered parts of plants or as teas. Teas were made into infusions or decoctions. When using the soft parts of a herb, like the flowers or leaves, you generally make an infusion. In an infusion, you do not boil the herb. You pour boiling water over the herb, cover it, and let it stand for 10–20 minutes. Usually, you use one teaspoon (5g) of dried herb per cup of water or one ounce (see the following Measurement Conversion chart) of herb per pint of water. Sometimes a cold-water infusion is used, in which cold water is poured over the herb instead of hot.

If you need to draw the ingredients out of a harder part of the plant, like the root or bark, you will usually need to make a decoction. To decoct a herb, put the herb in a stainless steel or glass pot and pour cold water over it. Cover. Bring the water to a boil, turn it down to simmer and let the tea simmer, covered, for about 20 minutes to an hour. Traditional herbalists will often combine herbs to make a formula specific to one individual.

What do you do if the formula contains both soft parts that need to be infused and hard parts that need to be decocted? Simply decoct the hard parts and then strain the tea and pour it over the soft parts, cover and infuse it for 10–20 minutes.

Pills and Liquids

In addition to teas, herbs can be taken as pills or in liquid form. The pill may contain just the crude, powdered herb so that the whole herb can be swallowed easily. Liquids can be tinctures or extracts. Tinctures usually contain one part of the herb to five parts of the liquid solvent that the herb is in (i.e., a 1:5 concentration). A fluid extract is a stronger liquid, containing one part of the herb for each part liquid solvent – usually around a 1:1 concentration. The most concentrated form of a herb is called a solid extract. Solid extracts are usually at least 4:1 concentrations. This means that the solid extract is four times more potent than the crude herb. Some solid extracts are concentrated as high as 50:1 or more.

Standardization

Sometimes herbs are said to be "standardized." Standardization means that a certain ingredient, believed either to be the active ingredient or a reliable marker for other ingredients believed to make the herb work, has been standardized, or guaranteed to be present, in a certain amount. Scientists like standardization because it assures the buyer that the herb he or she is buying is the same as the herb scientists used in the studies. Traditional herbalists are less enthusiastic. They may prefer to use the herb in its natural state, with all its complexly balanced components in their natural proportions. We often like to use products that contain both and have had good results in clinic doing so. We have given dosing information for both approaches where appropriate.

The Language of Herbalism

Though we have tried to use plain English throughout the book, it is sometimes easier to describe what a herb does by referring to its herbal properties, or actions, and it will be useful to become familiar with a few of these.

Analgesic	relieves pain
Antispasmodic	prevents or relaxes muscle spasms or cramps
Astringent	has a contracting or tightening effect on tissue and stops the loss of body fluids like haemorrhages and other secretions
Carminative	relieves gas and gripping
Demulcent	are taken internally to soothe damaged, irritated or inflamed tissue
Diaphoretic	induces sweating
Diuretic	increases the flow of urine
Expectorant	encourages the expulsion of excess mucous from the throat and lungs
Nervine	calms and nourishes the nervous system
Sedative	strongly calms the nervous system

Dosage

Herbalism is a living tradition. With new experiences and new research, things will change. With *Healthy Herbs* we have tried our best to reflect the most current information. Material on dosing, contraindications and drug interactions is especially difficult. Dose information is offered as a general guideline. It could change according to age, weight, condition and other factors. The doses given are for an average size adult. A general guideline for converting the doses to children's doses is to divide the child's weight by 150, the average weight (in pounds) of an adult. For example, if the child weighs 75 pounds, then give him or her half the adult dose (75/150=1/2). At around age twelve, the child is ready to receive an adult dose. Always remember that doses might have to be altered for the individual. (Traditionally, these herbs are often combined, which could also affect dosing, but that is beyond the scope of this work.)

Approximate Measurement Conversions

This measure ...	Equals approximately ...
1ml of a tincture or extract	20–30 drops
1 dropper full	40 drops
1 teaspoon of a tincture or extract	4–5ml
1 teaspoon of a dried herb	5 grams
1/4 teaspoon of a dried herb	1 gram
1 tablespoon of a tincture or extract	10-12ml
1 tablespoon of a dried herb	12 grams
1 ounce	30 ml
1 pint	500ml
1 pound	455grams

Contraindications and Drug Interactions

As for contraindications and drug interactions, we have tried hard to make this book as accurate and up to date as possible. Drug interaction is a relatively new field and not part of the tradition of herbalism, which long predates the use of manufactured drugs. Opinions sometimes differ and knowledge advances. You should never rely on any one source for this information, especially with regard to pregnancy and drug interactions. A good herbalist who is aware of your history should be consulted about making choices that are right for you. For safety information on each herb, including side effects, contraindications, drug interactions and appropriateness for pregnancy and breast feeding, we have consulted, in addition to recent studies, several of the most authoritative sources available. We have also, where appropriateness for pregnancy is debated in these scientific texts, included the traditional wisdom of several respected women's herbals. A list of some of the authoritative texts on safety is provided at the end of the book.

Finally, this book is offered as a guide to the wonders of the plants that grow and thrive alongside us and to some of their healing powers; it is not intended for self-diagnosis or treatment nor is it meant to replace a qualified practitioner. That a particular herb is listed as helping arthritis does not mean that – in the absence of dietary and lifestyle changes and without being combined with other herbs or nutrients – it will, by itself, heal you.

Healthy Herbs

Alphabetical Listing

Alfalfa

(Medicago sativa)

Alfalfa has been used for centuries for its nutritional value. Aboriginal people of North America used the seeds of the alfalfa plant to make bread or mush and the branches were boiled and the greens were eaten. It was considered a very healthy addition to the diet. And still today, this herb is highly prized. It is considered a superlative restorative tonic that is used to treat all chronic and acute digestive weaknesses. It does this by helping the body assimilate nutrients. Alfalfa is also rich in many nutrients, including calcium, potassium, iron, phosphorus, betacarotene, and vitamins C, D, E and K, making it a wonderful supportive herb that restores strength to the sick and the weak. It works to build strength and vitality and can be used to increase weight.

Its cooling properties make alfalfa ideal for disorders related to aging problems that include too much heat and inflammation. Traditionally, this herb has been used for cystitis, burning urine, prostatitis, insomnia, increasing mother's milk, lowering fevers, lowering cholesterol, diabetes, ulcers, arthritis and rheumatic problems, lower backache, jaundice, asthma, hay fever, and to encourage blood clotting.

Clinically, we find alfalfa is also wonderful for those suffering from toxicity, chronic fatigue immune dysfunction syndrome (CFIDS or CFS), weak bones, sluggish bowels, or general weakness.

There is no absolutely established dose for alfalfa. A standard infusion is often suggested at a dose of one cup three times a day. Some experts recommend 500–1,000mg of the dried herb a day or 1–2ml of the tincture three times a day.

At the recommended doses, alfalfa is extremely safe. It should not be used, however, by people with lupus. Alfalfa is safe to take while pregnant or breast feeding, though one source says to avoid the seeds while pregnant. Brinker speculates that you should avoid extensive use while pregnant: no one else lists this concern, and Amanda McQuade Crawford, in her women's herbal, endorses alfalfa herb as a safe alterative during pregnancy.

It is possible that alfalfa's high vitamin K content could reduce the effectiveness of warfarin and other anticoagulants. It is also possible that, because of its phytoestrogens, it could have an additive effect if taken with estrogen replacement therapy or the birth control pill.

Aloe vera *(Aloe vera)*

This incredibly versatile herb is used for all kinds of digestive problems, to regulate female hormones, to counteract wrinkles, for constipation, liver problems, ulcers, to heal the gut and to stop bleeding from the intestines, HIV, and to cleanse and remove parasites and unwanted material from the digestive system. As a juice, it is one of our favourite herbs to use when there is irritation or inflammation in the intestines.

In India, women drink aloe vera every day to counteract the signs of aging. It also has been used for thousands of years for skin problems such as infections, acne, eczema, psoriasis, stings, poison ivy, and wounds. Topically, the gel is one of the best treatments for healing burns, sunburns, injuries and wounds.

In the West, aloe is used to cleanse the liver and, when combined with turmeric, to relieve PMS. It is also used to enhance the menstrual flow.

Aloe is valued for its ability to heal peptic ulcers, enhance the immune system, for allergies, for diabetes (*Phtyomedicine* 1996), and asthma. Aloe has antiviral and antibacterial properties and is antifungal. Traditionally, it has also been used for dental disease and viral, bacterial and fungal infections. Today, it is used to fight problems such as *E. coli*, herpes, feline leukemia, *klebsiella pneumonia*, *streptococcus*, and *candida*.

Aloe is a wonderful anti-inflammatory, and it can also help with pain.

It contains vitamin C, E and zinc: useful nutrients for healing. Aloe can also be used to heighten enzymes.

In India, women drink aloe vera every day to counteract the signs of aging.

The optimum dose of aloe juice or gel is not known. Some sources recommend about 2 tablespoons three times a day. Bottles of the juice sometimes recommend drinking 1–8 ounces a day. The dose of the dried leaf as a laxative is 50–300mg at bedtime for no more than ten days. *Do not exceed this dose.*

Simply put, aloe vera juice or gel is very safe; dried aloe leaf isn't. Freely use the juice or gel; don't use the dried leaf at all.

Aloe juice or gel is safe to use even when pregnant or breast feeding. It should not be used externally on deep vertical wounds like those from laporotomy or caesarean section. Aloe juice has no negative drug interactions, but it does have one positive one: it improves the effect of the diabetes drug Glyburide (*Phytomed* 1996).

The dried leaf of the aloe plant is an extremely potent laxative. It should not be used while pregnant or breast feeding. It should not be used by anyone with intestinal obstruction, intestinal inflammation (like colitis, Crohn's, irritable bowel syndrome or appendicitis), inflamed haemorrhoids, profuse menstruation or bleeding between periods, or kidney disorder. It should not be used at all in children under twelve. In fact, as a glance through the rest of this book will show, there are much safer laxatives, and you probably just shouldn't use dried aloe leaf at all. As for drug interactions, the dried leaf can increase potassium loss caused by diuretics or corticosteroids, and it can reduce the absorption of oral drugs.

Andrographis (*Andrographis paniculata*)

Andrographis is an exciting herb that is still barely known in the west. This herb hails from India and deserves a warm welcome in North America as it is excellent for both preventing and treating colds. Andrographis has no direct antibacterial or antiviral properties: it does its work by stimulating the immune system. And it has some incredible studies to back it. One double-blind study found that after four days, cold symptoms significantly improved when people were given andrographis than when they were given a placebo (*Phytother Res* 1995). A year later, researchers again found that people suffering from colds and sinusitis improved more significantly when given andrographis than when given a placebo (*Phytomed* 1996). In an impressive double-blind study, 208 people with upper-respiratory-tract infections were given either andrographis or a placebo. By only the second day – and that's incredibly fast – the andrographis group showed a significant improvement in cold symptoms like runny nose and sore throat compared to the placebo group. By day four they also showed significant improvement in cough, headache, earache and fatigue (*Phytomed* 1999).

But that's not all. Andrographis is not only one of the best herbs to take if you catch a cold, it is also a great herb to take in the winter to prevent colds. When 107 healthy children were given either 200mg of standardized andrographis extract or a placebo for three months during the winter, by the third month the children on the herb had a significant 2.1 times lower risk of catching a cold (*Phytomed* 1997).

In the most recent study on treating colds, 1,020mg of andrographis was combined with 120mg of eleuthero (formerly known as Siberian ginseng). The people in the study were suffering from acute upper-respiratory infections – laryngitis, bronchitis, common cold – or sinusitis. They were given either the herbal combination or a placebo for five days. The herbs brought about a significantly greater improvement in headache, sore throat, runny nose and fatigue (*Phytomed* 2002). In the most recent study, the combination of andrographis and eleuthero again flexed its muscle. When combined with conventional cold therapy, it was more effective than conventional therapy alone or conventional therapy with echinacea in children with colds (*Phytotherapy Research* 2004).

By only the second day – and that's incredibly fast – the andrographis group showed a significant improvement in cold symptoms like runny nose and sore throat compared to the placebo group.

Traditionally, andrographis has been used for a lot more than just colds. It is a powerful bitter that increases the production and flow of bile, making it good for indigestion, gas, strengthening digestion, as an appetite stimulant, and as a laxative. It has been used for dysentery and hepatitis and is a good herb for round worm (*ascaris lumbricoides*). Andrographis has also been proven effective for fighting fevers and inflammation and has painkilling and antioxidant properties.

Andrographis is often used as an extract standardized for andrographolides. Take 400mg three times a day to fight a cold. As an unstandardized dried herb, take 500–3,000mg three times a day. As a liquid extract, take 4–6ml a day for prevention of colds and 12ml a day for treating them. If you are using andrographis to treat indigestion, then unfortunately you'll have to drink the bitter tea: sorry. Infuse one teaspoon (5g) per cup.

Andrographis has no adverse effects at the normal dose. High doses may cause gastrointestinal upset. There are no adverse drug interactions, although one source says that because andrographis inhibits platelet aggregation, it should possibly not be taken with anticoagulant medications. Don't use andrographis if you are pregnant.

Anise *(Pimpinella anisum)*

This herb, best known as a flavouring in cooking, is an aromatic used by ancient cultures in many parts of the world. It is a wonderful herb to both prevent and treat gas and cramping in the digestive tract. Because of its soothing properties, anise is useful for nausea, belching, colic and bloating. It is also of value in treating colds, coughs, flus and even bronchitis, whooping cough and asthma, due to its expectorant and antispasmodic properties. By helping to increase body heat, anise helps the immune system to fight off infections, and it can be used to keep the body warm in winter. Anise can also be used to help bring on or to increase mother's milk in nursing mothers. A 1990 study showed that anise can help improve the absorption of iron. The authors of the study recommended that it be used to help both adults and children fight iron deficient anemia. One of our favourite uses for anise is as a flavouring for medicinal herbal teas that don't taste very good. The seeds have also been shown to have insecticidal properties.

The *German Commission E* (an authoritative German government body that decides which herbs to approve) gives the dose of anise as 3g, although herbalist Michael Tierra suggests 3–9g. As a tea, infuse 1–2 teaspoons crushed seeds and drink two to three cups a day.

 Anise is safe. There are no drug interactions. Although no women's herbal we consulted says not to use anise while pregnant, and one actually recommends it as a safe carminative during pregnancy, Brinker speculates that its use should be avoided, and the American Herbal Products Association's *Botanical Safety Handbook* flatly contraindicates it.

Arnica (*Arnica montana*)

This analgesic and antiseptic herb is primarily used externally for the pain and inflammation that is associated with injuries, aches, strains, rheumatism, phlebitis, joint problems, post-operative surgery, insect bites, and bruises. Arnica is also good for inflammation of the throat and oral cavities. It has a history of use for sprains, wounds, sores, abscesses, for depression, typhoid, pneumonia, anemia, diarrhea, and cardiac weakness, and, as a topical tincture, to stimulate hair growth. Some studies have also shown it to have antimicrobial, anti-inflammatory and immune-stimulating properties. It may also have some respiratory stimulant and uterine activities.

Arnica comes as a gel, cream or oil for topical use. Or the oil can be made at home, using fresh or dried arnica leaves and flowers that have been crushed and left in warm sesame or olive oil for three days. Squeeze through a cloth and use externally. Arnica is only used internally in small homeopathic dosages.

 Use freely externally as an oil, gel, liniment or cream.

 Do not consume arnica internally unless it is a homeopathic preparation. Long-term use may cause allergic dermatitis and eczema. Do not use on open wounds or broken skin.

Artichoke

Artichoke is most often thought of as a food, and with good reason. It is both healthy and delicious. But although it is less well-known than the other great liver herbs, artichoke is no less amazing. According to herbal authority Rudolf Fritz Weiss, M.D., and others, artichoke has similar liver protecting and detoxifying talents as its close, but more famous, relative, milk thistle. Daniel Mowrey, Ph.D., says that it protects the liver from the same wide range of poisons as milk thistle. And, like milk thistle, artichoke has the ability to stimulate regeneration of the liver and repair damaged livers.

Artichoke is able to increase both the production and the secretion of bile, making it valuable in aiding detoxification, digestion, including the digestion of fatty food, easing constipation, and preventing parasites. In a truly impressive study of people with digestive disorders, artichoke was able to reduce vomiting in 88.3% of them, nausea in 82.4%, abdominal pain in 76.2%, loss of appetite in 72.3%, constipation in 71%, gas in 68.2% and fat intolerance in 58.8% (*J Gen Med* 1996).

Other studies done on people with digestive problems have found similarly remarkable results. In one study, artichoke reduced vomiting in 95% of people as well as nausea in 85% and abdominal pain in 75% (*Phytother* 1995). A third study also found that artichoke significantly reduced nausea, abdominal pain, gas and bloating (*Phytomed* 1997). Artichoke appears to be an effective herb for the whole constellation of problems associated with indigestion, and it is endorsed for this use by the *German Commission E*. As these symptoms suggest, artichoke is also a good herb for irritable bowel syndrome.

The versatile artichoke is able to increase the good HDL cholesterol while lowering total cholesterol, the bad LDL cholesterol and triglycerides. In a double-blind study, 143 people with high cholesterol were given either 200mg dry artichoke extract or a placebo twice a day. Total cholesterol dropped by 18.5% in the artichoke group, but only 8.6% in the placebo group. The bad LDL cholesterol dropped by 22.9% in the herb group versus only 6.5% in the placebo group (*Arzneimittelforschung* 2000). Research has also shown artichoke's ability to lower triglycerides by 12.5% (Fintelmann, 1996).

And artichoke can contribute to heart health in another way. Its antioxidant powers stop the dangerous LDL cholesterol from oxidizing, an important factor in preventing atherosclerosis (*Phytomed* 1997). Artichoke can also be used as a diuretic.

As a dried leaf, take 2g of artichoke three times a day. As a tincture, take 6ml three times a day. As an extract, take 2ml three times a day. Artichoke can be taken as a pill standardized for 13–18% caffeylquinic acid at a dose of 160–320mg three times a day.

Artichoke is an extremely safe herb. There are no side effects, and the herb is safe for women who are pregnant or breast feeding. There are no drug interactions, though it could possibly enhance cholesterol-lowering drugs.

Artichoke is contraindicated in obstruction of the bile duct and the warning is often given that it should only be used for gallstones after consulting with a health practitioner. Despite the frequent warning in the scientific literature that herbs that increase bile should not be used for gallstones without consulting a practitioner, Colin Nicholls says in the foreword to Brinker's important interaction book that many herbalists consider these herbs to be significant in the treatment of gallstones. Weiss agrees, calling artichoke an important treatment for gallstones and says that it has long been used this way in Europe. Mowrey echoes these claims, while giving the conventional recommendation for care. In the *Textbook of Natural Medicine*, Murray and Pizzorno, N.D.'s, recommend herbs that increase bile for treating gallstones and specifically recommend artichoke, as well as dandelion, milk thistle, turmeric, and boldo.

Artichoke is able to increase both the production and the secretion of bile, making it valuable in aiding detoxification, digestion, including the digestion of fatty food, easing constipation, and preventing parasites.

Ashwagandha

(Withania somnifera)

This remarkable herb is often referred to as Indian ginseng. It has been used for over 2,500 years and comes from Ayurvedic medicine, where it has a long history of use as a vitalizer, which is similar to what we would today call an adaptogen. Ancient healers used ashwagandha as a rejuvenative tonic with the ability to restore strength to an emaciated body. It is reputed to give strength and vigour and increase stamina. Being an adaptogen, it is able to help the body increase nonspecific resistance to disease. It is useful for arthritis, asthma, bronchitis, cancer, candida, fever, inflammations, nausea, rheumatism, diabetes, leucoderma cancer, and to improve cognitive function and stress. Ashwagandha is considered a sedative, a hypotensive, an antispasmodic, is anti-tumour, is an analgesic, and an anti-inflammatory.

Ashwagandha is a nervine that helps relieve stress and anxiety. It is especially good for nervous exhaustion caused by stress, including improving sexual function and libido when the problem is caused by nervous stress or adrenal exhaustion.

Research has confirmed ashwagandha's ability to stimulate the immune system (*Phytomed* 1994), to act as an anti-inflammatory (*Indian J Exp Biol* 1981), to improve memory (*Phytother Res* 1995), and to ease anxiety (*Acta Nerv Super* 1990).

> *Ancient healers used ashwagandha as a rejuvenative tonic with the ability to restore strength to an emaciated body. It is reputed to give strength and vigour and increase stamina.*

1 teaspoon of the dried root bark per 1 1/2 pints of water, decocted for 1/2 hour. Drink 1 cup 2 times a day. Another source suggests 3–6 grams of the root decocted for fifteen minutes and drunk three times a day. Ashwagandha can also be taken as a pill at a dose of 1–2 grams of the whole herb per day. As a tincture, try 2–4ml three times a day.

Ashwagandha is very safe and has no side effects. It should not be taken by pregnant or breast-feeding women. Because of its own sedative powers, ashwagandha may potentiate the sedative effects of barbiturates.

Astragalus   *(Astragalus membranaceus)*

Astragalus is one of our favourite herbs for deeply toning the immune system. We usually suggest that it be used in cycles, on and off, over a period of time to help build up a weak immune system. We are not alone in loving this herb: it has been in use for as long as two thousand years. This very ancient Chinese herb is one of nature's most venerable tonics and has long been used by the Chinese to enhance the body's natural defence systems. It strengthens the body's defensive energy. It enhances resistance to weakness and disease. Astragalus strengthens the immune, cardiovascular and glandular systems and can help when disease affects any of these systems.

Astragalus has warming properties and is a tonic to the spleen, kidneys, blood and lungs. It is useful for all immune breakdowns from the common cold to AIDS. In addition to enhancing and building the immune system, astragalus has antibacterial, antiviral and anti-inflammatory powers. It fights flus, colds, fevers, and bronchitis. It is used to increase the body's *qi*, or energy, and can help to overcome fatigue, control diabetes, overcome poor appetite and help with anemia.

Astragalus has been used to fight cancer. Two very authoritative books on natural approaches to cancer say that the herb fights cancer by boosting immunity and possessing anti-tumour activity. Furthermore, astragalus protects against the horrible side effects of chemotherapy and radiation.

Astragalus helps the heart, lowering blood pressure and increasing the heart's contractions. It is also a valuable diuretic. It balances the energy of the internal organs and improves digestion. According to herbalist Lesley Tierra, it has also been used for diarrhea, prolapse of the uterus, stomach or rectum, uterine bleeding caused by weakness, sweating, numbness of the limbs, and even paralysis.

Astragalus is often taken as a decoction. The usual recommendation is to decoct 9–18g of the dried root. A larger dose of 10–30g, or even higher, is sometimes recommended. In pill form, take 1–1.5g three times a day. Or take 2–6ml of the tincture three times a day.

Astragalus is very safe, including during pregnancy and breast feeding. There are no side effects or drug interactions, though it could potentially enhance interferon and interleukin. Some sources say not to use it during acute infection.

Most Commonly Seen Conditions in a Herbal Clinic

- Pain: back, neck, migraine, arthritis, sciatica, toothache, headache
- Sleep disorders
- Depression / anxiety
- Women's health problems: menopause, P.M.S., endometriosis, fibroids, cysts, breast cancer, infertility, menorrhea, dysmenorrhea, amenorrhea
- Men's sexual health: impotence, lack of desire, low sperm count
- Digestive problems: IBS, Crohns', colitis, diverticulitis, ulcers, diarrhea, constipation, nausea, food allergy, acid reflux, ulcer, candida, hiatus hernia, parasites
- Immunity: cold, flues, HIV, allergies
- Skin problems: acne, rashes, eczema, psoriasis, rosacea, vitiligo, hives
- Weight loss
- Heart and circulatory issues
- Cancer
- Diabetes

Bilberry

Unlike its close relative, the North American blueberry, this European blueberry is actually blue on the inside too. If ever a berry should be called "blue," this is it, but it'll settle for "Bil." Bilberry is nature's answer to diseases of the eye – it is an eye specialist. Bilberry is loaded in antioxidant flavonoids called anthocyanidins that have a special affinity for the eyes. The world first took notice of this affinity during World War II when RAF pilots began to report that their vision on night bombing raids improved when they ate bilberry jam. Since then, all kinds of studies have brought the promise of bilberry to light.

How does a simple berry have such an enormous effect on something as complex as vision and the eye? It seems to improve vision in a number of ways. Vision depends on a large amount of blood flow through the eyes. Bilberry improves that flow of blood and oxygen to the eyes and works as a potent antioxidant to protect the eyes from damage. It also works in another peculiar way. Light-sensitive pigments in the eye called retinol purple, or rhodopsin, are necessary for impulses to be sent from the retina in the eye to the brain. Bilberry protects against the breakdown, and accelerates the regeneration, of retinol purple.

Bilberry is the herb to take for virtually any disorder of the eye, including the biggies: cataracts, macular degeneration, glaucoma, and diabetic retinopathy. It has also been recommended for simple eye strain, helping the eyes adjust more quickly to light and dark, and nearsightedness. Several early studies on improving night vision using bilberry were all positive, although recent results have been mixed.

Cataracts are the leading cause of impaired vision. Most people over sixty will have some degree of cataracts. They occur because of free-radical damage to the lens of the eye. So it is not surprising that a herb that is loaded in free-radical-fighting antioxidants and that has a special affinity for the eye should offer such promise in the battle against cataracts. In a double-blind, placebo-controlled study, people with cataracts were given either a placebo or bilberry and vitamin E. The vitamin E was synthetic and so may have contributed nothing. After four months, a remarkable 97% of the people on bilberry had no progression of their cataracts, compared to 77% in the placebo group (*Ann Ottalmol Clin Ocul* 1989).

Macular degeneration is the leading cause of blindness in people over fifty-five. Since it is caused by free-radical damage and reduced blood and oxygen supply to the eye, from what we have already seen of the way bilberry works, it is again no surprise to find bilberry is effective. Michael Murray and Joseph Pizzorno, N.D.'s, say that the flavonoid-rich herbs, bilberry, ginkgo biloba and grape seed extract, have all been shown in studies to stop the progression of, and perhaps even improve the vision in, macular degeneration. And of these three, they say bilberry is the best.

Glaucoma is another significant cause of blindness. Behind glaucoma lays poor collagen, which normally offers support to the structures of the eye. Another important capability of the flavonoids in bilberry is their ability to strengthen collagen. People with glaucoma given a single dose of bilberry showed improvement on electroretinography measurements (*Arch Med Int* 1985).

Retinopathy can be caused by diabetes or high blood pressure. Among diabetics, retinopathy is the leading cause of blindness. Several studies have proven bilberry's benefit in this eye disorder. A remarkable 77% of people with retinopathy from diabetes or high blood pressure either improved or greatly improved when they were given bilberry, while there was only slight improvement in 6% of those given a placebo (*Ann Ottalmol Clin Ocul* 1987).

Bilberry can also help people who are nearsighted (*Boll Ocul* 1986; *Boll Ocul* 1990).

Though bilberry is best known as an eye specialist, people with vein problems can benefit from bilberry's powerful ability to decrease the permeability and fragility of veins and to keep them flexible. Bilberry is able to protect the small blood vessels known as capillaries from damage, to repair and strengthen them, and even to stimulate the formation of new, healthy ones. The flavonoids in bilberry also improve circulation through the larger blood vessels. All of these effects on blood vessels make bilberry a valuable herb for varicose veins (*Min Cardioangiol* 1978), capillary fragility (*J Mal Vasc* 1980; *Min Ginecol* 1980), venous insufficiency (*Fitoterapia* 1988), and Reynaud's disease (*Min Angiol* 1982). Because bilberry can strengthen fragile capillaries, it can help people who bruise easily and who are prone to nosebleeds. It has even been used before surgery to minimize bruising and excessive bleeding (*Ann Ottalmol Clin Ocul* 1989). Bilberry anthocyanidins are also able to prevent blood from clotting and to break down plaque deposits on artery walls. Bilberry may prevent angina attacks.

Bilberry also has a number of less known benefits. It is an astringent herb that can be used for diarrhea. It is also anti-inflammatory. One study found that bilberry significantly reduced the symptoms of dysmenorrhoea, or painful menstrual periods (*G Ital Obsted Gionecol* 1985). Another intriguing benefit of bilberry anthocyanidins is their ability to decrease the leakiness of the blood-brain barrier (*J Med* 1977; *Clin Physiol Biochem* 1986), which protects the brain from drugs, pollution and other harmful things. Since multiple sclerosis involves immune cells crossing the blood-brain barrier and attacking the myelin sheath, bilberry, and other flavonoid-rich herbs like ginkgo biloba, may have a role to play in treating MS.

If you are using the dried fruit or making a decoction of the dried fruit, take 5g four to twelve times a day. You could also take an extract at a dose of 2–4ml three times a day. Bilberry is usually taken as a dry extract in pill form, standardized for 25% anthocyanidins: the dose is 80–160mg three times a day.

Bilberry is extremely safe. There are no side effects, contraindications or drug interactions. It has been speculated that very high doses – 170mg of anthocyanidins a day – could interact with blood thinners; however, this is far above the amount in the recommended dose of bilberry.

Bilberry is perfectly safe to take while you are pregnant or breast feeding. In fact, it might even be a good idea. Pregnant women suffering circulatory disorders in the legs, which is common in the third trimester, had significant relief when they took bilberry. The herb helped with pain, tingling, tiredness, heaviness, itching, cramps, swelling, varicose veins, skin pigmentation, ulceration, and burning. It also improved haemorrhoids (*Quad Clin Ostet Ginecol* 1987).

Black Cohosh
(*Cimicifuga racemosa*)

Although it doesn't get the same media spotlight as St. John's wort, echinacea or Ginkgo, one of the most exciting herbal stories is black cohosh. At a time when the case for hormone replacement therapy (HRT) has crumbled as the evidence mounts that it causes heart disease, stroke, and breast and other cancers, what could be more exciting news for women than a herb that has been shown over and over again in studies to work better than hormones with none of the side effects of HRT?

The is black cohosh, a herb that has been put up against estrogen repeatedly and has never lost. The first time black cohosh challenged the hormones was in a large study of 629 women . Within six to eight weeks on black cohosh, 80% of the women experienced an improvement. Two hundred and four of those women had been on estrogen replacement therapy before, and, for 72% of them, the herb had advantages over the hormone. What was also exciting was that the black cohosh was able to help not only the physical symptoms of menopause but the psychological ones as well. Hot flashes improved in 86.6% of the women, sweats in 88.5%, and heart palpitations in 90.4%, but there was also improvement of depression in 82.5% and of nervousness and irritability in 85.6% (*Gynecology* 1982).

Two years later, women were given either black cohosh, estrogen or valium in a double-blind study. Amazingly, the herb beat both drugs. And again, black cohosh also beat both drugs for the psychological symptoms of depression and anxiety. On the Kupperman menopausal index, after twelve weeks, the valium produced a drop

> *Black cohosh . . . has been put up against estrogen repeatedly and has never lost. The first time black cohosh challenged the hormones . . . [w]ithin six to eight weeks on black cohosh, 80% of the women experienced an improvement . . . Hot flashes improved in 86.6% of the women, sweats in 88.5%, and heart palpitations in 90.4% . . . there was also improvement of depression in 82.5% and of nervousness and irritability in 85.6%.*

in score from 35 to 20, the estrogen a slightly better result of 35 to 16 and the black cohosh a still better result of 35 to 14 (*Med Welt* 1985).

In 1987, black cohosh went head to head with estrogen again. In this double-blind study, the herb again did better than the hormone on menopause and anxiety scales. In the black cohosh group, hot flashes dropped from five a day to only one, but the estrogen was able to produce a drop to only three and a half from the original five. What is more, while estrogen provided little help for the vaginal lining, black cohosh dramatically improved it (*Therapeuticum*). This last advantage is important because the thinning and drying of the vaginal lining that can occur with the drop in estrogen at menopause can make intercourse painful and also increase the susceptibility to infection, itching and burning.

A later 1991 double-blind study which demonstrated the ability of black cohosh to significantly improve menopausal symptoms, including hot flashes, also demonstrated significant improvement in the vaginal lining (*Planta Medica* 1991).

More recent information about black cohosh can also be seen as an exciting new breakthrough. While the herb has proved superior to the hormone for the symptoms of menopause, it still left the problem of osteoporosis, another concern for menopausal women. But now a new study suggests that although black cohosh is not estrogenic, it may still be able to address the osteoporosis aspect of menopause. In this double-blind, placebo-controlled study, black cohosh was again shown to be as effective for menopause as estrogen despite having no estrogenic effect. But the big surprise was on bone markers. Markers for bone loss went down in both the hormone group and the herb group, but while markers for bone formation were not improved by estrogen, they went up significantly in the black cohosh group (*Maturitas* 2003). This small study suggests that black cohosh may be even more perfect for menopause than we thought, since it seems to protect against osteoporosis as well.

Black cohosh is useful not only at the end of menstruation, but is also valuable for painful or absent menstruation. It may also be helpful for PMS. Clinically, we have seen black cohosh to be remarkably effective in preventing the symptoms of PMS.

Using black cohosh for women's health issues is not new. First Nations people of North America used this herb so often for women's health issues that they named the root "squawroot."

But black cohosh's uses extend beyond women's health. Because of its anti-inflammatory power, black cohosh is also useful for rheumatism and rheumatoid arthritis, and its antispasmodic properties are helpful in cases of bad coughs like whooping cough, as well as asthma and bronchitis.

The form of black cohosh used in most of the studies is an extract that is standardized to contain 1mg of the triterpene 27-deoxyacteine in each tablet. In this form, two tablets, or 40 drops of extract, are taken twice a day.

Traditionally, this herb has also been used as a tea: decoct 1 teaspoon (5g) per cup and drink three cups a day.

If you are using a nonstandardized form, doses are less precise. As an extract, try taking 2–3ml per day. As a tincture, recommendations vary from as low as 1ml twice a day to as high as 4–6ml a day; as a powder doses again vary, but try 0.5–1g three to four times a day.

The great advantage of black cohosh over estrogen is not only that it works better, but that, unlike estrogen, it is perfectly safe. No serious side effects have ever been reported. Contrary to what is often said about black cohosh, the herb is not estrogenic (*Menopause* 1998), freeing it from the dangerous side effects of the hormone. And, unlike estrogen, black cohosh not only does not stimulate breast tumours, it actually inhibits them (*Arch Gynecol Obstet* 1993). A recent study again clearly showed that the herb does not stimulate the proliferation of estrogen receptor-positive breast cancer cells and concluded that black cohosh is not contraindicated in women with a history of breast cancer. A very recent study has once again confirmed that black cohosh is not only effective for menopause but that it is safe, easing menopausal symptoms without having any estrogenic effect (*Journal of Women's Health & Gender Based Medicine* 2002).

Because it stimulates the uterus, Black cohosh should not be used during pregnancy, except during the last week to prepare the uterus for childbirth or to stimulate a long overdue pregnancy. There are no other contraindications. There are no drug interactions.

Black walnut

(Juglans nigra)

This herb is so powerful that when it grows outside and the nut falls on the ground, it can kill pretty much everything around it around it. This is what makes black walnut such a powerful antiparasite herb, but it has many uses.

Black walnut is antiseptic, a vermifuge (kills worms) and is astringent. Different parts of the walnut are used in herbal medicine, including the fruit, the leaves and bark. The fruit is used to increase strength and weight gain. The extract of the hulls is used for all kinds of skin diseases, such as herpes, psoriasis, eczema, and skin parasites. An infusion of the leaves is also used for various skin diseases, while the bark is used to purify the blood and to relieve constipation. Black walnut is considered a mild laxative that does not cause nausea, irritation or pain and does not impair the digestive function. Many North American Aboriginal people used black walnut for various digestive purposes.

Because of its antiparasitic properties, walnut is used to treat amoebic and bacterial dysentery and fungal infections like *candida*. It is especially good for tapeworm. It is often combined with other herbs, like goldenseal, wormwood, garlic, chapparal, and cloves for this purpose. Other uses of walnut include treatment of abscesses, anaemia, blood poisoning, and eye inflammation. In the 1960s, scientists at the University of Missouri found that black walnut had anti-cancer properties.

Not much information is available here. Herbalist Michael Tierra says to take a standard infusion or 10–20 drops of the tincture of the hulls. The fruits can be used freely.

Some preparations may lead to yellowing of the skin when applied topically. One of the ingredients in walnut, juglone, has been found in animal studies to be a mutagen; prolonged use is, therefore, contraindicated. In the major works on contraindications, black walnut is not contraindicated during pregnancy or breast feeding, although one text on parasites says to avoid its use in children or infants.

Bromelain
(Ananas comosus)

Bromelain comes from pineapple and is a well-known herb for digestive problems, helping users to digest proteins and aiding in pancreatic insufficiency. This herb is also used for acute postoperative swelling, to heal surgical inflammation and bruises (*J Dent Med* 1964; *J Dent Med* 1965; *J Obstet Gynecol Br Common* 1972; *Obstet Gynecol* 1967).

It is also used to heal injuries (*Practitioner* 1960) and burns, as a smooth muscle relaxant, for angina, as a natural antibiotic, for perirectal abscesses, for painful menstruation (*Obstet Gynecol* 1957), arthritis, thrombophlebitis (*Angiology* 1969), varicose veins (by helping to break down fibrinigin), edema, prevention of ulcers, inhibiting appetite, shortening of labour, and as an adjunct to cancer therapy.

A few studies have shown that bromelain may help increase the effectiveness of chemotherapy in cancer treatment (*Kreebsgeschehen* 1976). Bromelain may help break down the tumour cells' coating, allowing the immune system to target the cancer cells more effectively. Other studies have shown that patients with cancer who took bromelain had a greater reduction in cancer cells than those on standard therapy alone (*Agressologie* 1972). The results hold the promise that bromelain may exert some effects against cancer on its own.

Bromelain is also useful for both rheumatoid and osteoarthritis and can be used to reduce the amount of corticosteroids used. Bromelain possesses a wide range of actions, including anti-inflammatory and antispasmodic activity, that make it suited to a wide range of uses.

This herb is also wonderful for respiratory congestion and infections, sinusitis (*Headache* 1967), pneumonia, and bronchitis. When it is used for coughs, bromelain seems to work by suppressing the cough and thinning the mucous. When patients were put on bromelain for chronic bronchitis, they showed increased lung capacity (*Drugs Exp Clin* 1978).

Bromelain improves the absorption and action of antibiotics.

When bromelain is used as a digestive enzyme, it should be taken with meals. As an anti-inflammatory or in its other uses, it should be taken between meals on an empty stomach. Bromelain is often standardized in the range of 1,800–2,000 mcu (milk clotting units). Take 500 mg three times a day.

Bromelain is very safe, even long term. There are no side effects or contraindications, including during pregnancy and breast feeding. Allergic reaction is possible. One source says to avoid it in cases of bile duct obstruction.

Bromelain improves the absorption and action of antibiotics. It can also improve the workings of some chemotherapy drugs, including 5-fluorouracil and Vincritine (*J Ethnopharmacol* 1988). It may also enhance the action of aspirin and cortisone. Bromelain could potentiate blood thinners.

Buckthorne *(Rhamnus catharticus)*

Buckthorne has been used since the Middle Ages. Today it is highly valued as a remedy for one of our most common health problems: constipation. Since so many people suffer from constipation, this is a welcome and safe remedy. Buckthorne is an excellent herb for stubborn constipation that can be used for longer periods of time than better known herbs like senna and cascara sagrada. It is a mild laxative that relieves colic, hemorrhoids and liver congestion. Buckthorne can also be helpful in treating obesity.

Buckthorne extract has also been found to kill several species of fungi. Applied externally, it is effective against herpes. It is known to have antiviral activity against influenza virus A2 and other viruses. It also has anti-cancer activity against HELA cancer cells. In 1991, a study found buckthorne to be effective against *candida* and *staphylococcus*.

Buckthorne can be taken as a decoction at a dose of 0.5–2.5g, one cup morning and/or bedtime. As a tincture, take 1–2ml twice a day.

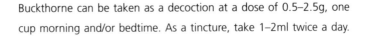

As an extract, recommendations range from 0.5–2.5ml at bedtime to 2–4ml twice a day.

Although buckthorne is safe for extended periods of time, it is not a good idea to rely on any laxative on a permanent basis. The cause of the constipation should be determined and alleviated.

Do not use buckthorne if you are pregnant or breast feeding. This herb should not be used if you have an intestinal inflammatory condition like Crohn's, colitis, irritable bowel syndrome or appendicitis, according to the authoritative texts on contraindications, although highly respected herbalist Michael Tierra specifically recommends it for ulcerative colitis and appendicitis. You also should not use buckthorne if you are suffering from abdominal pain of unknown origin, and use it with caution if you have kidney stones. Don't give it to children under twelve.

Overuse of buckthorne could cause a loss of potassium which could worsen the toxicity of antiarrhythmia drugs and cardiac glycosides. It could also increase potassium deficiency when taken with diuretics and corticosteroids. Because of its laxative effect, buckthorne could reduce absorption of oral drugs.

Burdock *(Arctium lappa)*

Burdock is a common plant found both in Europe and the United States. It has been widely consumed as a vegetable for at least hundreds of years and is highly valued for its herbal properties. Burdock is an especially good detoxifier for the blood, kidneys, skin, liver, stomach, and lungs. It is found in most herbal formulae for purifying the skin and is used for eczema, psoriasis, acne, boils and other skin problems. Burdock's high concentration of minerals, including iron, makes it a wonderful tonic to the blood and a good blood purifier, where it can be used for conditions like sciatica, rheumatism, gout, lumbago and arthritis. It is also used to cleanse the kidneys, helping to expel harmful acids, and as a diuretic. The oil of burdock helps to expel toxic matter form sweat glands and is often used to clear excess heat from the body, such as in fevers, carbuncles, canker sores, and infections. Burdock is also used for complaints of the gastrointestinal tract.

And that's not all: Burdock may have anti-tumour properties and has been an ingredient in at least two famous herbal cancer treatments. Some experiments have also found burdock to have antibacterial properties, antifungal properties, and that it may be useful for diabetes and for a variety of female problems, such as uterine fibroids, ovarian cysts, endometriosis, P.M.S., and fibrocystic breast disease.

In pill form, take 1–2g of the dried root three times a day. As a tea, decoct 1 teaspoon (5g) of the dried root in a cup of water, and drink it three times a day. Suggested doses of the tincture range from 2–4ml a day to 2–4ml three times a day.

Burdock is very safe: there are no risks, no side effects and no drug interactions. It is safe to take while breast feeding. Brinker speculates that you should avoid excessive internal use while pregnant, but his caution is only speculative, applies only to "excessive" doses, and he is the only one who gives this caution. A survey of women's herbals produced no contraindications during pregnancy and one passionate endorsement of it.

Butcher's Broom *(Ruscus aculeatus)*

Butcher's broom has been used in Europe for over two thousand years as a laxative, diuretic, and for gastrointestinal and reproductive problems. This is one of the best herbs for treating and preventing circulatory problems. Butcher's broom is used for swelling of the feet and legs, for varicose veins, pain and heaviness of the legs, leg cramps, itching, and swelling. It is also used for urinary obstruction, urinary tract stones, healing fractures, hemorrhoids, arthritis, clearing phlegm from the lungs, and to improve breathing. For treating hemmorrhoidal pain, a topical ointment is used.

Make a decoction of the root and take three cups a day. Mix the decoction with honey to aid in clearing mucous from the lungs. Or take butcher's broom in pill form at a dose of 1,000mg three times a day. There are also standardized butcher's broom pills available: these extracts are standardized for 9–11% ruscogenin. One source gives the dose as 100mg three times a day; another gives a larger dose of 50–100mg ruscogenin a day.

Butcher's broom is perfectly safe. There are no drug interactions or contraindications, including for pregnant and breast-feeding women. In very rare cases it may cause gastrointestinal upset or nausea.

Butterbur *(Petasites hybridus)*

A recent flurry of research might put this forgotten traditional cough remedy back in the herbal medicine chest: but not for cough.

Butterbur, also known as purple butterbur, is an almost entirely unheard of herb. It is almost never mentioned in herb books. But it will be. Recent studies are bringing this herb back into the limelight in a whole new role: the prevention of migraines, hay fever, allergies and asthma.

In a study that was recently released, butterbur was found to be equally effective as the antihistamine fexofenadine (Allegra) and significantly better than a placebo in relieving the symptoms of allergies (*Phytotherapy* 2005). And it has also proven effective as the antihistamine cetirizine for relieving hay fever (*BMJ* 2002). Actually, the herb had an unexpected advantage over the drug. Unlike most antihistamines, this one is supposed to be nonsedating. But some people who took it still experienced drowsiness and fatigue. No one in the butterbur group did, though. So why not take the herb instead of the drug?

You might want to consider butterbur if you have asthma too. When butterbur was given to asthmatics, 2/3 had a clinically significant increase in air flow: they could breathe better. Chest tightness, wheezing and coughing improved, and the number and severity of asthma attacks went down. Overall, 95% said that butterbur was effective in treating their asthma. What's more, 43%-48% of those who were also taking pharmaceuticals were able to reduce their dose when they were also taking the herb (*Alternative Medicine Review* 2004).

At least four studies have now shown butterbur to be a valuable treatment for migraines. In the first, migraine sufferers were given either 50mg of standardized butterbur extract or a placebo twice a day for twelve weeks. The butterbur gave them a significant decrease in the frequency of migraines and in the number of migraine days. It also significantly reduced nausea and vomiting. There were no side effects (*Inter J Clin Pharmacol Ther* 2000).

The second study gave either 50mg or 75mg of standardized butterbur extract or a placebo twice a day to migraine sufferers for twelve weeks. There was a significant reduction in the frequency of migraines in the group getting the larger amount of butterbur compared to the placebo. The intensity of the headaches was also better in this group (*Neurology* 2002).

In the third, 75mg of butterbur twice a day for four months reduced the number of migraines by 45% compared to only a 28% reduction with a placebo. Significantly more people on the butterbur had a greater than 50% reduction in monthly migraines. The authors said that butterbur's effectiveness is comparable to migraine drugs, but has the advantage of being safer to use (*Neurology* 2004).

The fourth study is important because it found that children who suffer from migraines are also helped by butterbur. Seventy-seven percent had at least 50% fewer headaches, and 91% experienced at least some improvement. Like adults, kids tolerated the herb well (*Headache* 2005).

Butterbur is a powerful antispasmodic and pain killer. It is also an anti-inflammatory herb. Because it is an antispasmodic, butterbur is also helpful for kidney stones, digestive tract spasm, whooping cough and asthma. It is also good for lower back pain, including back pain caused by slipped discs. Also, as an antispasmodic, butterbur might be useful for menstrual cramping, and in one of the migraine studies, a number of women did report that while using the herb for headaches, their menstrual pain got better.

Butterbur is also used for preventing ulcers and for irritable bladder, urinary tract spasm and gastritis.

The *German Commission E* lists a dose of 4.5-7g of the root. Recent research, though, has focused on an extract of butterbur standardized to 15% petasin and isopetasin. The dose of this extract is 50mg two to three times a day. Donald Brown, N.D. limits this dose to people over the age of twelve.

 The butterbur safety issue has focused on a potentially liver toxic component known as pyrrolizidine alkaloids, or PA's for short. In the migraine and hay fever studies, the butterbur extract had the PA's removed. You should only use butterbur supplements that have had this ingredient removed or that contain no more than 1mcg a day of PA's; 1mcg a day is the upper limit set by the *German Commission E*. As long as this is the type of butterbur you use, the herb is very safe with no serious side effects. When rare side effects do occur, they usually involve mild gastrointestinal complaints. Butterbur should not be used if you have liver disease or if you are pregnant or breast feeding. There are no drug interactions.

Want to Know Just How Popular Herbal Medicine Is?

The World Health Organization estimates that 80 percent of the world's population relies on herbs for their primary health care needs (*Bulletin World Health Organization* 1985). And herbs are not only used in developing countries: 30 to 40 percent of all medical doctors in France and Germany rely on herbal medicines as their primary medicine. Herb sales world wide are exploding. For example, over 4 billion dollars are spent on herbal products each year in Germany. In Japan even more is spent (Michael Murry, *The Healing Power of Herbs*).

Why are herbs so popular? Because they have been used for thousands of years, safely and effectively, and over the last twenty to thirty years, scientific information about herbs has exploded.

calendula   *(Calendula officinalis)*

Calendula is better known as the beautiful orange and yellow marigold. This herb was very popular in the Middle Ages. It is native to the Mediterranean countries. Calendula is one of the best herbs for all kinds of skin problems and it works in many ways to heal the skin. It possesses skin regenerating properties and is antibacterial, antiviral, antifungal, immune stimulating, anti-inflammatory, and astringent. It can be used as an oil, salve or as a poultice to treat burns, stop bleeding, soothe pain or injuries and irritation, and promote the healing of wounds and tissues. Calendula is so effective at stopping irritation and inflammation that even those suffering from shingles can get relief using a strong infusion or juice of the petals applied topically. Creams for dry skin or psoriasis, cracked nipples, rashes, boils, skin ulcers, or eczema often contain calendula.

Taken internally, an infusion can be used for fevers, inflammation of the ear and throat area, ulcers, menstrual cramps, and eruptive skin diseases like measles. Some early research suggests it may help with HIV (*Biomed Pharmacother* 1997). An old remedy for curing earache is to use one or two drops of the oil of calendula and place it directly into the affected ear.

Dried calendula flower can be taken in pill form at a dose of 1–2g a day. Calendula can also be made into a tea by infusing 1–2 teaspoons (5–10g) in a cup of water three times a day. You can also take 1–4ml of the tincture three times a day or 0.5–1ml of the extract three times a day.

Calendula is very safe. There are no side effects, contraindications or drug interactions. As for pregnancy, the jury is split on this herb. The most authoritative texts on contraindications give it a thumbs up: two declare it safe and one says to avoid it only in early pregnancy. However, a survey of women's herbals and other books also produced two contraindications and a caution. What does all this mean? It's hard to say. No one seems to have any problems using calendula when breast feeding.

Cascara sagrada *(Rhamnus purshiana)*

This herb, along with buckthorne, is one of our favourite herbs for treating constipation. Cascara sagrada is one of the best tonic laxative herbs that there is. Many herbalists believe that it can be used on a daily basis, if necessary, for chronic constipation. Its properties affect the entire digestive system, including the stomach, pancreas, gallbladder and liver. Its ability to clear the decaying matter from the intestines makes cascara especially useful for those with colitis, anal fissures, hemorrhoids, liver failure, and jaundice. When cascara is used alone, it can cause gripping pains and is, therefore, best combined with carminative, antispasmodic herbs like peppermint or ginger, anise or fennel.

Use only dried bark that has been aged for one year. In pill form, take 300–1,000mg a day in a single dose. Infusions should be made from 1–2.5g a day. If you use a tincture, take 1–5ml a day; if you use an extract, take 1–2ml a day. Take the smallest dosage that is necessary to produce a laxative effect.

Do not use cascara sagrada when pregnant or breast feeding, and don't give it to children under twelve. Don't use cascara if you have intestinal obstruction or acute intestinal inflammation, as in Crohn's, colitis, appendicitis, irritable bowel syndrome, ulcer, or if you have abdominal pain of unknown origin. Herbalist Michael Tierra, however, says that this herb is useful for colitis. Some say not to use cascara during menstruation or if you are generally debilitated. Cramping is a possible side effect of this laxative herb.

Chronic use or abuse of this laxative could lead to potassium loss and can increase the potassium loss of diuretics and corticosteroids if used together with them. The loss of potassium could increase the toxicity of cardiac glycosides and antiarrhythmia drugs. Its laxative effect could reduce absorption of oral medications.

catnip *(Nepeta cataria)*

Although this herb is best know as a treat for cats, it is also a very useful herb for people. Catnip is famous for its ability to sedate the central nervous system by gently relieving nervous congestion from built-up emotional tension. And so it is often used to relieve insomnia, hyperactivity in children, stress and anxiety. The gentleness of catnip makes it an ideal herb for children and babies.

The gentleness of catnip makes it an ideal herb for children and babies.

But catnip is also wonderful for treating colds, fevers and diarrhea. It is such a gentle herb and good cure for diarrhea that it is frequently used in enemas to help relax and restore tone to the bowels. Catnip's soothing properties also make it of value in treating colic and gassy intestines. Other uses of catnip include treating iron-deficiency anemia, menstrual disorders, chronic coughs, and toothache.

Catnip is best taken as a tea: infuse 1–2 teaspoons (5–10g) in a cup of boiling water and enjoy it three times a day, including a cup before bedtime. Take it every half hour for fever, until the fever breaks. Catnip is often combined with other relaxing herbs like lemon balm or passion flower for insomnia.

Catnip is safe and has no side effects, drug interactions or contraindications. It will not cause daytime drowsiness. This is another herb whose safety for pregnancy is not agreed upon. We couldn't find a women's herbal that contraindicated it, and one actually endorsed it. But the authoritative contraindication books do not allow this herb during pregnancy. With the variety of herbs available to treat insomnia and stress, it may be better to choose another one.

cat's claw *(Uncaria tomentosa)*

This herb has not yet caught on in the North American mainstream. But in Peru, the home of this vine, cat's claw, or *una de gato*, is found everywhere. When we were in Peru, we were surprised to find cat's claw pills in every drugstore where we looked for it, sometimes on the shelf right beside the prednisone, revealing one of this great herb's traditional uses: as an anti-inflammatory. We found cat's claw in packages of shredded bark ready to be made into tea. We even saw a woman from the Amazon sitting in the streets of Cuzco selling strips of the bark along with the jewellery she had made from Amazonian beans and small oranges. She was sipping a cold tea, made from cat's claw mixed with a herb with the fantastic name *sangre de drago* (blood of the dragon), as people have done for thousands of years for serious illness.

In his book *Cat's Claw: Healing Vine of Peru*, Kenneth Jones says that cat's claw has been used by the Aboriginal people of Peru for at least two thousand years. Traditionally, it has been mainly used for treating inflammatory conditions, including arthritis, rheumatism and urinary tract inflammation, as well as cancer, ulcers, and as a contraceptive. But it was also traditionally used for diabetes, fevers, "loose stomach," abscesses, bone pain, haemorrhages, menstrual irregularities, skin eruptions, weakness, deep wounds, "normalizing the body," preventing disease, cleansing the kidney, and aiding in recovery after childbirth.

If this long list of traditional uses for cat's claw seems incredible, what is more remarkable is that it is being borne out by science. Research in laboratories has been able to demonstrate cat's claw's anti-inflammatory, anti-cancer and immune-stimulating properties.

Many of cat's claw's traditional uses revolve around its anti-inflammatory power. And in 1989, Jones reports, scientists in Peru and Italy found that cat's claw contained the anti-inflammatory beta-sitosterol. However, the herb didn't contain enough beta-sitosterol to account for all of its anti-inflammatory ability. Shortly after, Italian researchers found a rare group of glycosides that were working as the main anti-inflammatory force in cat's claw. But it was found that there must still be more to this mysterious herb, because when scientists isolated those glycosides and compared them to a simple cat's claw tea, the simple tea was very nearly as powerful an anti-inflammatory as the isolated glycosides.

Then German researchers found that cat's claw contained another group, called alkaloids, that were also very powerful anti-inflammatories. This new discovery explained not only the powerful anti-inflammatory effect of cat's claw, but also explained its traditional use as an immune herb. German researchers discovered that alkaloids found only in cat's claw had a major effect on the immune system. They enhanced the white blood cells' ability to engulf and destroy bacteria, tumour cells and dead matter, a process known as phagocytosis.

So scientists in European laboratories were able to prove what healers in South American jungles had already known for two thousand years: cat's claw is able to fight inflammation and boost immunity. They also found two kinds of flavonoids in cat's claw: catechin tannins, the ingredient family that made green tea famous, and proanthocyanidins, the powerful family found in such herbs as grape seed extract, bilberry, Ginkgo, and hawthorn. These powerful antioxidants also explain a lot of cat's claw's traditional power and versatility.

Cat's claw has been found to have some anti-cancer properties and may help with chemotherapy. It is claimed that cancer patients seem to tolerate conventional treatment better and to recover faster when cat's claw is used.

More recent research has continued to emerge and lend support to cat's claw's traditional résumé. One very small study showed the herb's ability to support the immune system (*J Ehnopharmacol* 2000). Another found that cat's claw significantly decreased the amount of damage done to DNA and increased DNA repair – more evidence that the herb from Peru increases immune response (*Phytomed* 2001).

Science is also confirming one of cat's claw's most important traditional uses: treating arthritis. In a double-blind study of people with osteoarthritis of the knee, a species of cat's claw known as *Uncaria guianensis* significantly reduced the pain associated with activity – though not with resting – and disease activity compared to a placebo. The herb was also found to be well tolerated and safe. The researchers concluded that cat's claw is an effective treatment for osteoarthritis (*Inflamm Res* 2001).

Another group of scientists came to the same conclusion for the other major arthritis. They added 60mg a day of cat's claw to the drugs that forty rheumatoid arthritics were on. The number of painful joints were reduced by 53.2% in the herb group, but only 34.1% in the placebo group. The herb group also had significantly less morning stiffness. As in the other arthritis study, this study found the herb to be safe (*J Rheumatol* 2002).

In a non-traditional use, cat's claw is showing some promise against AIDS, though Peruvian experts caution that the preliminary research is inconclusive. One study, however, has led Kenneth Jones to cautiously exclaim that there is good reason for hope. In this study, people lost their symptoms using a standardized extract of cat's claw. Jones says that the group with CD4 counts between 200 and 500 fared the best. Their CD4 counts increased significantly in the first year and continued to rise for three years. They remained stable for four to five years and none of them dropped below 200 during the study. After six months, those using both the herb and AZT showed the same improvement as those using the herb alone (Keplinger U, 1993).

Cat's claw also seems to be an effective treatment for ulcers and digestive problems. Practitioners say it is useful against ulcers, parasites, and candida, and that it promotes intestinal healing. We have found that it is also very useful for Crohn's and colitis sufferers.

If you use cat's claw as a pill, Blumenthal, in the American Botanical Council's *Clinical Guide to Herbs*, cites 350–500mg 1 to 2 times a day as the dose. McAleb *et al* list the dose higher, at 500mg up to nine times a day. If the cat's claw in the pill is a dry standardized extract, take 20–60mg a day. As a tincture, take 1–2ml two to three times a day. If you prefer to take a traditional cat's claw tea, decoct one gram, or about a quarter teaspoon, for fifteen minutes and drink it three times a day. Some sources seem to suggest a longer decoction time of forty-five minutes.

As with the dosage information, the scientific research on this herb is in its infancy, and the safety information can be a little confusing. Generally, for most people, cat's claw is very safe. It is nontoxic and no serious side effects have ever been reported. It should not be used by women who are pregnant or breast feeding and its safety in children under three years of age is unknown.

Cat's claw has been both contraindicated and recommended for people who have recently had or who are planning marrow or organ transplants. The contraindication is based on the herb's immune-enhancing properties and is only speculative. Caution is advised for people who have multiple sclerosis or tuberculosis. Brinker says speculatively to avoid long term use if you have an autoimmune disease until more information becomes available. Cat's claw is also contraindicated if you are taking thymus extract or if you are a hemophiliac and have been prescribed fresh plasma. Although the contraindication also appears for people using insulin, hormones or, simultaneously, some vaccines, Heather Boon, Ph.D., and Michael Smith, Ph.D., say that the rationale behind this concern is unknown.

As for drug interactions, very few are reported. One study suggests that it may raise blood levels of certain drugs. Cat's claw significantly enhanced immunity in people given pneumococcal vaccine (*Phytomed* 2001), and it enhanced the effectiveness of Sulfasalazine and hydroxychloroquine in rheumatoid arthritis in the study discussed above (*J Rheumatol* 2002).

---

cayenne *(Capsicum anuum)*

This incredibly useful plant originally comes from South and Central America, where the indigenous people have been using it for over nine thousand years for scores of diseases as well as for food. Today it is cultivated in many countries. The most potent form comes from Africa.

Capsicum includes red and green peppers, cayenne, paprika, and bell peppers. It is a stimulant, astringent, carminative, and antispasmodic that is considered a first-aid remedy for most conditions. It is used for diarrhea, cramps, muscle spasms, pains in the stomach and bowels, pain, shingles, sore throats, colds, flus, fevers, cluster headaches (*Cephalagia* 1993), neuralgia (*Anesth Analg* 1992), haemorrhages, rheumatism, arthritis, psoriasis (*J Am Acad Dermatol* 1993), constipation, indigestion, depression, asthma, energy loss, diabetic neuropathy pain, frost bite, and for weight loss.

It is also used for heart and circulatory problems: for preventing heart attacks, strokes and to treat high or low blood pressure. Cayenne is an excellent antioxidant herb, and it reduces atherosclerosis by reducing bad cholesterol and triglycerides. It also reduces platelet aggregation (blood stickiness) and increases fibrinolytic activity, helping to break down clots.

Some herbalists use cayenne for almost any illness in crisis and will use it alone or in combination with other herbs, as in pleurisy, pneumonia or in heavy bleeding. When uncooked, cayenne powder is supposed to be non-irritating. Externally, cayenne is used for toothache, swelling, inflammation, to stop thumb sucking, to prevent nail biting, arthritis, neuralgia, rheumatism, and backache. When combined with plantain, cayenne can be used externally to draw out embedded foreign objects.

One of cayenne's main uses it to stop pain, and it seems to do this in several ways that are not fully understood. It is thought that cayenne works to block substance P, a substance which normally helps give pain signals to the brain, and as an anti-inflammatory. Cayenne has been clinically shown to reduce pain when used topically in osteoarthritis and rheumatoid arthritis sufferers (*Ann Pharmacother* 1993). It is possible that cayenne may fare better in arthritis sufferers that do not already have heat or inflammation.

Some evidence suggests that it may prove useful for ulcers.

Although cayenne is spicy, eating cayenne actually helps to cool the body by stimulating the hypothalamus, the cooling centre of the brain, to lower body temperature. This makes it ideal for hot days or for travelling to hot places.

When I have a cold, [we] soak hot pepper flakes in orange juice and take it by the tablespoonful. Boy does that burn a cold out!

In acute cases of illness, herbalists sometimes use one teaspoon (5g) of cayenne powder every fifteen minutes. Normally, though, the dried, powdered fruit is taken in doses of 30–120mg three times a day. Taking cayenne as a pill is the least painful way of ingesting it. It can be infused and taken diluted: infuse 0.5–1 teaspoon (2–5g) in a cup of water, mix one tablespoon of the tea in hot water and take it 3–4 times a day or as needed. Tinctures can be taken at a dose of 0.25–1ml three times a day. (When I have a cold, Linda sometimes makes me soak hot pepper flakes in orange juice and take it by the tablespoonful. Boy, does that burn a cold out!)

Externally, creams containing 0.125–0.075 capsaicin can be used up to four times a day.

Cayenne is a safe herb. No side effects are expected, and it is safe to take while pregnant or breast feeding. There are rare cases of hypersensitive reaction. You should not use cayenne if you suffer from excessive acid or acid reflux, from chronic irritable bowel, or from pulmonary tuberculosis. Don't inhale it. Excessive doses may cause GI irritation in sensitive people.

The cream should not be applied to injured skin. Unless it is being used in an eye-wash formula, do not get cayenne near your eyes. That's a mistake you'll only make once: it stings! Wash your hands really well after using it so that you don't accidentally rub your eyes later and experience that eye-closing burn.

Cayenne can interfere with antacids and may interfere with monoamine oxidase inhibitors and blood pressure-lowering therapy. It may also increase the metabolism of drugs by the liver.

chamomile

German Chamomile (*Matricaria recutita, Chamomilla recutita*)
Roman Chamomile (*Chamaemelum nobile, anthemis nobilis*)

Chamomile is one of the most popular and widely used herbs in the world. Even people who are not familiar with herbs know chamomile and almost everyone has enjoyed a relaxing cup of chamomile tea. Strangely, though, despite its popularity, researchers have almost entirely ignored this herb; there are very few clinical studies done on chamomile. But the versatility of this valuable and gentle herb is no secret.

Chamomile's versatility comes from its perfect arrangement of properties. It is anti-inflammatory, antispasmodic, sedative, carminative, wound healing, and antibacterial. Put these together, and the huge list of conditions it helps begins to make sense.

As a calming herb, chamomile is wonderfully relaxing. It is great for insomnia, nervousness and anxiety. Chamomile's gentleness makes it a perfect herb for calming children. By the way, it is also a perfect herb for colicky babies, and applying the tea to the gums every two to three hours is a wonderful relief for teething.

Next to its use as a calming tea, the next best known use of chamomile is for digestive problems. Here its anti-inflammatory, antispasmodic and carminative properties dominate. The *German Commission E* approves chamomile for gastrointestinal spasm and inflammatory diseases of the gastrointestinal tract. It is a good herb to include in your treatment of irritable bowel disease, Crohn's and colitis. More simple stomach complaints like indigestion, gas and upset stomach are quickly relieved by this gentle but powerful herb. Chamomile is a good herb for diverticulitis and diarrhea, and James Duke, Ph.D., says that it is excellent for heartburn.

One prominent use of chamomile that is not well known in North America is in the treatment of ulcers. Leading German herbal authority Rudolf Fritz Weiss, M.D., calls chamomile the remedy of choice for ulcers and says that there is "no other remedy more tailor-made" for ulcers, including drugs. He says that chamomile does not merely provide symptomatic relief from ulcer pain but, used in sufficient quantity over sufficient time, it actually heals the ulcer by addressing the inflammation, spasm and ulceration. For healing ulcers, Weiss suggests a strong tea infused from two to three teaspoons (10–15g) of the flower or thirty drops of the fluid extract taken throughout the day.

Topically, chamomile cream has been shown to be useful for wound healing and for eczema. One study found it to be 60% as effective as cortisone cream for eczema (*Meth Find Exp Clin Pharmacol* 1983), while others have found it to be equally effective (*Z Hautkr* 1985).

Chamomile has many other uses. It is good for menstrual cramps and can help bring on absent periods. It is good for colds and flus, and its antifungal properties make it useful for *candida*. It can be gargled several times a day for sore throat, canker sores and gingivitis. It is helpful for the

Rudolf Fritz Weiss, M.D., calls chamomile the remedy of choice for ulcers and says that there is 'no other remedy more tailor-made' for ulcers, including drugs.

pain of a slipped disk, sciatica and gout. Try chamomile for cramps, headaches and neuralgia. Chamomile is also a good herbal source of calcium. Cosmetically, it is often used in skin products and makes a good rinse for blond hair.

 Chamomile is most commonly and pleasantly taken as a tea. Infuse 3g of the flowers and drink a cup at least three times a day on an empty stomach. If you are using chamomile pills, take 2–4g three to four times a day. As a tincture, take 3–10ml three times a day, and as an extract, take 1–4ml three times a day.

Chamomile is a very safe and gentle herb. There are no side effects, contraindications or drug interactions. It is perfectly safe to use chamomile long term. Some sources say to avoid applying the infusion near the eyes.

Although Brinker speculates that you should avoid excessive use of German chamomile in early pregnancy, Aviva Jill Romm gives this warning only for women with a history of miscarriage or who are spotting in the first four months. For these women she suggests no more than one cup a day. No other authoritative source lists any contraindications for pregnancy or lactation. A survey of women's herbals in our home library revealed no general warnings for pregnant women. On the contrary, many of the women's herbals endorse its use. Romm says it is one of her two favourite herbs when she is pregnant, and Rosemary Gladstar calls chamomile "a must for pregnant women." Roman chamomile, on the other hand, should be avoided during pregnancy.

The only other concern frequently heard for chamomile is the possibility of allergic reaction. This concern, though, has been grossly overstated. Again, although the risk may be there for Roman chamomile, there is really very little risk with the German chamomile more frequently found in stores. Even though chamomile is one of the most commonly used herbs in the world, between 1887 and 1982, only five cases of allergic reaction to German chamomile have been reported world wide (Robbers and Tyler, 1999). You may want to avoid chamomile if you are allergic to plants in the asteraceae (compositae) family to be safe but, even here, clinical evidence does not support this caution.

Chastetree berry
(Vitex agnus-castus)

Chastetree berry, or Vitex, is probably the most valuable and versatile of all the women's herbs. It has been widely used since ancient times for regulating and controlling the female reproductive system.

Legend has it that in Roman times women used this herb to reduce sexual desire while their husbands were away at war. In the Middle Ages, it was known as monk pepper because it was used by monks to reduce sexual desire. This history is what led to the name chastetree berry. Of course, none of this is true. But chastetree berry was, and still is, one of the most important herbs for female reproductive health. This wonderful herb was used, and is still used, for problems like amenorrhoea, dysmenorrhoea, menopause, and for certain pregnancy issues. Today it is also one of the most important herbs for premenstrual syndrome (PMS).

For PMS, it is simply the best treatment there is. Huge numbers of women have found relief with this herb. One massive study of 1,542 women found that chastetree berry totally eliminated symptoms of PMS in 33% of cases and partially eliminated them in another 57%. Only 4% of the women were not helped by the herb. That means that 90% of women were helped by chastetree berry and a third of them were completely symptom free (*TW Gynakol* 1992).

Similar results were found in another large study of 1,634 women who were given chastetree berry for three menstrual cycles. Ninety-three per cent of them had total or partial elimination of symptoms. This time, 42% were totally free of PMS, while another 51% had their symptoms improve; 81% were either much or very much better (*J Women Health & Gender-Based Med* 2000). By the way, nineteen women who had not been able to conceive became pregnant while on the chastetree berry – a power of chastetree berry often noted in the studies.

> *Several large studies have found that when women suffering from PMS or a wide variety of other menstrual irregularities are given chastetree berry, about 90% of them get satisfactory, good or very good results, with about a third of them getting complete relief.*

Another group of researchers wanted to see how chastetree berry would stack up against vitamin B6, another natural remedy frequently used for PMS. While 60.6% improved on the vitamin, 77.1% improved on the herb. Chastetree berry was superior over the whole range of PMS symptoms, from breast swelling and tenderness to tension, headache, constipation, and depression (*Phytomed* 1997).

Most recently, chastetree berry was tested in its first placebo-controlled study. One hundred and seventy women with PMS were given 20mg of chastetree berry extract or a placebo for three menstrual cycles. There was a significantly greater reduction in symptom scores in the herb group, including symptoms of breast tenderness, headache, mood swing and irritability; 52% of the women reduced their symptoms by 50% or more, compared to only 24% of the placebo group (*BMJ* 2001).

But chastetree berry helps more than just PMS. It helps the whole range of menstrual irregularities from absence of periods to infrequent periods to too frequent periods to too heavy periods. Several large studies have found that when women suffering from PMS or a wide variety of other menstrual irregularities are given chastetree berry, about 90% of them get satisfactory, good or very good results, with about a third of them getting complete relief (*Therapeutikon* 1991; *Der Frauenarzt* 1991; *Gynakol* 1994). In several of these studies, the ability of chastetree berry to overcome infertility was again seen. In one study, 56 out of 145 women who were trying to become pregnant, did (*Therapeutikon* 1991). In another, 42% of thirty-three women with fertility problems became pregnant (*Gynakol* 1994). And in a third study, in which 63% of women with menstrual irregularities normalized their cycle, 29% of them became pregnant (*Therapiewoche* 1993).

Another study has again found this result. It gave either a placebo or a homeopathic combination featuring chastetree berry to sixty-six women who had been trying unsuccessfully to become pregnant for one to three years. After three months, ten women became pregnant while on chastetree berry compared to half as many on the placebo (*Research in Complementary Med* 1998). Several women's herbals recommend chastetree berry for infertility.

Chastetree berry is able to help such a wide variety of problems at both extremes of the menstrual spectrum because of its remarkable ability to regulate hormones in whatever direction they need regulating.

British herbalist David Hoffmann says that chastetree berry "will always enable what is appropriate to occur," and herbalist Rosemary Gladstar praises chastetree berry's power of restoring and regulating the estrogen / progesterone balance. This balancing act is what allows chastetree berry to help, no matter what hormonal problem is being treated. In addition to menstrual problems and infertility, chastetree berry is also able to help endometriosis, fibrocystic breast disease, fibroids, and corpus luteum insufficiency. It is an excellent herb for menopause. Chastetree berry is also valuable for its ability to regulate the menstrual cycle after coming off the birth control pill.

Chastetree berry does not contain hormones. It regulates the hormones by working in the pituitary gland. Specifically, chastetree berry seems to increase progesterone while decreasing estrogen and prolactin.

Since it decreases prolactin, you would think that chastetree berry should be avoided during breast feeding, since prolactin is essential for the production of breast milk. And yet, many traditional herbalists specializing in women's health recommend this herb for encouraging breast milk. Several studies have confirmed this traditional use. We found references to at least five studies on chastetree berry and lactation that reported this positive result.

In addition to a wide range of women's health benefits, chastetree berry has still other benefits. At least seven uncontrolled studies have found that it helps acne. Herbalist Christopher Hobbs says that chastetree berry is effective for teenage acne in both girls and boys. We have found clinically that it is especially helpful for acne related to PMS.

One more possible and totally unexpected potential use currently remains theoretical. Ernest Hawkins reports in *HerbalGram* that chastetree berry bonds to dopamine-2 receptors. These receptors control a system that might be involved in addictive behaviour, raising the possibility that chastetree berry may one day find a use helping people with addictive personalities.

There is a wide range of recommendations for the dose of chastetree berry because different European countries seem to use different doses. If you are using the tincture, take 2–6ml (about 40–120 drops) a day. If you are using the extract, take 2–4ml a day. If you are taking the herb in pill form, German sources suggest 30–40mg of dried herb a day, while others suggest 500–1,000 or even as high as 650mg up to three times a day. If you are using a standardized extract in the form of a pill, take 175–225mg standardized for 0.5% agnuside one or two times a day. The consensus seems to be to take chastetree berry in one dose before breakfast.

Chastetree berry works by balancing the hormones, so although its benefits may be felt as soon as the second menstrual period, it works best when taken long term. When used for a year to a year and a half, chastetree berry can even put an end to PMS permanently.

Chastetree berry is very safe. Side effects are very rare, occurring in only 1–2% of cases and include occasional minor rash with itching and mild upset stomach. One source lists the very rare possibility of hair loss, agitation, dry mouth, and tachycardia. These warnings do not usually appear in the literature or in clinical studies.

There are no contraindications for chastetree berry. It is possible that chastetree berry could interact with dopamine antagonists and so should be avoided by people on those drugs. It is sometimes said that because of its effect on hormones, chastetree berry should be avoided by those on the birth control pill or hormone replacement therapy. However, this warning is speculative and has not been borne out clinically. At least two recent studies have noted that there was no negative interaction between the herb and the birth control pill (*Arch Gynecol Obstet* 2000; *BMJ* 2001).

Chastetree berry should not be used while pregnant, although it has been used in the first trimester to prevent miscarriage by women with progesterone insufficiency. Some sources theorize that this herb should be avoided during breast feeding, but chastetree berry has been shown to safely enhance the production of breast milk.

chickweed *(Stellaria media)*

Fortunately for us, chickweed is a very common wayside weed that is readily available to many people. And this is extremely lucky since chickweed is one of the best herbs for soothing itchy, burning rashes. Chickweed contains saponins, which exert powerful anti-inflammatory properties, like those of cortisone, but without the harmful side effects of cortisone. This soothing ability of chickweed makes it extremely valuable in treating rashes. It is one of our favourite herbs clinically when there is any sign of rash or redness on the skin, especially if there is itching involved. Usually, a chickweed oil, salve or cream is used for skin problems, including rashes, eczema and psoriasis.

But chickweed is used for many other purposes. It is used to treat blood toxicity, fevers, sore throats and lung problems, inflammation and other diseases where there is too much heat, for boils, abscesses, for weight reduction, and as a mild diuretic and laxative.

Chickweed cream should be applied generously several times a day. Macerate the whole herb in olive oil for four days, squeeze through a cloth, and apply. A strong infusion of the fresh plant can also be added to bath water to ease itching. To make a tea, infuse two teaspoons (10g) of dried herb per cup of water and drink a cup three times a day. The dose of the tincture is 1–5ml three times a day.

There are no side effects, drug interactions or contraindications, including while pregnant or breast feeding.

cinnamon *(Cinnamomun zeylanicum, cinnamomun verum)*

When most people think of cinnamon, they think of desserts and other delicious food. Yet cinnamon is also a wonderful herb that has been in use for thousands of years for all kinds of healing. It was used by the ancient Greeks, Egyptians and Chinese. Cinnamon is warming to the system and is used to warm the internal organs, helping to treat stubborn diarrhea, indigestion, gas, bloating, dysentery, abdominal pain, loss of appetite, cramping and spasming in the digestive tract, coughs, wheezing, lower back and heart pain. Its astringent properties also make it useful for stopping bleeding from the uterus. In addition, cinnamon has antibacterial and antifungal activity, including powerful activity against *candida*. Traditionally, cinnamon has also been used for respiratory complaints such as asthma and bronchitis and to increase blood circulation.

Preliminary studies suggest cinnamon may help balance blood sugar levels, making it useful for diabetics and hypoglycemics. Most recently, a placebo-controlled study highlighted the enthusiasm over cinnamon for reducing the risks of diabetes and heart disease in type II diabetics. Cinnamon was able to significantly lower the subjects' glucose levels as well as their total cholesterol, harmful LDL cholesterol and triglycerides (*Diabetes Care* 2003). Expect to hear more about this herb.

The dose of the ground cinnamon bark is 2–4g a day. If you want to take cinnamon as a tea, infuse or decoct 1/2–1 teaspoon (2–5g) per cup of water three times a day. Be sure to keep the pot covered so the volatile oils do not escape. Dose recommendations for the tincture range all over the place: one source says as low as 1ml three times a day, one says 2–3ml three times a day, and another goes as high as 3.3–6.7ml three times a day. The dose of the extract is 0.7–1.3ml three times a day.

Allergic reactions of the skin are possible with cinnamon, so it should not be used by people with allergies to cinnamon or to Peruvian balsam. It should possibly also be avoided by people with ulcers or acid reflux. Though women's herbals do not contraindicate cinnamon in pregnancy, all the authoritative contraindications texts do. Cinnamon does not seem to be contraindicated while breast feeding. Cinnamon may potentiate insulin.

Cleavers
(Galium aparine)

Cleavers is a very effective diuretic that also cleanses the blood while being perhaps the best tonic for the lymph system. It is used to treat all urinary and reproductive organ inflammations, including cystitis. It also treats hepatitis, venereal disease, enlarged lymph glands, tonsillitis and adenoid problems, psoriasis, fevers, skin eruptions, and skin diseases. We have seen this herb work well when it is combined with uva ursi and buchu for men with inflamed and infected prostate glands.

Externally, it is often used in a poultice to treat scalds, burns and rashes.

 Infuse 2–3 teaspoons (10–15g) of the dried herb in a cup of water three times a day or more. Alternatively, you can take 2–5ml of the tincture three times a day.

 There are no side effects, drug interactions or contraindications, including while pregnant or breast feeding.

Coltsfoot
(Tussilago farfara)

In coltsfoot, nature has combined soothing, expectorant, antispasmodic and cough suppressing actions to make a truly valuable herb for coughs and most respiratory problems. It can be used for irritating coughs, emphysema, asthma, and bronchitis.

 Coltsfoot is taken as an infusion, using 1–2 teaspoons (5–10g) of the dried flowers or leaves only. It should be drunk as hot as possible, three times a day. If you use a tincture, take 2–4ml three times daily. Coltsfoot should be taken for no more than one month.

 Coltsfoot provides a classic example of the clash between science on the one hand and tradition and nature on the other. Science has condemned this established herb because it has detected minute amounts of an ingredient, called Pyrrolizidine alkaloids (PA's), that could cause liver cancer. While it may be true that, when given to animals over prolonged periods of time in doses hundreds of times greater than those used medicinally, it may cause damage, this concern is not applicable to humans.

Recently, however, concern has been raised over reports that PA's could cause liver damage: a condition known as hepatic veno-occlusive disease. For this reason, use of the root of coltsfoot internally has fallen out of favour, with a number of authorities advising against taking it. Brinker, in his authoritative book on contraindications, still allows the internal use of coltsfoot, but only for four to six weeks per year. The leaves, however, contain a much smaller amount of PA's and are allowed by these authorities to be taken internally for up to one month. No coltsfoot preparation should be taken while pregnant or breast feeding or by people with liver disease. The external use of coltsfoot is still fine, but it should not be applied over broken skin.

One study found that after decocting coltsfoot for half an hour, there was no detectable amount of PA. Other research has found that the mucilage in this plant negates whatever small amount may be there. Though clearly still controversial, the recommendations given here should be followed until more is known.

Comfrey   *(Symphytum officinale)*

Comfrey is a remarkable herb for any kind of wound healing. Its old, traditional names, "knitbone" and "boneset," point to its use in the healing of broken bones as well as wounds.

The wound healing powers of comfrey are so great that we are sometimes cautioned to be careful when applying it externally to very deep wounds in case tissue forms over the wound and heals the surface before it has a chance to heal deeper down. Its incredible ability to soothe while promoting fast healing makes it an ideal herb for ulcers, wounds and fractures. It can be used internally or applied externally to the skin, through which it is easily absorbed. In addition, the same soothing properties, coupled with its expectorant properties, also make comfrey useful for irritating coughs and bronchitis.

Externally, creams from the root or leaf can be applied several times a day. If you are going to use comfrey internally, only the mature leaf should be used – not the root and not the fresh leaves. Infuse 1–2 teaspoons (5–10g) of the leaf in a cup of water and drink three times a day for no more than one month. You can also use a tincture of the leaf by taking 2–4ml three times a day for no more than one month.

Comfrey is another herb that has come under attack for the same reason as coltsfoot: minute amounts of Pyrrolizidine alkaloids (PA's), which may cause liver cancer, have been detected. When rats were fed a diet consisting of 30–50% comfrey, they developed tumours. No kidding. The same objections raised about the coltsfoot findings apply here: the relevance of animal research, the relevance of the dose, the minuscule presence of the ingredient and the ignorance of other balancing components in the herb. One of the few studies that looked at the whole plant found no cancer causing properties. In fact, they found the opposite.

But, like coltsfoot, comfrey has become controversial because of reports that the Pyrrolizidine alkaloids (PA's) can lead to hepatic veno-occlusive disease. For this reason, the internal use of the root and the fresh leaves of comfrey is contraindicated. The mature leaves contain very little if any PA's, which is why their limited internal use is permitted in the dosage section.

Francis Brinker, N.D., an expert on the safety of herbs, has said recently that the blanket contraindication for the internal use of comfrey has been challenged based both on experience and on insufficient scientific investigation. Nonetheless, until the PA controversy is cleared up, the reports should be taken seriously.

Comfrey in any form should not be taken if you are pregnant or breast feeding. Don't give it to children and don't use it if you have liver disease. If you use the mature leaf, don't use it for more than a month.

PA's do not contribute to the medicinal value of herbs, and they can be removed, as in the case of butterbur. PA-free tinctures are available: they are the best bet, and they can be taken long term.

Many of the great values of comfrey are attained through its external use for wound and bone healing. And topically, it is still perfectly safe to use comfrey as long as you do not apply it to broken skin (though even here, one lone source says not to use it topically for more than four to six weeks).

Cramp bark *(Viburnum opulus)*

Cramp bark is one of our favourite herbs for the relief of menstrual cramps, and we have given it to scores of women with great success. For this purpose, we like to use a very strong liquid tincture or even an extract.

The herb's name says it all. Cramp bark is wonderful for muscular cramps, but especially for the cramps of menstruation. It is considered one of the very best herbs for menstrual cramps. It is also excellent for excessive menstrual bleeding. But that is not all it does. The same uterus-relaxing properties that alleviate menstrual cramps make cramp bark one of the best herbs for preventing miscarriage, especially miscarriage brought on by stress or anxiety. When combined with ginger, dong quai and chamomile, it is very useful for PMS. Because of its nervine and sedative properties, cramp bark is also used for heart palpitations, asthma, and rheumatism. Cramp bark is a sedative, nervine, antispasmodic, and astringent herb.

Decoct one tablespoon of the dried bark in a cup of water for 10–15 minutes and drink 3–4 times a day or as needed. As a tincture, use 4–8ml three times daily. For menstrual pain, try taking 1/2 teaspoon (2g) every 2–3 hours.

Cramp bark is remarkably safe and can be used even long term with no side effects or toxicity. It is perfectly safe during pregnancy and breast feeding and can be used over an extended period of time if miscarriage is a potential problem. There are no drug interactions.

Cranberry
(Vaccinium macrocarpon)

Cranberry is usually taken as a juice. Cranberry juice is one of the most important herbs for urinary tract infections, and it works in a novel and ingenious way. Cranberry juice has the amazing ability to prevent *E. coli* (the cause of about 90% of urinary tract infections) from adhering to the walls of the urinary tract (*J Urol* 1984; *New Engl J Med* 1991). If the bacteria can't hang around, it can't do its dirty work. This ability to take care of the bacteria and treat urinary tract infections without actually killing anything makes cranberry a very safe and gentle way to treat infections.

Several studies have shown how well cranberry juice works. Sixteen ounces of cranberry juice helped 73% of people with urinary tract infections in one early study (*Southwest J Med* 1968). More recently, women who had just recovered from a urinary tract infection caused by *E. coli* were given either 50ml of concentrated cranberry juice in 200ml of water or a placebo or nothing. After six months, only 16% of the women on cranberry suffered a recurrence of the infection compared to 39% on the placebo and 36% who took nothing (*BMJ* 2001).

Cranberry juice can even overcome *E. coli* that is resistant to antibiotics. In a study of women with urinary tract infections caused by *E. coli* which was, in most cases, antibiotic resistant, urine was collected before and after drinking 8 ounces of cranberry juice. In 80% of the women, the juice prevented the bacteria from adhering to the bladder wall (*JAMA* 2002).

Like so many other powerful herbs, the latest research shows that it is a group of flavonoid antioxidants known as proanthocyanidins that are responsible for preventing the bacteria from adhering to the urinary tract walls (*New Engl J Med* 1998). It is not entirely surprising then that other proanthocyanidin rich juices may frustrate *E. coli* as well. Blueberries are another excellent source of these flavonoids and blueberry juice

Cranberry juice has the amazing ability to prevent E. coli (the cause of about 90% of urinary tract infections) from adhering to the walls of the urinary tract.

does work (*New Engl J Med* 1991). A recent study showed that drinking one to three glasses a week of any of cranberry, raspberry, strawberry or current juice lowered the risk of urinary tract infection (*Am J Clin Nutr* 2003). Make sure the juice is pure and unsweetened, since sugar can contribute to, instead of resolve, the problem.

Because the proanthocyanidins in cranberry are powerful antioxidants, cranberry may have uses other than in the treatment of urinary tract infections. It inhibits the oxidation of the dangerous LDL cholesterol, an important step in preventing cholesterol problems. It may also be useful in cancer treatment. Recent research has found that in the same way as cranberry stops the bacteria from adhering to the walls of the urinary tract, it also stops bacteria in the mouth from sticking together and forming dental plaque (*Journal of the American Dental Association* 1998). So cranberry could turn out to have a role to play in dental health.

Always use pure, unsweetened cranberry juice diluted in water. For treatment, drink 16 ounces a day; for prevention, drink 4–16 ounces a day. If you prefer taking a pill, take 10 to sixteen 400–500mg pills a day or, more conveniently, one 400mg pill of concentrated cranberry extract two to three times a day. Remember, if you have a urinary tract infection, drinking plenty of fluid is important. If you take a pill instead of drinking 16 ounces of the juice, you will have to drink more water to make up for the fluid.

Cranberry juice is perfectly safe. There are no side effects or contraindications. It is safe to use long term and is safe during pregnancy and breast feeding. There are no drug interactions, including with antibiotics. Very recently, however, there was a report of five cases of cranberry possibly increasing the effect of warfarin (*Curr Prob Pharmacocovigil* 2003).

Though cranberry has traditionally been used to prevent kidney stones, the information on this use is confusing and conflicting. Some sources contraindicate cranberry in people who have or are prone to some types of kidney stones. Two small studies, however, found the herb to reduce the incidence of kidney stones (*NY State J Med* 1968; *Urology* 1973).

Dandelion

Dandelion is the most ironic herb in nature. If herbs can laugh, this one is laughing at us. Each spring, home owners spend a fortune on herbicides to rid their lawn of dandelions. These herbicides contribute greatly to the chemical load our livers need to detoxify to keep us healthy. And one of the greatest liver detoxifiers to be found is the root of the very weed we just used all those chemicals to kill.

In many natural medicine traditions, spring is the time to cleanse the body and detoxify. And when all else is struggling to grow green once more, the dandelion waves its golden head in the air, calling out for us to take notice of its cleansing and healing properties. Considered a weed by most, by those who are still close to nature, it is a beautiful yellow flower and one of nature's most valuable offerings to the liver. We always leave our dandelions in our lawn and wait until they can be harvested. Then we pick them, leaves and roots, and enjoy a healthy – and free – natural detox. The leaves go into our salads, adding a wealth of vitamins and minerals. The roots, however, are the most prized because of their liver detoxifying properties. We dry them, use them in teas and tinctures and enjoy their benefits all year round.

The leaves are valuable bitter greens, great for the digestive system and for loss of appetite, whether eaten in a salad or taken as a supplement. They are also one of the most powerful and safest diuretics around. Dandelion leaf is at least as strong as any pharmaceutical diuretic, without the side effects. While diuretics cause loss of potassium, dandelion, being loaded with potassium, replaces what the body loses.

And dandelion leaf isn't just loaded in potassium. This herb is a nutrient treasure chest. The leaves are very high in vitamins A, B and C. They are a rare plant source of vitamin D and are rich in choline. They are also packed with the minerals calcium, magnesium, iron, boron, zinc, copper, manganese, phosphorus, and potassium.

> *. . . the dandelion waves its golden head in the air, calling out for us to take notice of its cleansing and healing properties.*

Looking at this list, it comes as no surprise that James Duke, Ph.D., recommends dandelion as an osteoarthritis herb that strengthens the bones. Its iron content also makes it a good herb for anemia.

But don't stop with the leaf. Hidden below the ground is what herbalist David Hoffmann calls one of the most widely applicable, gentle liver tonics: the root of the dandelion is a safe treatment for many liver conditions. Herbalist Rosemary Gladstar calls dandelion the liver herb par excellence and recommends it for all liver disorders, gall bladder problems and digestive upsets.

Because it increases bile and stimulates saliva and gastric juices, dandelion root is a valuable aid to digestion. Dandelion increases bile in two ways: it increase the production of bile in the liver and the release of bile by the gall bladder. This greater efficiency of bile flow helps hepatitis, gallstones, bile duct inflammation and jaundice, according to Michael Murray, N.D. Herbalist David Hoffmann adds inflammation and congestion of the liver and gallbladder. As a digestive bitter, it is also used for loss of appetite.

Dandelion root is a fabulous herb for cirrhosis, jaundice, liver congestion and hepatitis. Herbalist Michael Tierra says that even the most severe cases of hepatitis can be cured quickly with dandelion. Tierra also says that dandelion is good for clearing obstructions of the spleen, pancreas, gall bladder, bladder, and kidneys.

As for some of the more unusual uses of dandelion, its iron content makes it good for anemia; it is recommended for high blood pressure, hypoglycemia, morning sickness, rheumatism, and colitis; and it is said to be a good herb for pneumonia, bronchitis and upper respiratory infection.

Gladstar says that dandelion is a valuable herb for women. She says that as a liver herb that acts as a diuretic and helps regulate hormones, it is a wonderful herb for menstrual bloating, PMS and menopause.

The leaf can be eaten in salads. As a diuretic, infuse 4–10g of the leaf and drink it three times a day. As an extract, take 4–10ml three times a day.

The doses for the root are 2–8g three times a day as a decoction, 5–10ml three times a day as a tincture, 4–8ml three times a day as an extract.

Dandelion is a very safe, gentle herb. It has no side effects or drug interactions. It is safe for women who are pregnant or breast feeding. Some say that dandelion should not be taken by people with intestinal or bile duct obstruction or gall bladder empyema. Brinker contraindicates it in cases of intestinal spasm and liver cancer. Some contraindication books say not to use dandelion if there is gall bladder inflammation, but Hoffmann specifically recommends it for this use, and Gladstar recommends it for all gall bladder problems. The texts also say only to use dandelion for gallstones after consulting a practitioner. This caution is the usual one for herbs that increase bile (see the section on artichoke for a fuller discussion). Herbal authority Rudolf Fritz Weiss, M.D., calls dandelion a specific for people who have a disposition toward gallstones and Mills and Bone also recommend it for gallstones in their authoritative text, as do Murray and Pizzorno in theirs.

Devil's claw *(Harpogophytum procumbens)*

When we first started working in a health food store several years ago, devil's claw was one of the herbs most talked about. Echinacea for immunity, ginkgo for memory, valerian for insomnia, ginseng for energy, and devil's claw for rheumatoid arthritis. Then devil's claw fell out of favour, and for a long time very little was heard about it. Well, it's time to start talking about it again.

Devil's claw probably fell out of favour because it was mostly recommended as an anti-inflammatory herb for rheumatoid arthritis, but the research on its anti-inflammatory action has been conflicting, which is why people stopped recommending it.

Devil's claw fares better as an anti-inflammatory in chronic cases than it does in acute cases, as Tankred Wegener says in an article in *HerbalGram* #50. He also says that when the results are positive, it's usually a water extract of devil's claw given orally that is used, as opposed to an alcohol extract or an isolated component of the herb.

Whether this African herb is an anti-inflammatory or not, several recent studies are regenerating enthusiasm for this once prominent herb because they are proving it able to reduce pain and improve mobility in people suffering from arthritis.

A double-blind study conducted in 1992, for example, found that when people suffering from rheumatic joint pain were given devil's claw for two months, there was a significant decrease in the intensity of their pain and a significant increase in their mobility.

But, surprisingly, the real promise is showing up not in rheumatoid arthritis studies as always thought, but in osteoarthritis studies. In a double-blind 1984 study, people with osteoarthritis who were given devil's claw had significantly reduced pain compared to a placebo group. In 1997, significant improvements in mobility and morning stiffness were experienced by forty-three people with both osteo and rheumatoid arthritis.

Most recently, 122 people with osteoarthritis were given either devil's claw or a drug. Not only did the devil's claw group suffer significantly fewer side effects, but 65.3% of them had good or very good results – better than the 60% in the drug group (*Phytomed* 2000).

Devil's claw is also good for gout, another kind of arthritis. Elevated uric acid levels cause gout, and devil's claw lowers uric acid levels.

Recent studies have also suggested that devil's claw may have a role to play in relieving back pain for at least some people. In one double-blind study, people with chronic low back pain were given either devil's claw or a placebo. Nine of the herb group became pain free compared to only one in the placebo group: a significant difference. Pain improved by 20% in the herb group and 8% in the placebo group: a nonsignificant difference (*Phytomed* 1996).

When people suffering low back pain were given either devil's claw or a nonsteroidal anti-inflammatory drug, 32% of the herb group were pain free after four weeks compared to 23% of the drug group. After six weeks, 29% of the herb group were pain free and 45% of the drug group. Pain improved by 20% in both groups and changes in mobility were also the same in both groups.

In a more recent study, 197 people with back pain were given either 600mg or 1,200mg of devil's claw or a placebo for four weeks. The number of people who were pain free at the end were 5% in the placebo group, 9% in the 600mg group and 15% in the 1,200mg group. Only those whose back pain did not radiate to the legs benefited (*Eur J Anaesthesiology* 1999).

Aside from joint and back pain, devil's claw also has many other benefits. Rudolf Fritz Weiss, M.D., says that devil's claw is one of the most powerful bitter tonics. This property makes it an excellent herb for indigestion and loss of appetite, two uses of the herb approved by the *German Commission E*. Herbalist David Hoffmann adds a related benefit: he says devil's claw is good for liver and gallbladder problems.

Weiss and Daniel Mowrey, Ph.D., both report that devil's claw also lowers cholesterol.

As a tea, decoct for fifteen minutes and drink three cups a day. In pill form, use 1–2 grams of the dried powdered root three times daily. As a tincture, take 15–30ml a day, and as an extract take 6–12ml a day. If you are using standardized devil's claw in tablet form, take 600–1,200mg a day. For loss of appetite, a smaller dose of 1.5 grams of dried root powder is sufficient. Devil's claw should be taken between meals.

Devil's claw is an extremely safe and well-tolerated herb. There are a few cases of mild gastrointestinal complaint, but no reports of serious adverse effects. Devil's claw may be contraindicated for people with ulcers.

There are no side effects or interactions with drugs. Devil's claw is safe for pregnant or breast feeding women.

Devil's club
(Oplopanax horridus)

Many people confuse this herb with devil's claw, the better-known herb, and so devil's club is not as well known. Yet devil's club is one of the best herbs for controlling blood sugar. It is, therefore, useful for diabetes and hypoglycemia. It also helps to reduce sugar cravings.

Though little known to most of us, devil's club is probably the most revered herb of the First Nations people of the Pacific Northwest. Its traditional uses include treatment of diabetes and infection, and its spiritual uses include purification, luck, protection against supernatural entities, and warding off witchcraft (*HerbalGram* #62).

Its traditional uses include treatment of diabetes and infection, and its spiritual uses include purification, luck, protection against supernatural entities, and warding off witchcraft.

Devil's club is antibacterial, antiviral and antifungal, and it is sometimes used as a respiratory stimulant and expectorant.

Most sources do not even mention this herb, and so little information is available. Try 1 ounce simmered for 30 minutes in a pint of water, drunk 3 times daily.

Again, little information is available. But devil's club seems to be perfectly safe, even for pregnant and breast feeding women.

Dong quai *(Angelica sinensis and related species)*

In Asia, dong quai has a reputation as being second only to ginseng and is considered a supreme herb, especially for females. Dong quai is used to treat almost every gynecological problem. It has especially been used to treat menopause, although it does not seem to do this through estrogen since it is now known that it is not a phytoestrogen; however, it still helps with menopausal symptoms, especially hot flashes. Dong quai is not used alone for menopause. Mixed with other herbs, it helps by toning the uterus and perhaps by helping women to better use their own existing estrogen. Dong quai tones the uterus and has antispasmodic and alterative, or blood purifying, properties. Dong quai can be used for painful menstrual periods since it such an effective herb for treating menstrual cramps. It can also be used for irregularity; for amenorrhoea, or lack of a period; for abnormal menstruation; PMS; delayed flow and weakness during the period; but it should not be used when there is a heavy menstrual flow or during pregnancy. In Asia, however, it has a reputation for fostering a healthy pregnancy and easy delivery.

This herb's antispasmodic properties make it of value in treating insomnia, high blood pressure, and abdominal and uterine cramping.

It is used to treat anaemia and nourish the blood and is warming to the circulation. It can also be used to treat constipation that is caused by dry intestines.

Historically, dong quai has also been used to treat migraine, asthma, arthritis, injuries, and abdominal pain. Angelica's analgesic activity has been shown to help with pain conditions like arthritis, headache, cramps, and trauma.

Clinically, dong quai, has also been shown to have many useful actions for the circulatory system. It lowers blood pressure by its ability to dilate blood vessels; it has antiarrhythmic action; it inhibits blood platelet aggregation; and it increases blood flow to the extremities.

Angelica has also been found to have anti-allergy activity and has long been used in Asia for this purpose. It seems to work by reducing elevated antibody levels, helping to stop an allergic response. Angelica also offers cancer-fighting properties by stimulating white blood cells, which can destroy cancer cells and prevent their spread. A compound of angelica called coumarin and the polysaccharides of the water extract of Japanese angelica offer immune modulation activity in several ways. This ability to modulate the immune system makes angelica a useful agent in the fight against cancer.

Dong quai has also shown antibiotic activity against both gram-negative and gram-positive bacteria.

According to Michael Murray and Joseph Pizzorno, N.D.'s, for use as an expectorant, an antispasmodic and carminative, you should use the *Angelica archangelica* and *Angelica atropurpurea* species; for cancer, menstrual problems, menopause, and smooth muscle spasms like headache, cramps and abdominal spasms, you should use the *Angelica sinesis* or *Angelica acutiloba* species. *Angelica sinensis* is the one that is commonly used and commonly found in health stores.

A wide range of doses are given for dong quai. If making a tea, decoct anywhere from 1–5g and drink it three times a day. In pill form, take 1–4g three times a day. You can also take dong quai as a tincture at a dose of 2–4ml three times a day or as an extract at a dose of 1ml three times a day.

Dong quai is a very safe herb. It should not be used, however, if you are prone to bleeding or are experiencing heavy menstruation. If you want to use dong quai for painful menstruation, it's best to take it as a tonic for several months, beginning fourteen days after the first day of your period and taking it until the first day of the next period. That way, you will treat the pain but not enhance the bleeding.

Don't use dong quai during a cold or flu or if you have diarrhea.

Dong quai can enhance the activity of warfarin.

The pregnancy and breast feeding question is complicated. Several texts say not to use this herb during pregnancy and one even says not to use it while breast feeding. Chinese herbals, though, apparently do not include this contraindication or include it only for the first trimester. Some sources refine the warning, saying not to use dong quai during the first trimester or if you have a history of miscarriage.

Do Herbs Really Work?

The results we have seen with herbs are remarkable. And that's not surprising. Herbs have been used, and herbal knowledge has been refined, for thousands of years. We evolved beside the plants we use. And despite the frequent claim that herbs have not been studied, many of them have been studied very well. Several have been shown to be as good or better than the drugs that are used for the same conditions, while being safer. Some examples are St. John's wort for depression, black cohosh for menopause, saw palmetto berry for enlarged prostate, kava kava for anxiety, Ginkgo biloba for Alzheimer's, valerian for insomnia, peppermint oil for IBS, hawthorn for congestive heart failure and butterbur for hay fever.

Echinacea

(Echinacea purpurea, Echinacea angustofolia, Echinacea pallida)

That beautiful flower growing in your garden that looks like a huge purple daisy just might be one of the most powerful and important immune supporters in the world. And in this day of antibiotic resistance and side effects, and apparently unstoppable viruses, that just might make your garden an important part of the pharmacy of the future.

This magical herb does not fight infection the way antibiotics do. Although it has mild antibiotic and antiviral properties, echinacea does its work by helping you do yours: it doesn't kill the bacteria and viruses, it helps your immune system to fight off bacteria and viruses the way it's naturally supposed to. We grow an echinacea in our front garden that we make into a tincture that can knock the cold out of anyone!

Echinacea helps your immune system in three main ways. First, it stimulates the production and activity of immune cells. Echinacea increases your immune cells' capacity to engulf and destroy cancer cells and invading pathogens: literally, to devour them, a process called phagocytosis. Echinacea also has an interferon-like effect. Interferon is your body's own immune-enhancing virus and cancer fighter.

Secondly, echinacea activates a secondary system, called the alternate complement pathway, that is triggered when antibodies go to work, and destroys invaders.

The third way that echinacea helps your immune system is really unique. Your immune system's first line of defence is a protective barrier called hyaluronic acid. Germs spread through your body by eating their way through this barrier by means of an enzyme called hyularonidase. Once through the barrier, germs can spread throughout the body and attack your cells. Echinacea has the ability to inactivate hyaluronidase and lock invaders out. First Nations healers have long used echinacea to treat snake bite. Most snake venom permeates the body via hyularonidase.

Some past studies have questioned echinacea's ability to prevent colds, while confirming its ability to treat them. However, a recent meta-analysis of high quality double-blind, placebo-controlled studies found a 55% higher chance of catching a cold when taking a placebo than when taking echinacea, showing that echinacea does prevent colds (*Clin Ther* 2006).

Healthy Herbs 57

Many studies have confirmed echinacea's ability to support the immune system. Just as importantly, clinical experience by herbalists and by the many people who use it overwhelmingly testifies to echinacea's power over colds and flus.

Whether echinacea prevents or treats colds may depend on the kind of echinacea you use. Canadian herbalist Terry Willard, Ph.D., says that the whole herb or the powdered root taken as a pill is an immune system modulator and is an excellent preventative for people exposed to viruses, while echinacea tincture or extract is an immune booster that is effective when taken at the very first signs of a cold. Herb expert Daniel Mowrey, Ph.D., agrees. He says that echinacea is actually an immune tonic that brings an underachieving or overactive immune system into balance. Like Willard, though, Mowrey says that the extract is a pure immune stimulant. Another respected authority on herbs, Kerry Bone, also calls echinacea an immunomodulator used for weakened, suppressed or imbalanced immunity.

In addition to whether echinacea stimulates or balances the immune system and treats or prevents colds, there are other related areas of confusion that have led to highly popularized but false claims about this remarkable herb. For example, it is almost always claimed in the popular literature that echinacea should never be used long term because it will overstimulate the immune system. This claim is simply false. Long term use of echinacea is safe and no evidence exists to suggest otherwise.

It has also been claimed that echinacea should not be used for progressive conditions or autoimmune diseases like tuberculosis, collagen disorders, multiple sclerosis, AIDS and HIV. However, these contraindications, too, are false. Bone points out that no clinical studies document adverse effects in any of these conditions (*Eur J Herb Med* 1997-8). Bone and Mills, as well as herb expert Paul Bergner and the American Botanical Council (Blumenthal, *et al*, 2000, 2003) go on to add that not only is echinacea not harmful in autoimmunity, scientific data and a large body of clinical observation support long term use of echinacea for autoimmune disorders.

There is another special immune use of echinacea that is worth mentioning. Intense exercise can suppress immunity. But a placebo-controlled study found that when echinacea was given to triathletes for four weeks prior to competing, the herb prevented the usual immune suppression. No one in the echinacea group got an upper respiratory tract or other infection, but several of the athletes not on echinacea did. While the placebo group missed a total of twenty-four training days to colds, not a single day was missed in the echinacea group (*J Clin Res* 1998).

There are also other uses for echinacea. When 203 women with recurrent vaginal yeast infections were given either an antifungal cream alone or in combination with oral echinacea, there was a 60.5% recurrence rate in the drug group compared to only 16.7% in the group taking echinacea (*Therapiewoche* 1986). In a more unexpected role, echinacea is also useful for healing ulcers, wounds and skin infections. An echinacea ointment was 85% effective in treating 4,598 people with wounds, inflammatory skin conditions, eczema, leg ulcers, burns, or herpes. Echinacea is an anti-inflammatory herb, and herbalist Michael Tierra and others note that it may even prevent wrinkles. Echinacea is a good herb for people who suffer recurrent infections, including children with recurrent ear infections.

Overall, echinacea is a remarkable, even magical, herb for supporting your immune system.

Echinacea can be used in many ways. The root can be taken as a pill or decocted as a tea and taken at a dose of one gram three times a day. Echinacea tinctures should be dosed at 2–5ml three times a day and extracts at 0.5–2ml a day. If you are using the expressed juice of the fresh plant, take 2–3ml three times a day. For acute conditions, you can take higher doses short term. Willard and Mowrey suggests using 250–500mg a day of the whole herb or powdered root if you are using echinacea preventatively. When fighting an active infection, make sure you start taking echinacea at the very first sign. Some herbalists like to give about 30 drops of echinacea every two hours at the first sign of a cold.

Different active ingredients are found in different parts of the echinacea plant and are drawn out either better or worse by alcohol or water. So which part should you use? The best advice seems to be to use an alcoholic extract or tincture made from the whole plant, including the roots and the above ground parts of the plant; a pill made from the whole plant or the roots; or a tea made from the roots.

Echinacea is remarkably safe. Most of the reported warnings for this herb are not true. An additional warning not to take echinacea with immune-suppressing drugs is also based only on theory and lacks any clinical documentation. In fact, there are no known drug interactions for echinacea. There are also no adverse effects. Echinacea is even perfectly safe to take while pregnant or breast feeding – there is no increased risk (*Arch Intern Med* 2000).

Elder *(Sambucus nigra)*

This is one of our favourite herbs for preventing colds and flus. And so far it has rarely failed. Clinically, we also see amazing results. Though this herb is still seldom mentioned and little known, it is emerging as an extremely important antiviral.

Elder's primary role is in fighting colds, flus and fevers. Traditionally, the flowers have been used most. They induce sweating, which helps the immune system fight infection, while acting as an expectorant and anti-inflammatory, making it a perfect tea to drink when you feel a cold or flu coming on. Similarly, it can be used for any respiratory tract problem, like sinusitis and hay fever. It combines well with yarrow and peppermint as a tea.

But it is the berry that is one of our favourite remedies for fighting colds and flus. And recently, the berry has moved out of the flower's shadow to emerge as a leading herb for colds and flus. Elderberry extract has the amazing ability to stop viruses from penetrating into your cells, which stops them from replicating (*J Alt Comp Med* 1995). That is why this herb has proven so remarkable against colds and flus. In fact, it has been proven effective against ten strains of flu virus (*J Altern Compliment Med*), a record, herbal expert Paul Bergner has pointed out, that could make elderberry a more effective preventative than the flu shot.

Elderberries are also a concentrated source of anthocyanidins, which are powerful

[F]lu sufferers took six days to get better while taking a placebo, while 90% of the elderberry group was better in just three days.

antioxidants (*J of Ag Food Chem* 1998, *Eur J Nutr* 1999). In fact, antho-cyanidins in elderberry have been shown to enhance immune function (Watzl *et. al.*, 2000). Most recently, Dr. Vivian Barak and her associates have published research showing that elderberry extract activates a healthy immune system by heavily increasing inflammatory (*European Cytokine Network* 2001) and anti-inflammatory (*IMAJ* 2002) cytokine production. Cytokines are tiny proteins put out by immune cells that communicate messages to other immune cells to modulate the immune response. These immune cell messengers are one of the many exciting and important new topics in immune system research.

So just how well do these berries work? In one study, flu sufferers took six days to get better while taking a placebo, while 90% of the elder-berry group was better in just three (Mumcuoglu, *J Alt Comp Med*). And in a recent double-blind placebo-controlled study, when people with the flu were given either elderberry or a placebo four times a day for five days, there was a significant difference on a scale that ranked improvement from 0-10. By the third or fourth day, most of the elderberry group had improved to near 10, while the placebo group did not achieve that level until after seven or eight days. By the fourth day, scores for aches and pains, sleep quality, respiratory tract mucous and nasal congestion had all climbed to over 9 in the elderberry group but were still at or below 1 in the placebo group (*J International Med Res* 2004). Pretty impressive!

And now a potentially exciting and very timely new use of elderber-ry extract has been suggested. Preliminary laboratory research conduct-ed at the Kimron Veterinary Institute in Israel has found that a standard-ized extract of elderberry immediately neutralized cell damage induced by the West Nile virus. This research suggests the possibility that elder-berry extract, taken during the mosquito season, may be useful in pre-venting West Nile virus. In discussing this exciting study with us, Dr. Mumcuoglu, a leading elderberry researcher, said that, though the results are very encouraging, since the study was a test tube study and not a clin-ical study on people, no recommendations can yet be given for the pre-vention or treatment of West Nile virus.

In addition to the herb's own action against the virus, elderberry extract can also strengthen the immune system's ability to fight the virus.

As well as being a great antiviral herb, elderberry is a good blood purifier and is good for arthritis and rheumatism.

Make a tea from the flowers by infusing 2 teaspoons in a cup of water for 10 minutes. Drink it three or more times a day, as hot as possible. You may want to drink a very hot cup or two, get in a hot bath and then go to bed under lots of warm covers to help the flower do its work. If you are taking the flower in pill form, take 3-5g three times a day.

If you are using the elderberry liquid extract, Dr. Mumcuoglu says to take two teaspoons daily as a preventative or immune enhancer and two teaspoons four times daily for antiviral effect if you are actually fighting off a cold or flu.

Both the flower and the berry seem perfectly safe. There are no side effects or drug interactions. The flower is safe to use when pregnant or nursing. However, Dr. Mumcuoglu told us in a personal communication that, since the berry has not been researched in pregnancy, she does not recommend it during pregnancy. She also said that since the berry stimulates the immune system, they do not recommend it for people with auto-immune diseases.

Elecampane *(Inula helenium)*

Elecampane is the stuff of myth and legends. According to the Weiners' *Herbs that Heal*, Helen of Troy was carrying elecampane when she was abducted by Paris (so be careful carrying this one around!). And so, of course, this herb was well know to the ancient Greeks and throughout folklore history. It was used to promote menstruation, as a diuretic, for lung and gastric complaints, and for colds.

Today elecampane is known as an effective herb to treat all kinds or respiratory complaints and coughs, but it is also used in digestive weakness. Its expectorant properties make elecampane an excellent choice for chronic mucous, coughs, asthma, and bronchitis. Clinically, evidence has suggested that elecampane may be useful against tuberculosis and other bacteria as well as *candida*. It may also possess anti-ulcer activity.

Elecampane's ability to soothe and reduce gassiness makes it excellent for the digestion and assimilation of food, and it also helps to prevent the formation of mucous in the digestive system. It is a tonifying herb, a diuretic, antiseptic, astringent (a herb that dries up mucous surfaces), stimulant, and vermifuge (a herb that helps to get rid of parasites). James Duke, Ph.D., says that it's worth giving elecampane a try for intestinal amoeba. Elecampane is also used for the urinary tract.

Make an infusion from 1g (1/4 teaspoon) of the ground root, and drink it three to four times a day. We have seen the dose of the tincture given as both 1–2ml or 3–5 ml three times a day.

Contact dermatitis is possible. Large dosages may cause diarrhea, cramps dizziness, nausea, and symptoms of paralysis; however, the dose would have to be way higher than the ones recommended here.

Eleuthero
(formerly Siberian Ginseng)
(Eleutherococcus Senticosus)

Although related to ginseng both botanically and in its use, Siberian ginseng is not a ginseng at all and is no longer officially known by that name. Meet eleuthero, the perfect herb for anyone who is under normal stress or feeling run down. Whereas ginseng is ideal when your energy has utterly collapsed or you are recovering from illness, eleuthero is just the thing when you are simply stressed. Compared to the true ginsengs, eleuthero is more neutral and balancing, and less stimulating.

Traditionally, eleuthero has been used as a tonic for vigour, stamina and general health; to improve appetite and memory; and to fight heart disease, bronchitis and rheumatism.

Eleuthero is the perfect adaptogen. Adaptogens are remarkable herbs that have three properties. First, they are safe. Second, they have the ability to increase your resistance to a wide range of things that negatively stress the body. And third, they have the amazing ability to normalize body functions in either direction: to bring them up when they are down and to calm them when they are too high. Eleuthero supports the adrenal glands and helps the body to withstand all kinds of stressful conditions, from heat and noise to increases in work load. It also helps to improve the quality of your work when under stress (*Econ Med Plant Res* 1985).

The adaptogenic properties of eleuthero make it not only an ideal herb for stress, but also for improving mental and physical work performance. Several studies show that it is effective for brightening mental alertness, increasing productivity and improving athletic performance. Eleuthero has been widely used by athletes, including Russian Olympians.

While eleuthero is building up performance and resistance to stress, it is also building up resistance to disease. Eleuthero strengthens the immune system (*Rastit Resur* 1978; Shadrin A. *et. al.*, 1985; *Arzneimforsch* 1987; *Int J Altern Comp Med* 1995; Phytother Res 2000). It is a good herb to take to prevent getting sick and missing days at work. In a double-blind study, one thousand factory workers were given eleuthero every other month. During that year, there was a 50% reduction in illness and a 40% reduction in lost work days (*Adaptation & Adaptogens* 1972). Another study found exactly the same results. Thirteen thousand Russian auto workers took eleuthero in November and December and reduced their colds, flus and other infections by 40%. Eleuthero is also able to improve well-being and lung capacity in bronchitis and pneumonia. Eleuthero also improves immunity. It enhances the effects and decreases the side effects of conventional cancer treatment. It is a great herb for chronic fatigue immune dysfunction syndrome (CFIDS or CFS).

Eleuthero shows off its extraordinary adaptogenic powers by regulating hormones, balancing blood sugar in either direction, and by normalizing blood pressure in cases of both high and low blood pressure. In addition to raising or lowering blood pressure as needed, eleuthero also lowers cholesterol and helps atherosclerosis and angina as well as improving kidney function (*Econ Med Plant Res* 1985). Eleuthero can also protect against toxins and radiation.

Although European and North American sources list the dose in the 1–4g a day range, the traditional dose is a much higher 5–15g a day and even higher. Michael Murray, N.D., also puts it in the higher 2–4g three times a day range, and the American Botanical Council, while going with the lower dose for the root in pill form, gives the higher 9–27g dose for the decoction. If using the tincture, herbalist Christopher Hobbs in his book, *Ginseng: the Energy Herb,* recommends two droppers (roughly 3–4ml) morning and evening. Murray and others put the tincture dose at 10–20ml three times a day. If using the stronger liquid extract, the dose is 2–4ml one to three times a day.

Some sources recommend cycling eleuthero by taking it for six to weeks and then discontinuing it for two weeks before starting up again. Hobbs says that it can be taken for longer than *Panax ginseng* and likes to use it for two to three months, and even up to eight months. Mills and Bone, in their authoritative text, say to cycle six weeks on, two weeks off for maintenance but to take it continuously during illness.

Eleuthero is extremely safe. There are no side effects, with the possible exception of people with rheumatic heart disease. Though eleuthero is sometimes contraindicated in high blood pressure, Brinker says this contraindication only applies to high blood pressure over 180/90. We already know that eleuthero has a balancing effect on blood pressure. The American Botanical Council's *Clinical Guide to Herbs* says there is no literature to support the contraindication for people with high blood pressure. Some say to discontinue eleuthero during an acute infection. Eleuthero is safe to take while pregnant or breast feeding.

Although there are no negative drug interactions for eleuthero, there are some positive ones. Eleuthero prevents and treats diarrhea that is caused by antibiotics (*Med Welt* 1997). It makes the antibiotics monomycin and kanamycin work better against *shigella dysentery* and *Proteus enterocolitis* (*Antibiotiki* 1982). It may potentiate the radioprotection drug adeturone (*Acta Physiol Pharmacol Bulg* 1987). Eleuthero may also enhance the effect of insulin and diabetes drugs.

In the middle ages herbs were often associated with women healers. These women faithfully served the population using herbs to heal illnesses. The political and social concerns at the time often caused these healers to be looked at with fear and suspicion, largely because they were so skilled they began to be seen as very powerful: too powerful for the comfort of many men at the time. The result: many of these women were frequently believed to be witches and persecuted – even murdered as such.

Eyebright *(Euphrasia officinalis)*

A very well-named herb, eyebright is a specific for eye problems. And it has been used for a very long time for just that purpose. Even the poets Milton and Shenstone mention the virtues of eyebright in their poetry.

Eyebright is an excellent herb to use to improve conditions of the eyes such as conjunctivitis, strained and tired eyes, cataracts, irritation, inflammation, inflammation of the eye lids, and for improving eyesight. According to the Weiners, it has the reputation for begin able to restore the sight in people over seventy years old. Eyebright has soothing, cooling and anti-inflammatory properties that make it ideal for treating problems of both the eyes and sinuses. It can be used either internally or as an eyewash. Use as a standard infusion and allow to cool for an eye wash. It is often combined equally with other herbs like goldenseal, bayberry, raspberry, and one-half part cayenne pepper for an eyewash.

Make an eyebright tea by infusing one teaspoon (5g) of the dried herb per cup of water, and drink it three times a day. If using the infusion as an eyewash, make it the same way, but be sure to allow it to cool. You can also use the dried herb in pill form at a dose of 2–4g a day. If you prefer the tincture, take 2–6ml three times a day.

A very safe herb, eyebright has no side effects, contraindications or drug interactions. It is safe during pregnancy and breast feeding.

Fennel   *(Foeniculum vulgare)*

Fennel is a very valuable spice. It was well known to ancient healers like Hippocrates and Dioscorides who used it to increase milk in nursing mothers.

Fennel has antispasmodic, carminative, diuretic, expectorant, and stimulant properties. It is used to treat colic and is especially useful for relieving children's colic. In a recent study, 121 infants with colic were randomly assigned to receive 5 to 20ml of a 0.1% fennel seed oil emulsion or placebo up to four times per day for one week. Symptoms were recorded in diaries for one week before starting the study, during the study, and for one week following cessation of the treatment. The researchers found that the colic symptoms decreased significantly, by 45% in the infants taking the fennel formula, compared with only a 5% reduction in symptoms in those taking the placebo formula. In the overall findings, the researchers reported that colic was eliminated in 65% of the infants taking the fennel. No bad side effects were observed in infants receiving the fennel (*Alternative Therapies* 2003).

Other studies have also shown that fennel reduces intestinal spasm and increases the motility of the small intestines. These properties make it an excellent herb for constipation and for anyone with irritable bowel syndrome. Another study has found a herbal combination which includes fennel to be extremely useful for those with colitis (*Vutr Boles* 1981). It is also wonderful for cramps, spasming gastrointestinal tract, gas, to get rid of mucous, as an eye wash, to prevent gripping in laxative formulae, for coughs, for flavouring in herbal formulae, and to encourage breast milk.

Fennel makes a nice licorice-flavoured tea. Infuse or decoct 1–3g of the crushed seeds in a cup of water; keep it covered. Drink three cups a day. Some sources recommend a higher dose of 1–2 teaspoons (5–10g) three times a day. For the tincture, the dose is 2–4ml three times a day. Some sources suggest a higher dose of 5–15ml two to three times a day. The extract can be taken at a dose of 1–3ml two to three times a day.

There is no need to worry about the discrepancies in doses for fennel because it is an extremely safe herb. There are no side effects, contraindications or drug interactions for fennel seed. Allergy to fennel is rare but possible, including in people with allergies to celery or carrots. The *German Commission E* says not to use fennel seed for more than several weeks without consulting a practitioner, but Brinker qualifies this caution as "speculative," and Mills and Bone say that it is perfectly safe for long term use despite this unexplained caution.

Fennel seed is safe during pregnancy and breast feeding, especially as an infusion, but the fennel oil is not. Brinker alone says not to use fennel seed at these times; no other source we could find had this warning, and several women's herbals allow it and even recommend it for relieving gas during pregnancy. Fennel has long been known as a good herb to use while breast feeding to enrich and increase the flow of milk.

Fenugreek *(Trigonella foenum-graecum)*

Fenugreek is one of the oldest recorded plants used for medicinal purposes. It has been used in Greek, Arabian and Indian medicine for thousands of years and is recorded as being used in Egypt as early as 1500 BCE. It has also been used by the Chinese for thousands of years. It is also extremely valuable. Although fenugreek has many uses, it has mainly been used for mucous congestion and lung congestion because of its excellent expectorant, astringent and demulcent properties. But that's not all. Fenugreek is also used for ulcers, inflammation in the stomach and intestines, loss of appetite, and gout.

> *Fenugreek is one of the oldest recorded plants used for medicinal purposes.*

But the recent excitement over fenugreek has been caused by the discovery that it is an effective herb for diabetes and cholesterol. Fenugreek has been shown to reduce blood sugar levels in both type I (*Eur J Clin Nutr* 1990) and type II (*Nutr Res* 1996; *Phytother Res* 1996; *J Assoc Physicians India* 2001) diabetes. And it has also been shown to improve cholesterol and triglycerides in diabetics (*Eur J Clin Nutr* 1990; *Phytother Res* 1996; *J Assoc Physicians India* 2001) and in nondiabetics (*Indian J Pharmacology* 2000).

Some believe that fenugreek is an aphrodisiac. It has also been used for breast enlargement and is one of the very best herbs for promoting breast milk.

Externally it can be used in poultices and packs to treat skin conditions like inflammations, boils, and carbuncles.

Make a decoction by simmering 1.5 teaspoons (7.5g) of seed in a cup of water for ten minutes three times a day. Or take 6g a day of the crushed seeds, 6ml of the extract or 30ml of the tincture. The dose used for diabetes and cholesterol in the studies has ranged from as low as 12.5g to as high as 100g. For external use, use 50 grams, powdered, with one litre of hot water.

Fenugreek is safe. There are no contraindications and the only side effect is the possibility of a skin reaction with repeated external applications. Brinker says to avoid excessive use during pregnancy; most sources say not to use it at all while pregnant. It is perfectly safe to use while breast feeding, however, and has long been used to enhance breast milk.

Because of its positive effect on insulin and cholesterol, it is possible that fenugreek could enhance the effect of insulin and cholesterol-lowering drugs.

Feverfew *(Tanacetum parthenium)*

Feverfew is nature's answer to the unbearable pain of migraine headaches. This powerful little flower has a long tradition of use for headaches and a number of studies back its use specifically for migraine headaches. But don't take it just when you have a headache, like aspirin. If you are prone to migraines, take feverfew every day.

In one small study, half the people who reported being helped by feverfew continued to take the herb, while half of them were given a placebo. Those who were on a placebo had almost a 300% increase in migraines. They also had a significant increase in the severity of the headaches and of nausea and vomiting. Those who continued on the feverfew had no change in their freedom from migraines (*Br Med J* 1985).

A second double-blind study also found feverfew reduced both the number and the severity of headaches as well as nausea and vomiting (*Lancet* 1988). More recently, feverfew brought about a significant reduction in pain intensity, vomiting, nausea, and sensitivity to noise and light (*Phytother Res* 1997).

Feverfew also has anti-inflammatory properties.

Traditionally feverfew has also been used for fever – where it gets its name – and for rheumatism.

It used to be thought that the parthenolide in feverfew was the active ingredient, so dosing information was always given based on parthenolide content. But recent research suggests that parthenolide is not really the active ingredient. A Dutch study tried using a dried alcoholic extract of feverfew leaf instead of the whole leaf used in the other studies. The extract contained easily enough parthenolide to be effective, but it wasn't (*Phytomedicine* 1996). Since we know feverfew works, this study suggests that some components in the whole leaf not extracted by the alcohol – and not the parthenolide, which was captured by the alcohol – are doing the work on migraine. A later Israeli study (*Phytother Res* 1997) found that feverfew with a lower parthenolide content than the other studies did work, suggesting again that something other than parthenolide is doing the work. So it is advisable to use a feverfew supplement that contains the whole leaf and take 50–150 mg a day. To be effective, feverfew must be taken on a daily basis and will take four to six weeks to really start working.

Feverfew is very safe. In some sensitive people, chewing the fresh leaf instead of buying a dried leaf pill, may cause mouth ulcers. The occasional person might experience mouth ulcers or gastric disturbance even with feverfew pills, but this happens only rarely and only in the first week. There are no long term side effects.

Feverfew should not be used during early pregnancy because of its ability to bring on menstruation. Use the minimum dose if you are using it through the rest of your pregnancy. All major sources but one agree that feverfew is safe to use while breast feeding (and that one does not list a source or a reason).

Feverfew should be avoided if you have an allergy to it or to members of its family, like ragweed. It should not be used by children under two. There are no drug interactions for feverfew. If you are about to undergo surgery, discontinue feverfew because of the possibility that it could act as a blood thinner. For the same reason, you should avoid feverfew if you have a bleeding disorder. It has been speculated that feverfew may be best avoided if you are using blood thinners like aspirin or warfarin, but this contraindication has not been proven. Large numbers of people taking feverfew with medications experienced no adverse side effects (ESCOP 1996).

Fo ti, Ho shou wu (Polygonum multiflorum)

Fo ti ought to be one of the most popular herbs, since it is considered an anti-aging tonifying herb. According to legend, a fifty-eight-year-old Tang dynasty man who was unable to father a child was advised to eat fo ti and did. He then had several children and his grey hair turned black. He went on to live to 160 and his child to 130. His grandchild was named Ho Shou Wu, the name Fo ti is known by in China. Not bad for one little herb!

> *Fo ti [is] an anti-aging tonifying herb. According to legend, a fifty-eight-year-old Tang dynasty man who was unable to father a child was advised to eat fo ti and did. He then had several children and his grey hair turned black. He went on to live to 160 and his child to 130. His grandchild was named Ho Shou Wu, the name Fo ti is known by in China.*

Fo ti is considered a rejuvenating tonic that will restore energy, increase fertility and give strength even to those who are in their advanced years. This remarkable herb is also of extreme value in strengthening the kidneys, liver and blood and so plays a role in all deficiency diseases. It is used to treat hypoglycemia and diabetes, since it helps to balance blood sugar; it prevents premature aging; restores hair colour after it has gone grey; and it strengthens muscles, ligaments, tendons, and bones. Clinically, we have found it to be a wonderful herb when used in combination with herbs like ginger root, bromelain, valerian, and astragalus for those who suffer from low backache due to kidney weakness. Traditionally, it has also been used for replenishing sperm, for gout, colic, to reduce high blood pressure, to lower cholesterol, for enteritis, and hemorrhoids. Fo ti is of extreme value to those who consume a typical western diet that stresses the kidneys and liver because it strengthens these organs.

 Decoct 5–15g of fo ti per cup of water, and drink three cups a day. You can also take 2.5g of fo ti in a pill three times a day.

 Fo ti may cause diarrhea and should not be used if you have diarrhea. Other than that, fo ti is a very safe herb with no contraindications or drug interactions. It can safely be used during pregnancy and breast feeding and, who knows, maybe your baby will live to be 130!

Garlic   (*Allium sativum*)

From pesto and Caesar salad to colds and cancer, garlic is as valuable in the medicine chest as it is in the kitchen. This incredible herb can do it all, and it has been for a long time. Records testifying to garlic's use go back over five thousand years. Because it is so gentle – it's a food after all – and can do so much, garlic is often discussed as a player in the treatment of many conditions and the star of none: a sort of utility player who's always valued but never the superstar. But don't let garlic's safety or versatility fool you. It's one amazing herb!

Garlic is a perfect treatment for atherosclerosis and one of the very best herbs for preventing heart disease. Garlic is excellent for heart disease because it leaves nothing out: it is capable of addressing virtually every causal factor of heart disease. It lowers cholesterol and, as a powerful antioxidant, prevents the dangerous oxidation of the harmful LDL cholesterol. It prevents blood platelets from becoming sticky and clumping together and acts as a blood thinner. Garlic lowers blood pressure and it keeps the arteries elastic and not stiff. With all these properties in one little clove, you've got yourself one powerful heart herb.

Although not every study has found garlic to be a great cholesterol lowerer, most have. And based on the findings of several studies, garlic can lower total cholesterol by 9% to 12%, the bad LDL cholesterol by 16%, triglycerides by 13%, and raise the beneficial HDL cholesterol by 10%. Its blood pressure lowering ability has been shown in many studies (*Br J Clin Pract Suppl* 1990; *Eur J Clin Res* 1992; *Am J Med* 1993; *Br J Clin Res* 1995) and James Duke, Ph.D, says that it contains more anti-clotting compounds than any other herb. When a recent study added the important ability to protect the aorta from age-related stiffening (*Circulation* 1997), the ideal therapy for atherosclerosis emerged. How good is it? Unbelievably good! A four-year double-blind study gave either 300mg of garlic powder or a placebo three times a day to people who had significant plaque build up and at least one other cardiovascular risk factor. Over the four years, the plaque increased by 15.6% in the placebo group, but in the garlic group, it actually decreased by 2.6%. Amongst the people who were over fifty, the plaque disappeared by 6–13% (*Atherosclerosis*

1999). These results suggest that garlic can not only prevent atherosclerosis – a leading cause of death – but even reverse it.

Garlic fights not only heart disease but cancer. A number of population studies show that garlic reduces the risk of cancer. Larger population studies have found that when people consume garlic, they have significantly less risk of getting stomach cancer (*J Natl Cancer Inst* 1989) and colon cancer (*Am J Epidemiol* 1996). One study found that the risk of colon cancer went down by 35% with as little as one or more servings of garlic per week. For those who ate more, the risk went down by a full 50% (*Am J Epidemiol* 1994). Garlic may also reduce the risk of laryngeal and endometrial cancers (Mulrow, *et al.*, 2000), as well as prostate and breast cancer. A very recent study revealed that men who eat more foods in the garlic family – especially garlic and scallions – have a significant reduction in the risk of developing prostate cancer of almost 50% (*J Natl Cancer Inst* 2002). In a test tube, garlic inhibited growth of melanoma cells, a difficult to treat skin cancer, by more than 50%. The cancer cells treated with garlic actually began to revert back to normal (Koon S, *et al*, 1990).

Garlic is also good for everyday ailments. It is a strong antimicrobial herb. Garlic is antiviral, antibacterial, antifungal, and antiparasitic. Perhaps this powerful ability to fight off the deadly things that attack our bodies was the basis of the legend of garlic's power to fight off the vampire. The little vampires that garlic does fight off include *strep*, *staph*, *E. coli*, *salmonella*, *candida*, roundworm, hookworm, tapeworm, pinworm, *giardia*, and herpes. Garlic is also a good treatment for amoebic and bacillic dysentery. And trust us – as we found out on a trip to Honduras – you'll want a treatment for that if you get it. Garlic can even fight off some of the bacteria that have become resistant to antibiotics.

Garlic's antifungal properties make it not only a good herb when treating *candida*, but also when used externally for athlete's foot.

In addition to being antimicrobial, garlic is also anti-inflammatory and expectorant and can be helpful for colds, flus, allergies, sinusitis, bronchitis, and pneumonia. It can also help diabetes and makes a good detox for lead poisoning.

Garlic eardrops are excellent for treating ear infections. Often combined with mullein, calendula and St. John's wort in olive oil, there is a long tradition, and now also solid science (*Arch Pediatr Adolesc Med* 2001; *Pediatrics* 2003), to prove how well it works.

Of course, the most delicious way of benefiting from garlic is in the diet. The recommended dose of fresh, minced garlic is 2,700– 4,000mg a day. To put that in perspective, 4,000mg is about one clove of garlic.

If you prefer to take garlic supplements, the dose is 200–300mg of garlic powder three times a day. Many of the studies used 900mg. The garlic powder is often standardized to 1.3% alliin (about 10mg) and 0.6% allicin potential (about 4,000–6,000mg).

If using a pill that is aged garlic extract, the dose is 300–800mg three times a day.

As one of the most ancient and common foods, garlic is extremely safe. It has an excellent safety record, and adverse effects are very rare, with occasional reports of gastrointestinal symptoms. Garlic is safe to use while pregnant and breast feeding. One source says that caution may be indicated while breast feeding. All other major sources give garlic the green light for breast feeding, and one study has even found that components of garlic transmitted to breast milk will improve the baby's breast feeding (*Pediatr Res* 1993). It is possible, however, that garlic could cause colic.

There are no real contraindications for garlic. Because garlic is a blood thinner, you should stop taking it at least one week before surgery. For the same reason, garlic could enhance the anticoagulant effects of blood thinners like warfarin and aspirin. Although the possibility of this caution should not be totally dismissed, when the garlic-warfarin (Coumadin) combination was tested in a double-blind, placebo-controlled study, there was no interaction and no bleeding (Rozenfeld *et al.*, 2000).

Garlic is excellent for heart disease because it leaves nothing out: it is capable of addressing virtually every causal factor of heart disease... Garlic's antifungal properties make it not only a good herb when treating candida, but also when used externally for athlete's foot.

Many times on our travels we have been whipping up a winding mountain or ferrying across a turbulent sea and been so grateful for the powers of ginger. Ginger is the anti-nausea herb extraordinaire for all kinds of nausea, from motion sickness to morning sickness.

Bring ginger with you whenever transportation means motion sickness. Three double-blind studies have proven ginger to be safer and as – or even more – effective than the motion sickness drug Dramamine (*J Travel Med* 1994; *Euro Phytother* 1999; *European Phytother* 1999). One of these studies (*J Travel Med* 1994) gave either ginger or one of seven motion sickness drugs to 1,741 people whale watching on the Norwegian high sea. Typically, about 80% of the passengers on this trip suffer sea sickness. On this voyage, however, 82–85.5% felt fine. The ginger group did as well as any of the seven drug groups even though the ginger was given in a very small dose. In another of these studies (*Euro Phytother* 1999), everyone using ginger had good results and none of them suffered any side effects, but only 31% of the Dramamine group had good results while 69% of them suffered side effects.

Ginger has a very long history of use for morning sickness. And now the first double-blind, placebo-controlled study has shown the tradition to be true: ginger does ease the nausea of pregnancy. When seventy pregnant women suffering from nausea were given either 250mg of ginger or a placebo four times a day, nausea was significantly reduced in the ginger group compared to the placebo, and only 37.5% of those on ginger reported vomiting, compared to 65.7% on the placebo. Of those on ginger, 87.5% said their symptoms improved, compared to only 28.5% on placebo (*Obstet Gynecol* 2001). A recently released second study has come to the same conclusion. It found that a ginger syrup improved or stopped the nausea and vomiting of pregnancy (*Atlern Ther Health Med* 2002).

Ginger even helps when the nausea of pregnancy goes beyond regular morning sickness to a severe form called *hyperemesis gravidarum* (*Eur J Obstet Gynecol Reprod Biol* 1990). This form of morning sickness is so severe that it often requires hospitalization.

Some, but not all, studies have also found that ginger can help with postoperative nausea (*Anaesthesia* 1993; *Anaesthesia* 1990).

This common kitchen spice has many other uses as well. It is a powerful antioxidant and anti-inflammatory that is useful in many inflammatory conditions. Though not all studies have found ginger to help with arthritis, the evidence is beginning to mount. One study found that 75% of people with either rheumatoid or osteoarthritis improved when they were given ginger (*Med Hypotheses* 1992). A double-blind study found that ginger reduced pain significantly more than a placebo: 63% versus 50% (*Arthritis Rheum* 2001). Most recently, a study showed that 250mg of standardized ginger extract given four times a day significantly increased mobility and reduced pain in people with osteoarthritis of the knee (*Osteoarthritis and Cartilage* 2003).

Ginger may also lower cholesterol and increase the production of bile, act as a heart tonic, lower blood pressure, and stimulate circulation. It is analgesic, carminative and antispasmodic. Ginger can be used to aid indigestion, colic and gas. It also inhibits diarrhea and may help migraine headaches and ulcers. Ginger has an ability to warm the body. It can be used as a diaphoretic in fevers. It also has antifungal and antibiotic properties.

If taking a ginger capsule or tablet, try taking 500mg two to four times a day. For arthritis and other inflammatory conditions, some sources recommend up to 2–4g a day. For morning sickness, use one gram of ginger. For motion sickness, take 500mg of ginger half an hour before heading out and then again every two to four hours while in motion. Ginger can also be taken as a tea, using either the fresh root or dried powder at the same dose as for capsules and tablets. If using a ginger tincture, take 1.25–5ml three times a day; if using the extract, take 0.25–1ml three times a day.

Ginger is very safe. There are no side effects or drug interactions. Used in high doses, ginger could cause heartburn. One gram a day of ginger is a safe and effective dose for the nausea of pregnancy.

Recently there have been claims that ginger is not safe for pregnant women, claims that are hard to believe if you consider how long ginger has been safely used all over the world for treating morning sickness. The confusion comes from studies that used isolated compounds of ginger and not ginger as a whole food. Two studies that were done using very high dosages of an isolated compound of ginger, not the whole herb, found that the isolated compound of ginger may cause birth defects. But the study ignores the fact that other parts of ginger contain equally powerful antimutagenic properties, so using the whole herb is not a problem.

A 1991 review found no reports in the scientific literature of miscarriage or birth defects from ginger (Bergner 1991). Another 1996 review of all the studies on ginger could find no evidence for contraindicating ginger for pregnancy, since there was no evidence that it could harm the mother or the child (Fulder, Tenne 1996). Furthermore, ginger has been safely used in China for pregnancy for centuries.

Ginkgo biloba *(Ginkgo biloba)*

Ginkgo biloba might be the most valuable herb in nature. *Especially for older people.* A Ginkgo biloba tree can live to be over a thousand years old. The species itself has flourished for around three hundred million years, making it the oldest surviving species of tree in the world. It is often said how fitting it is that this most elderly of herbs is a perfect fit for elderly people. But what is not so often remembered is that before it is old, every Ginkgo tree first must be young. And Ginkgo biloba may no longer be just for the elderly any more.

Ginkgo has so many uses it may just be the most versatile herb of them all. It is invaluable to people who suffer eye diseases, hearing problems, asthma, altitude sickness, strokes, heart attacks, intermittent claudication, Reynaud's disease, depression and sexual dysfunction, including the sexual dysfunction caused by Prozac and other antidepressant drugs. But it is this herb's powerful influence on memory and concentration that has won Ginkgo its fame.

Ginkgo is simply the best thing nature has to offer for the declining mental sharpness that may accompany aging. Tons of studies have proven it to help the elderly in mental functioning, mood and sociability.

The declining cognition of old age may be due to declining flow of blood and oxygen to the brain. Ginkgo is the best thing available for this condition known as cerebral insufficiency. Cerebral insufficiency can cause memory loss, depression and tinnitus: symptoms that Ginkgo can improve in as little as eight to twelve weeks (*Curr Med Res Opin* 1991). But what really makes Ginkgo such an exciting herb is its ability to help memory and cognition – even in people with Alzheimer's disease.

In 1994, a double-blind, placebo-controlled study found a significant improvement in memory and attention – but no side effects – in people with senile dementia of the Alzheimer's type who were given 240mg of Ginkgo for only one month (*Hum Psychopharmacol*). The effectiveness and safety of Ginkgo was exciting news. Two years later, 222 people with dementia caused either by mild to moderate Alzheimer's or by multiple strokes again significantly improved their cognitive function when they were given 120mg of Ginkgo twice a day for half a year. And again, the herb was completely safe (*Pharmacopsychiatry* 1996).

1997 was a big year for Ginkgo. One study gave 240mg of Ginkgo or a placebo for six months to people with presenile or senile dementia of the Alzheimer's type or from multiple strokes. Ten percent of the placebo group responded, but 28% of the Ginkgo group did (*Phytomedicine* 1997). Another double-blind, placebo-controlled study found significant improvement when people with Alzheimer's type dementia were given 240mg of Ginkgo for three months (*J Psychiat Res* 1997).

But Ginkgo really hit the mainstream news when the prestigious *Journal of the American Medical Association* published its 1997 Ginkgo study. Two hundred and two people with mild to severe Alzheimer's or dementia from multiple strokes were given either 120mg of Ginkgo or a placebo for one year. The Ginkgo group had a statistically significant improvement. Compared to the placebo group, they improved in not only cognitive function, but also in social behaviour and daily living skills. The Ginkgo was able to stabilize, and often improve, cognitive and social function, while those on the placebo continued to decline. As in all studies on Ginkgo, the herb was incredibly safe with negative side effects no different than those caused by placebo. This study may be even more encouraging when you consider its patients received only 120mg of Ginkgo, half the dose employed in the other studies discussed here. The results may be even better at 240mg.

In 1998, when researchers selected four really well designed studies from a large number of studies, they found there was strong evidence that Ginkgo helps people with Alzheimer's (*Archives Neurology*).

So how does Ginkgo stack up against the best the pharmacy has to offer? Researchers compared studies in which the herb was used to studies using two conventional cognitive drugs. They found that while all three produced statistically significant improvement, side effects were lowest with Ginkgo (*J Drug Dev Clin Pract* 1996). And when eighteen elderly people were given either 240mg of Ginkgo or the drug tacrine, more responded to Ginkgo (*Psychopharmacol Bull* 1998). Two years later, another study compared Ginkgo to four acetylcholinesterase inhibitors, the dominant class of drug for Alzheimer's, and also found Ginkgo to be better – and safer – than tacrine and comparable to the newer drug, donepizil (*Phytomed* 2000).

So there is no doubt that Ginkgo biloba is a valuable treatment for Alzheimer's. In a recently released review of thirty-three good quality studies, for instance, the respected Cochrane Collaboration at Oxford University concluded both that Ginkgo is safe and that there is "promising evidence of improvement in cognition and function" in elderly people with dementia. The question is – and here is where the media controversy really begins – can Ginkgo boost memory in healthy people. The exciting answer now seems to be yes. But that was not always the answer.

The controversy was kicked off by an intensely publicized study that found 120mg of Ginkgo did not improve memory in healthy elderly people. Unfortunately but more surprising, however, was that the media – and even the *Journal of the American Medical Association* – chose to focus all publicity efforts on this study while choosing to entirely ignore a second study that found that the herb did work on healthy elderly people at a slightly higher 180mg dose (*Human Psychopharmacol Clin Exp* 2002).

The media also ignored earlier placebo-controlled studies showing that Ginkgo can improve memory in healthy people, young (*Phytotherapy Res* 1999) or old (*J Altern Complement Med* 2000). And more recently, a double-blind, placebo-controlled study has shown that Ginkgo, yet again, benefits mental performance in healthy adults 50-65 years old (*Deutsche Apotheker Zeitung* 2002), while yet another found it to help healthy elderly people (*Human Psychopharmacol Clin Exp* 2002).

And the evidence continues to mount. In a new study, when 1,570 healthy elderly people were given Ginkgo every day for ten months, both their mood and their ability to perform daily activities improved significantly (*Phytother Res* 2004). A recent review concluded that the majority of studies found Ginkgo to help healthy people. It noted that there were only three studies that didn't find that it helped, and that, of these, two were of questionable validity and the third only lasted five days!

So it looks like Ginkgo can help you remember, whether you are young or old, healthy or not.

How does it do it? In lots of ways it seems. It increases the flow of blood and oxygen to the brain; it has powerful antioxidant activity that protects brain cell membranes from free radical damage; it improves the availability of acetylcholine, the neurotransmitter whose deficiency is linked to Alzheimer's, and normalizes acetylcholine receptors; and it increases the rate of nerve transmission.

But Ginkgo is for more than just memory.

Ginkgo is also good for the eyes: it has been shown to help against macular degeneration and glaucoma. And it is good for the ears. One study found that 40% of people who suffered hearing loss related to old age improved when they were given Ginkgo. Ginkgo can also help hearing loss when it is caused by reduced blood flow, head injury or sonic damage. And though research has shown mixed results, several studies suggest that Ginkgo could help people with tinnitus, or ringing in the ears. Most recently, one study found Ginkgo to be at least as effective as a drug in combating sudden deafness (*Acta Otalaryngol* 2001).

Since Ginkgo is great for increasing circulation, it is not surprising that it is also great for intermittent claudication, painful cramping in the legs caused by reduced blood flow. Several double-blind, placebo-controlled studies have shown that Ginkgo can significantly improve the distance people suffering from this condition are able to walk without pain (Blume *et al*, 1998; *VASA* 1998; *Arzneim-Forsch Drug Res* 1999).

Another complication of reduced blood flow is erectile dysfunction, the inability to attain or maintain an erection. When sixty men, whose erectile dysfunction had not been helped by papaverine injections, were given 60mg a day of Ginkgo (which is, by the way, a very low dose), 50% of them had regained potency after six months (*J Urol* 1989). When a more normal dose of 240mg was used in another study, Ginkgo once again proved itself effective (*J Sex Educ Ther* 1991).

A timely new use is also emerging for Ginkgo in the field of sexual dysfunction. Selective serotonin reuptake inhibitor antidepressants like Prozac and Zoloft are becoming more and more popular prescriptions, and sexual dysfunction is a very common side effect of these drugs for both men and women. Ginkgo can counteract this side effect. One study found that 240mg of Ginkgo successfully reduced SSRI induced sexual dysfunction in 76% of men and 91% of women (*J Sex Marital Therapy* 1998).

Research also shows that adding Ginkgo to the regimen of elderly people who are not responding to antidepressant drugs can turn their treatment around quickly (*Geriatr Forsch* 1993).

If you're lucky enough to be traveling to exotic places with high altitudes, then bring your Ginkgo along, because it has another surprising use. Several studies have now shown that Ginkgo prevents altitude sickness. In one study, men who had previously suffered altitude sickness took Ginkgo before ascending to over 14,700 feet (4,480 meters). While 41% of the placebo group suffered altitude sickness, none of the Ginkgo group did (*Aviat Space Environ Med* 1996). More recent studies have confirmed this result (*High Alt Med Biol* 2001; *High Alt Med Biol* 2002).

And Ginkgo has still other uses. It can help with blood clots, inflammation, nerve cell damage, vertigo, allergies and asthma. Another study has also found that Ginkgo can very successfully halt and even reverse the progression of vitiligo, a skin disorder which causes patches of skin to lose pigmentation (*Clinical and Experimental Dermatology* 2003).

Ginkgo should be standardized to 24% ginkgoflavone glycosides and 6% terpene lactones. The usual dose is 120-240mg a day.

In addition to its incredible versatility and effectiveness, another amazing thing about Ginkgo is its safety. Side effects with Ginkgo are very rare and mild. In fact, in double-blind studies when Ginkgo is compared to a placebo, the frequency of side effects is virtually identical for the herb as for the placebo (DeFeudis 1991). There have been no major side effects reported in the studies.

It is regularly said that Ginkgo is contraindicated for people with bleeding disorders or who are about to undergo surgery because chronic use can increase bleeding potential since, as one of its benefits, Ginkgo inhibits blood platelet aggregation. This same concern and a couple of case reports have led to the warning for caution with chronic use of aspirin or with anticoagulation drugs like warfarin and Coumadin. But the real science consistently says otherwise. Double-blind placebo-controlled studies have found no interaction between Ginkgo and Aspirin (Schwabe 2001) or between Ginkgo and warfarin (*Thromb Haemostat* 2002). Most recently, when Ginkgo was added to warfarin, it did not seem to interact with the drug, nor did it affect bleeding values, including platelet aggregation (*BritishJClin Pharmacol* 2005). And most interestingly, a study found that even very high doses of Ginkgo (480mg) given for fourteen days did not increase the risk of bleeding at all (*Clinical and Laboratory Haematology* 2003). Other careful research has found the same (*Blood Coagulation Fibrinolysis* 2004; *Perfusion* 2005).

There are no contraindications for pregnant or nursing women.

In a bizarre turn, American researchers, claimed to have found a toxin in the herb while doing research involving pregnant women. So, you may hear contraindications for Ginkgo for women who are, or are trying to become, pregnant. They are false. According to herb authority Kerry Bone, there were at least three problems with the researchers' work. First, the toxin cannot be found in that herb: it's a botanical impossibility. Second, given the amount of toxin claimed to have been found in the herb and the amount found in the women, the women would have had to have swallowed at least 40 and perhaps as many as 2,000 pills a day instead of the normal two to four. Third, if that amount of the toxin had been in the pregnant women, their babies would have been dead. No authoritative sources list any contraindications for pregnant or nursing women.

Ginseng, Asian *(Panax ginseng)*

Ginseng is probably the most revered herb of them all. It has been used by millions of people for thousands of years. Though many herbs try to win the marketing benefits of ginseng by appropriating its name, not all ginsengs are really ginsengs. The real ginsengs are the Panax ginsengs, and the most important of the Panax ginsengs are Asian ginseng (*Panax ginseng*), which includes Chinese and Korean ginseng, and North American ginseng (*Panax quinquefolius*), which is grown in both Canada and the United States. Siberian ginseng, though related to ginseng, is not truly a ginseng at all and should not be called by that name: its proper name is eleuthero, and it has been discussed separately under that name.

In traditional Chinese medicine, ginseng is rarely seen as a cure for a specific ailment as feverfew might be seen as a cure for migraine or valerian for insomnia. It is more important than that. It restores and revitalizes the vital energy, or life force, of the body, known in Chinese medicine as *qi* (pronounced chi). Ginseng balances and strengthens the functions of the whole body so that they return to their proper state and the body can heal itself. Ginseng is the great promoter of health and longevity.

You will find two types of Asian ginseng on the market: red ginseng and white ginseng. They are the same root. They are prepared differently and the preparation makes a difference. Red ginseng is steamed with the peel on and then dried. It is said to be warmer and more stimulating than white ginseng. Red ginseng is best for people over forty and people who are debilitated. Contrary to its most popular use in North America, red ginseng should not be used long term by young people for energy. It is the ideal herb for people who are suffering from long term debility and weakness and who are lacking vitality.

White ginseng is peeled and then dried. It is the cooler and less stimulating of the two. It is a general purpose herb for those who need help getting through the day both mentally and physically

Ginseng is the perfect adaptogen. Adaptogens are remarkable herbs that have three properties. First, they are safe. Second, they also have the ability to increase our resistance to a wide range of things that negatively stress the body. And third, they have the incredible ability to normal-

84

ize body functions in either direction: to bring them up when they are down and to calm them when they are too high.

As an adaptogen, ginseng helps the body cope with mental and physical stressors and enhances mental and physical performance. Several studies show that ginseng enhances the overall quality of life, improving things like alertness, relaxation, vitality, mood, appetite, sleep, resistance to colds, blood pressure, performance, and well being.

Several studies have shown ginseng to enhance both mental and physical performance. Recently, the results on physical performance have been more mixed. Several factors may explain the mixed results. According to an article in *HerbalGram* #52, the negative studies have been those with the poorest study design and the smallest treatment groups. In other words, they may have been bad studies. Low doses of ginseng may also have been a factor. S. Dharmananda points out in *HerbalGram* #54 that the doses traditionally used in Asia are much higher than those often studied in the west. Though several studies do support the use of ginseng in athletic performance, this is not the traditional use of the herb. Though *qi* is often translated as energy, it means life energy as opposed to the way we often use the word energy. Ginseng is a balancing, strengthening and nourishing tonic: it is not meant to provide a caffeine-like kick. Ginseng enhances the body's energy by toning it, not by pushing it. This property of ginseng has also been shown in studies to improve alertness, reaction time, coordination, and energy in the elderly.

At the same time as ginseng's revitalizing power is nourishing mental and physical energy, it is also invigorating the immune system. Ginseng may build up the body's resistance to viral infections like the common cold. It has also been shown to be very helpful in cases of severe chronic respiratory disease (*Schweiz Z Ganzheits Med* 1995) and bronchitis (*Internat J Immunother* 1994). Ginseng also improves the results when you get a flu vaccine. People who were given ginseng along with the vaccine had significantly fewer colds and flus than people given a placebo along with the vaccine. How many fewer? A total of fifteen com-

Several studies have shown ginseng to enhance both mental and physical performance.

pared to forty-two in the vaccine plus placebo group (*Drugs Exp Clin Res* 1996).

Even more excitingly, Korean red ginseng has been found to have positive long term effects on immunity in people with HIV (*Abstr Gen Meet Am Soc Microbiol* 1997). And it also seems to lower the risk of several kinds of cancer (*Int J Epidemiol* 1990; *Cancer Epidemiol Biomarkers Prev* 1995). The most recent study on ginseng and cancer found a 50% lower risk of cancer amongst ginseng users, including big benefits for smokers (*Int J Epidemiol* 1998).

Rounding out the big three, in addition to cancer and AIDS, ginseng can also benefit the heart. It reduces total cholesterol and triglycerides while increasing the good HDL cholesterol and reducing platelet adhesiveness (*Planta Medica* 1985). Herbalist Christopher Hobbs says that red ginseng is better than white for promoting circulation and reducing clotting. Ginseng has also been shown to help congenitive heart failure when given both with and without digoxin.

Another circulatory problem that ginseng can help is impotence, or erectile dysfunction. Ginseng was traditionally used as a treatment for impotence, but modern science has been skeptical of this use. Until now. In 1995, 1,800mg of Korean red ginseng was discovered to significantly improve erectile dysfunction compared to both a placebo and a drug (*Int J Impot Res* 1995). A year later, when thirty-five elderly men with erectile dysfunction were given either Korean red ginseng or a placebo, the herb once again defeated the placebo: ginseng helped a full 67% of the men, while only 28% of the placebo group improved (*Korean J Ginseng Sci* 1996). That same year, ginseng was shown to produce a rise in sperm count, motility and testosterone, suggesting a role in infertility as well as impotence (*Panminerva Med* 1996). In the most recent study, forty-five men with erectile dysfunction were given either 900mg of powdered Korean red ginseng or a placebo three times a day for eight weeks. Sixty per cent of the men on the ginseng had improved erections. Erection scores increased by 42% in the ginseng group compared to only 16% in the placebo group. Sexual function in the ginseng group improved by 36% versus 10.4% in the placebo group. Ginseng also improved their sexual desire (*Journal of Urology* 2002). So tradition was right again. Move over Viagra!

Ginseng has a long tradition of use in the treatment of diabetes and it has been shown to help type II diabetics (*Diabetes Care* 1995). Ginseng can also be a useful herb during menopause (*Br Med J* 1980). It protects against radiation damage (*Am J Chin Med* 1981); has antioxidant properties; supports the adrenals; helps, not surprisingly, with long term fatigue (*Phytotherapy Research* 1996); and, according to herbalist Michael Tierra, it nourishes the blood and is useful for anemia.

So venerated is this Asian herb that it finds its way into every form. In a recent transfer through a Korean airport, we saw powdered ginseng tea, ginseng extracts, ginseng slices, ginseng soap and even – we've got to try this one – ginseng chocolates. The airport even had – and this is great – an alcohol, tobacco and ginseng store.

Whatever the form, the roots should be at least three years old, and the best ones are six to twelve years old. Hobbs says that ginseng pills should be used within a year. Teas and extracts are both good. Hobbs suggests that they are equally effective at extracting the ginsenosides, the major active ingredient in the root, but that the alcohol extract may get more of the antioxidants. The tincture, he says, may be more stimulating and the tea more supportive and nourishing over the long term.

Many western sources peg the dose of ginseng root at 1–2g a day. This dose, according to Dharmananda, corresponds only to the lowest dose in traditional Eastern texts. In China, he says, 1–3g is considered an effective low dose, while 3–9g is often used short term. Hobbs agrees with the 1–9g dose. When discussing ginseng root as a decoction, the American Botanical Council's *Clinical Guide to Herbs* also gives a 3–9g dose. Other Western sources also go with the lower dose of the dried root and the higher dose of the dried root in a decoction. If you are using a ginseng extract in a pill form standardized to 4% ginsenosides, the dose recommended and used in much of the Western research is 100mg twice a day. Keep in mind again, though, that this standardized dose is the equivalent of 1g of the dried root, considered the lowest dose in traditional Chinese texts. The dose of the liquid extract is 1–2ml and 5–10ml for the tincture.

Ginseng is very safe, as testified to by millions of ginseng users for thousands of years and confirmed in large numbers of studies. The most common contraindication listed is high blood pressure. However, the story here is confusing. Some studies have found that while ginseng can raise blood pressure at lower doses, it can actually lower it at higher doses. Dharmananda says that in China, ginseng is used in doses of 3–9g to lower blood pressure. Two recent studies have found ginseng to lower blood pressure (*Am J Chin Med* 1998; *Ann Pharmacother* 2002). Some sources say not to use large amounts of ginseng for a long time with stimulants like caffeine: this caution applies to the red and not the white ginseng.

Some sources say that ginseng helps chronic asthma, but should not be used during acute asthma; that it increases resistance to infection, but shouldn't be used during acute infection. Since in Chinese medicine, ginseng is a heating herb, it is best to avoid it in certain kinds of headache, palpitations and insomnia. It should also be avoided during excessive menstruation and nose bleed and you should stop taking it one week prior to surgery.

Hobbs recommends avoiding ginseng if you are highly energetic, nervous, tense, hysterical, or manic.

Though ginseng does not contain estrogen, there are a few reports of breast pain or menstrual irregularity in women who use ginseng long term. Generally, however, ginseng has no unwanted side effects.

Ginseng is safe to use while pregnant or breast feeding. You may occasionally see a warning not to take it during pregnancy, but this warning is not consistent with the tradition or the research. In fact, using ginseng while pregnant is a long established tradition, according to Hobbs, McGuffin and others. Hobbs says that it is thought to supply energy for both the mother and baby. One study found that ginseng reduced preeclampsia, a serious condition characterized by increased blood pressure and fluid retention during pregnancy.

There are no negative drug interactions for ginseng, although there may be some positive ones. Ginseng may relieve some of the side effects of glucocorticoid drugs. It may enhance amoxicillin and clavulanic acid in bronchitis (*Clin Drug Invest* 2001). Because of its beneficial effects on diabetes, levels of insulin may need to be adjusted.

Ginseng, North American *(Panax quinquefolius)*

The other important true ginseng, North American ginseng, is the most balanced of the ginsengs. It is held in high esteem in Chinese medicine. It is more cooling than Asian ginseng and can be used by younger people and by people who are less debilitated. North American ginseng supports digestion and the adrenal glands and is one of the best herbs for stress. It is a perfect herb for overworked, overstressed people with weak adrenals. No wonder it's called "North American" ginseng: it's amazing there's ever any on the shelves.

Being a cooling herb, North American ginseng is sometimes used for cooling down in the hot summers and for fever. It has also been used to support the lungs in conditions like tuberculosis and bronchitis. Research is also pointing to North American ginseng for diabetes (*Arch Intern Med* 2000; *Diabetes Care* 2000). Traditionally, it is also used for thirst, chronic low-grade fevers and weakness.

The dosage of North American ginseng is 1–9g, according to Christopher Hobbs. The American Botanical Council recommends 3–9g as a decoction and 3g as a pill.

North American ginseng is perfectly safe. There are no side effects and no drug interactions, though diabetics should monitor insulin doses since this herb helps with blood sugar levels. North American ginseng is safe to take during pregnancy and breast feeding.

Goldenrod *(Solidago virgaurea)*

Most people associate goldenrod with allergy season, since in North America it comes out at about the same time as ragweed. Yet this pretty yellow flowering plant is an extremely valuable herb that has been used to treat urinary tract inflammations and infections. The *Commission E* approves goldenrod as irrigation for inflammatory diseases of the lower urinary tract and for the prevention and treatment of kidney stones. In other words, it can be used to treat stones, pain, and inflammation in the urinary tract. It is also used for bacterial infections and to increase the amount of urine for relieving inflammation of the kidneys and bladder. Traditionally, it has been used by the Aboriginal people of North America to treat liver and gastrointestinal problems.

The dose of goldenrod is 3g of the herb two to four times a day. You can also make an infusion of 3g of the herb per cup and drink it two to four times a day. Herbalist David Hoffmann recommends a higher dose of 2–3 teaspoons (10–15g) per cup three times a day. As an extract, take 3ml two to four times a day. Hoffmann recommends higher doses, suggesting 2–4ml of the tincture three times a day (tinctures are weaker than extracts).

There are no side effects or drug interactions. Some speculate that goldenrod should not be used in cases of edema due to impaired heart or kidney function: though some of these same sources admit that goldenrod works very well when edema is of kidney origin. It is safe to take goldenrod when pregnant or breast feeding.

Goldenseal (Hydrastis canadensis)

Goldenseal has been called everything from overrated to one of the most useful of all herbs. We agree with the latter. Linda uses it often in her clinic with great results.

Much of the research on goldenseal has actually been carried out on berberine, one of its active ingredients, but there is a good deal of clinical testimony for this herb too.

Goldenseal is most valued for its dominance over microbes: it is a powerful and wide-ranging antimicrobial. As an antimicrobial herb, goldenseal specializes in infection and inflammation of the gastrointestinal, respiratory and genitourinary tracts. Berberine is antimicrobial, antifungal, antiparasitic, and antibacterial. It has been shown to be active against a huge range of invaders, including *staph, strep, E. coli, salmonella, chlamydia, shigella dysenteriae, entamoeba hystolytica, trichimonas vaginalis, giardia*, and *candida*. The whole goldenseal extract has also been shown to be active against a wide range of microorganisms, including *staph, strep, E. coli*, and *candida* (*Fitoterapia* 1999; *Planta Med* 2001).

Its range makes goldenseal valuable in virtually any kind of diarrhea, including traveller's diarrhea (*E. coli*), food poisoning (*salmonella*) and *shigella dysentriae*. Traveller's diarrhea is a sneaky little trip stopper that strikes unannounced and won't let up. It was not an unfamiliar companion on our early trips. The discovery of goldenseal put an end to that. We now start taking goldenseal one week before travelling, throughout the trip, and for one week after returning. Our trips have gone a lot more smoothly since.

When berberine challenged antidiarrhea drugs in children, it compared well with the drugs and worked faster (*J Ind Med Assoc* 1970). When children under five years of age who were suffering from acute diarrhea from a variety of bacteria were given either berberine or antibiotics, the berberine worked better (*Infect Immun* 1982).

Giardia is an extremely common parasite; it is the single most common protozoa infection. When children with *giardia* were given either a placebo, the drug metronidazole or berberine, the berberine was not as good as the drug for eliminating the parasite but was considerably better than the placebo. Berberine, however, was better than the drug for getting rid of the symptoms. The study's authors felt that an increase in the dose or duration of the berberine would improve its effectiveness (*Ind Pediatr* 1972). When other researchers increased the dose and duration of the berberine, it was comparable to metronidazole and other antigiardia drugs – and without the side effects (*Am J Dis Child* 1975). More recent research has suggested that the whole herb may work even better than the isolated berberine (*Tokai J Exp Clin Med* 1990).

Goldenseal is an effective herb not only for gastrointestinal infections, but also for respiratory infections. Goldenseal

As an antimicrobial herb, goldenseal specializes in infection and inflammation of the gastrointestinal, respiratory and genitourinary tracts.

is a valuable part of a treatment for pneumonia, sinusitis and all mucousy or phlegmy problems. It is able to stop *streptococcus* bacteria from adhering to cells (*Antimicrob Agents Chemother* 1988). If the bacteria can't drop anchor, they can't stick around to do their harm. Michael Murray, N.D., says that goldenseal may be the ideal treatment for strep throat.

The urinary tract also is the recipient of goldenseal's anti-infective powers. Just as berberine blocks the adhesion of *streptococcus* bacteria, so it blocks the adhesion of *E. coli*, the most common cause of urinary tract infections (*Antimicrob Agents Chemother* 1988).

Goldenseal is also a valuable herb for treating *candida*. It is good as well for treating small intestinal bacterial overgrowth. There are not supposed to be bacteria in the upper part of the small intestine: when they get there, trouble results. Goldenseal helps. Goldenseal can help external fungi too. You can make a decoction of it and use it for athlete's foot. The decoction can also be used as a mouth rinse for canker sores. Goldenseal has been used externally as an eyewash for trachoma, an infectious eye disease (*Indian J Med Res* 1982; *Indian J Opthamol* 1982). Berberine inhibits the growth of *trichomonas vaginalis* (*Ann Trop Med Parasitol* 1991), making it a good herb for treating vaginitis. As a powerful astringent herb, goldenseal is also valuable for excessive menstrual bleeding and haemorrhaging.

As a powerful bitter and bile stimulator, goldenseal can also stimulate appetite and help digestion. Actually, it is good for any digestive problem, form gastritis to ulcers to colitis.

Goldenseal may also turn out to be antimalarial and to help diabetes.

And there's another surprising benefit from this anti-infection specialist. Goldenseal may also turn out to be a good heart herb. A review of the benefits of berberine on heart health suggests that it may be useful in the treatment of arrhythmias and heart failure (*Cardiovasc Drug Rev* 2001). In a recently released study, researchers added either berberine or a placebo to the conventional treatment of congestive heart failure. The people who were given the berberine had a significantly greater improvement and there were significantly fewer deaths during the long term follow up (*Am J Cardiol* 2003). It's an exciting new possibility for goldenseal that is virtually never mentioned in the herb books.

The doses that are recommended for goldenseal vary. If using the dried root and rhizome in a pill or decoction, 0.5–1g three times a day is a common recommendation. Some give a higher dose of 4–6g a day or even 2–4g three times a day. The same range exists for tinctures and extracts. The tincture dose recommendations range from 4–7ml a day to 2–4ml three times a day all the way to 6–12ml three times a day. The authors who recommend the lower dose say that higher doses may be necessary in acute conditions. Extract doses range from 0.3–1ml three times a day to 2–4ml three times a day. As if this isn't confusing enough, there is one more option. You can take a solid extract pill at a concentration of 4:1 or standardized to 8–12% alkaloids at a dose of 250–500mg three times a day.

Goldenseal is a very safe herb. Despite frequent warnings to the contrary, it is safe to use long term. Goldenseal should not be used by people with kidney disease or kidney failure, and it may be contraindicated for newborns with jaundice. One source says not to use goldenseal where there is acute stomach inflammation with reduced mucous secretion. Normally, goldenseal is a good herb for stomach infection and inflammation and is recommended for gastritis.

Goldenseal should not be used during pregnancy. Almost all of the most authoritative sources allow goldenseal while breast feeding; however, one good source suggests avoiding it until more research is done.

There are no negative drug interactions for goldenseal. It may, however, increase the effectiveness of sulphacetamide eyedrops for *Chlamydia trachomatis* and of penicillin and chloromycetin on some strains of intestinal bacteria.

Gotu kola
(Centella asiatica)

Gotu kola has been used in India since prehistoric times. It was also used extensively in Indonesia for healing wounds and for leprosy. In the nineteenth century, it was used for skin problems, like eczema and psoriasis, as well as lupus, leprosy, varicose ulcers diarrhea, fever, amenorrhoea, and diseases of the female reproductive tract. It has also been used for snake bite, fractures and strains. It is said to be a miracle elixir of life, increasing longevity. LiChing Yun, who reportedly lived 256 years, claimed it was a result of his regular use of gotu kola!

Today, gotu kola is still used for many of the same treatments. Several studies have confirmed its uses. It is used mainly for wound healing, cellulite, burns, varicose veins, scleroderma, and cirrhosis of the liver, for memory, anxiety, and to improve concentration. It seems to have an ability to heal, especially to heal connective tissue.

Gotu kola can also help to reduce leg edema and prevent circulatory problems during air travel. A recent study looked at the benefits of using gotu kola to help those with varicose veins when they travel by airplane. The subjects that used gotu kola fared better than those in the control group who used nothing. The gotu kola users had less leg swelling and decreased circulatory problems compared to those in the control group (*Angiology* 2001).

It is said to be a miracle elixir of life, increasing longevity. LiChing Yun, who reportedly lived 256 years, claimed it was a result of his regular use of gotu kola!

Gotu kola has been used for depression and anxiety in China and India as a part of their traditional healing systems. It has been found to have anti-stress, anti-anxiety and tranquilizing powers (*J Res Indian Med* 1970). A recent study looked at gotu kola for anxiety. The group who used the gotu kola fared better than those who used the placebo (*Journal of Clinical Psychopharmacology* 2000).

Take up to 6g a day of dried gotu kola leaves in pill form. Michael Murray, N.D., recommends the middle dose of 2–4g a day. If the pills are a standardized extract, use 60–120mg a day (40% asiaticoside, 29–30% asiatic acid, 29–30% madecassic acid and 1–2% madecassoside). If your gotu kola is in tincture form, take 10–20ml a day in three divided doses; if it's an extract, take 2–4ml a day. You can also infuse 1–2 teaspoons (5–10g) of the leaf per cup of water, and drink it three times a day.

Gotu kola has proven to be extremely safe. Though rare, it may cause contact dermatitis when applied topically. In her book on women's health, Tori Hudson, N.D., lists gotu kola as a herb to avoid during pregnancy. Brinker says that you only need to avoid it in early pregnancy, and even then it is only excessive doses that should be avoided. He also says that this warning is only speculative; several other very authoritative texts don't even include this warning.

Grape seed extract (*Vitis vinifera*)

Free radicals are some of the most dangerous destroyers in the body. These unstable molecules have an unpaired electron, and they can't stand it. So they try to stabilize themselves by ripping electrons from neighbouring molecules, destroying other molecules in the process. This free-radical damage is associated with a bewildering number of today's most common and serious conditions. And it continues to happen unless crucial antioxidants stop it.

The most famous antioxidants are the vitamin antioxidants: vitamin C, vitamin E and betacarotene. But, what most people don't know is that the flavonoids found in many herbs are much more powerful antioxidants, and work against a wider range of free radicals, than the better known vitamin antioxidants. You just have to look at the list of herbs that have flavonoids in them to realize how valuable they are: ginkgo biloba, St. John's wort, hawthorn, green tea, milk thistle, bilberry, and cranberry are just the beginning. But the most perfect antioxidant herb of them all is grape seed extract. For most people looking for a general antioxidant to take preventatively to promote good health, grape seed extract is the herb to take.

Grape seed extract is a rich source of proanthocyanidins: one of the best antioxidant flavonoids. One of the significant qualities of grape seed proanthocyanidins is their versatility: they protect against both fat-soluble and water-soluble free

> *For most people looking for a general antioxidant to take preventatively to promote good health, grape seed extract is the herb to take.*

radicals. Most other antioxidants don't. Vitamin C only protects against water-soluble free radicals and vitamin E only against fat-soluble.

In addition to being powerfully antioxidant, grape seed proantho-cyanidins are anti-inflammatory. Coupled with their anti-inflammatory power, grape seed proanthocyanidins' very potent ability to strengthen collagen and prevent its destruction makes this herb valuable for any kind of arthritis. Its anti-inflammatory properties also make grape seed extract valuable for allergic and other inflammatory conditions.

Grape seed extract's dominance over free radicals and collagen destruction accounts for its value in so many conditions. Collagen maintains the integrity of skin, blood vessels, tendons, ligaments, cartilage, and connective tissue. And free radicals are associated with everything from cancer and heart disease to AIDS, arthritis, Alzheimer's, and aging. But if this generally valuable herb has a specialty, it is veins and eyes.

Grape seed extract has been shown in studies to help near sightedness (*Ann Ottal Clin Ocul* 1988), to reduce sensitivity to glare and improve night vision (*J Fr Opthalmol* 1988), and to reduce visual stress and visual fatigue in people who spend a long time staring at computers (*Ann Ottal Clin Ocul* 1990). As for the biggies, grape seed extract also helps people with macular degeneration (*Ann Ott Clin Ocul* 1988) and diabetic retinopathy (*Bull Soc Opthalmol Fr* 1987).

As for disorders of the veins, grape seed extract strengthens veins by decreasing capillary fragility and permeability (*Semaine des Huitaux de Paris* 1981). It is also a good herb for varicose veins (*Prensa Medica Mexicana* 1973). A large number of studies show that grape seed is excellent for venous insufficiency (*Phlebologie* 1993). Venous insufficiency is a serious circulatory disease of the legs, which causes edema, pain, swelling, fatigue, itching, and cramps.

Grape seed extract is also good for reducing heart disease and may be able to work against cancer without harming healthy cells. It also protects against damage from UV rays (*Fitoterapia* 1998). You might also try adding grape seed extract when trying to heal sports and surgical injuries.

 To get all the benefits of grape seed extract as a general antioxidant support, take 50mg a day. If you are using it to treat a condition, increase the dose to 150–300mg a day. In either case, it should be standardized to 85%–95% proanthocyanidins.

This extract from the seeds of grapes is extremely safe. There are no side effects or contraindications. There are also no drug interactions. Another piece of good news is that it seems to protect the liver and kidneys from the damage caused by acetaminophen (Tylenol) (*The FASEB Journal* 1998; *J Am Coll Nutr* 1998).

Grapefruit seed extract (*Citrus X paradisi*)

The extract of the seeds from grapefruit is the most versatile antimicrobial in the world. Effective against around 800 strains of bacteria and viruses, 100 kinds of fungi and numerous parasites, grapefruit seed extract boasts a list of credits unlike any other antimicrobial. This powerful agent is one of the first-choice treatments for *candida* and other fungi, including external fungi like toe nail fungus, athlete's foot and dandruff. It is also effective against *giardia*. And it is good for yeast infections.

When researchers pitted grapefruit seed extract against 194 strains of bacteria and 93 strains of fungi, it was effective against all but one (*J Orthomolec Med* 1990).

We bring grapefruit seed extract with us on every trip. It is a powerful preventative for parasites and traveller's diarrhea and is great for washing fruits and vegetables both when travelling and at home.

> *The extract of the seeds from grapefruit is the most versatile antimicrobial in the world. Effective against around 800 strains of bacteria and viruses, 100 kinds of fungi and numerous parasites, grapefruit seed extract boasts a list of credits unlike any other antimicrobial.*

Grapefruit seed extract is extremely bitter and must be taken diluted. Mix about 8 drops in a full glass of water or juice and drink it 2–3 times a day. One or two drops, once or twice a day is sufficient as a preventative for traveller's diarrhea. If using the capsule form, take

100mg two to three times a day. You must also dilute grapefruit seed extract for external use. Use about 1/3 of the extract and 2/3 glycerin, water or oil, and keep it away from your eyes.

 Grapefruit extract is safe even for long term use. There are no side effects or contraindications. No data seems to be available for its use during pregnancy and breast feeding.

Gravel root (Eupatorium purpureum)

If you suffer from urinary tract stones or are susceptible to them, this is one herb you should know about. Gravel root gets its name because of what it does: it helps dissolve and prevent urinary tract stones. This herb is a specific for the urinary tract in that it is used to strengthen the nerves of the urinary tract, so it is used for gravel, stones, blood in the urine, frequent and night-time urination. For stones, we often combine gravel root with marshmallow root, to soothe the inflammation, and uva ursi to treat and prevent any infection and to flush the system out.

Gravel root is a diuretic, nervine, tonic, antirheumatic, and carminative as well.

 Decoct one teaspoon (5g) per cup of water, and drink it three times a day. If using the tincture, take 1–2ml three times a day.

 No known side effects. Gravel root should not be used while pregnant or breast feeding. In a contraindication that was totally unexpected, given the extensive traditional use of this herb for kidney stones and the number of respected herbalists who recommend it, The American Herbal Products Association's *Botanical Safety Handbook* says not to use this herb internally, and Brinker gives the same warning as speculative. The reason is because of the presence of pyrrolizidine alkaloids. However, herbal expert Paul Bergner has communicated to us that "there seems to be a lot of imprecision on the issue of PA in Eupatorium species." We are confused by this one.

Green tea

(Camellia sinensis)

Delicious, healthy and inexpensive, green tea just might save your life –
a prescription that's easy to swallow.

Green tea has been a favourite drink of the Orient for thousands of
years. In China, green tea is drunk every day by an estimated 88% of the
population. Many cultures believed green tea to have health benefits.
They were right.

Green tea is an important herb for cancer, heart disease, the liver
and, surprisingly, teeth and bones. The flavonoids, or polyphenols, in
green tea are very powerful antioxidants.

People who drink green tea regularly have less cancer. A huge nine-
year study of 8,552 Japanese people over the age of forty found that the
more tea you drink, the later the onset of cancer. The results were especially dramatic when more than ten cups (40 ounces) were drunk each
day (*Preventative Medicine* 1997).

Green tea has been shown to be beneficial for preventing all kinds of
cancer. It can protect against oral cancer (*Proc Soc Exp Biol Med* 1999),
stomach cancer (*Cancer Causes & Control* 1995; *Carcinogenesis* 2002), and
esophageal cancer (*J Natl Cancer Inst* 1994; *Carcinogenesis* 2002). A major
study found that the people who drank the most green tea had a lower
risk of colon, rectal and pancreatic cancer (*Int J Cancer* 1997). And
recently, test tube studies also found that a component in green tea may
be a powerful inhibitor of pancreatic cancer (*Pancreas* 2002), while a
green tea extract substantially limited the growth of colon cancer cells
(*Intentional Journal of Oncology* 2002). Green tea can also reduce the risk
of lung cancer (*Jpn J Canc Res* 1995) and may decrease some of the cancerous effects of smoking (*Cancer Epidemiology, Biomarkers and Prevention*
1995). It may also help prevent prostate cancer. A seven year study found
that drinking green tea benefited people with breast cancer (*Japanese
Journal of Cancer Research* 1998).

More recently, green tea extract stopped the growth of new
blood vessels needed for growth of breast tumour cells in a laboratory,
showing its potential use for treating and preventing breast cancer (*J
Nutr* 2002). And in an exciting study just completed, women who regu-

larly drank green tea had significantly lower incidence of breast cancer than women who rarely drank it. Just half a cup a day was associated with a 47% decrease compared to women who drank none (*International Journal of Cancer* 2003). A green tea extract applied as a cream or swallowed as a pill was effective in treating HPV infected cervical lesions (*Eur J Cancer Prev* 2003). Drinking green tea just might be one of the simplest, cheapest and tastiest ways of preventing cancer.

But green tea's benefits don't stop with cancer. It also helps the other major killer: heart disease. Green tea helps fight heart attack, stroke, atherosclerosis, blood pressure, and cholesterol. There's good cholesterol and there's bad cholesterol, and green tea helps both. Green tea lowers total cholesterol, the bad LDL cholesterol, the very bad VLDL cholesterol and triglycerides, while raising the beneficial HDL cholesterol (*Prev Med* 1992; *BMJ* 1995; *J Epidemiol* 1996; *Lancet* 1997;). Green tea also prevents disease promoting damage to LDL cholesterol (*Am J Clin Nutr* 1997) and is associated with lower blood pressure (*Journal of Nutrition* 2003). A study of Japanese women found a lower rate of stroke for those who drank green tea more frequently than for those who drank it less often (*Tohoku Journal of Experimental Medicine* 1989).

And here's a surprising benefit of green tea. Although caffeine is an important cause of osteoporosis, drinking green tea actually prevents osteoporosis. Something in the green tea is overpowering the caffeine. Tea drinkers have significantly greater bone mineral density (*Am J Clin Nutr* 2000). One study found that ten or more years of tea drinking causes significantly higher bone mineral density (*Arch Intern Med* 2002).

Green tea can also help with weight loss by stimulating thermogenesis (*Am J Clin Nutr* 1999). Thermogenesis turns up the body heat and literally burns calories. When sixty obese women were given 250mg of powdered green tea eight times a day in a double-blind, placebo-controlled study, they had a significant weight loss of 1.9kg in thirty days and a significant decrease in waist measurement (*Revue De L'assoc Mondiale de Phytother* 1985). When green tea extract was given to moderately obese people for three months, their weight decreased by 4.6% and their waist by 4.5% (*Phytomedicine* 2002). Green tea's weight loss powers go beyond its caffeine content.

And green tea also acts as a herbal dentist. In 1991 it was discovered that the flavonoids in green tea prevent tooth decay (*Caries Research*). A number of studies have now found that green tea prevents periodontal disease (Makimura *et al* 1993; Sakanaka *et al* 1996; *J Periodontal Res* 2002). A recently published study found that people who regularly drink or rinse their mouths with tea have fewer cavities (*Nutrition* 2002). Other studies have found the same thing: children who drink a cup of green tea right after a meal have significantly fewer cavities, and rinsing with green tea while brushing reduced plaque and cavities.

A recent study found that a component of green tea can affect hormones in a way that could help fight benign prostate hyperplasia, prostate cancer, acne, and balding (*Hong Kong Med J* 2001). And applying green tea extract to the skin protects against burning and DNA damage from the sun (*J Am Acad Dermatol* 2001). Green tea can also help dry up diarrhea.

A lot of the research done on green tea has studied Asian populations who drink it. The amount of green tea typically drunk in Asia is about three cups a day. Some studies suggest that doses coming closer to ten cups a day are more beneficial. If you prefer to take green tea as a pill, the amount of polyphenols found in the typical three cups of tea is about 240–320mg, so look for that daily amount in a pill.

The nicest way to take green tea is to drink it. Infuse one teaspoon (5g) in a cup. Here's an interesting fact about green tea. Caffeine dissolves quickly in hot water, so if you are using green tea as a stimulant, just infuse it for 3–5 minutes; but if you want the healthy antioxidants and not the stimulants, infuse it for 15–20 minutes.

Next to water, green tea is the most common drink in the world – it is extremely safe. Generally, green tea has no side effects. Because of the stimulating effect of caffeine, very large amounts of green tea could cause restlessness, irritability, nervousness, anxiety, insomnia, tremour, headache, and heart irregularities. However, Michael Murray, N.D., has pointed out that for some reason, green tea does not usually cause these caffeine effects, even though it does contain caffeine. When green tea does cause these effects, it usually requires more than ten cups a day to do so.

There are no real contraindications for green tea. You may want to avoid large amounts of caffeine and be cautious if you have kidney disease, heart disease, duodenal ulcer, depression or anxiety, an over-active thyroid, or susceptibility to spasm.

Brinker speculates that green tea should be avoided during pregnancy and breast feeding because of the caffeine. Other authorities do not echo this warning, though one says that you should probably not drink more than five cups a day because of the caffeine. Brinker also says that young children should probably not drink green tea (but that's okay, they probably won't want to).

The drug interactions listed for green tea are all interactions between drugs and large amounts of caffeine: 250mg of caffeine may counteract the relaxing effects of barbiturates and benzodiazepines, may increase blood pressure if you are on phenylpropanolamine, and may interfere with the arthritis pain killing ability of methotrexate. To get that much caffeine, you'd probably need to drink around eight cups of green tea. If you are on a monoamine oxidase inhibiting anti-depressant, you should not consume excessive amounts of caffeine. Caffeine should not be consumed twelve hours before taking adenosine. Caffeine could also increase blood pressure in people on beta-blockers. When consumed at the same time, caffeine could inhibit iron absorption.

Caffeine can increase the absorption of Aspirin. Green tea may impair absorption of the asthma medication theophylline and could work synergistically with sulindac and/or tamoxifen and may reduce their side effects.

Brinker says that you may want to avoid alcohol extracts of green tea.

Green tea helps fight heart attack, stroke, atherosclerosis, blood pressure, and cholesterol. There's good cholesterol and there's bad cholesterol, and green tea helps both.

Hawthorn

(*Crataegus laevigata, Crataegus monogyna, Crataegus oxyacantha*)

Hawthorn is a herb that has been used for a very long time. It was first used by the Greek herbalist Dioscorides for heart problems. An extremely valuable herb, Hawthorn is nature's offering to the heart. Like Ginkgo biloba, bilberry, grape seed extract, milk thistle, green tea and others, hawthorn is rich in flavonoids called proanthocyanidins. Like these herbs, hawthorn has a variety of uses but, just as Ginkgo specializes in memory and bilberry specializes in the eyes, so hawthorn has a specialty – the heart. It is the best cardiovascular herb nature has to offer. The most remarkable thing about hawthorn is its versatility and its ability to seek out what the body needs. For example, hawthorn is able to address both high and low blood pressure.

Hawthorn has been shown in studies to be effective for high blood pressure, angina, cholesterol, arrhythmias, atherosclerosis, and congestive heart failure. Simply put, if you have a heart problem, you should probably be taking hawthorn.

Though most people talk about the hawthorn berries, most of the research has actually been done on the leaves and flowers of hawthorn. And most of that research has been done on a condition known as congestive heart failure. Congestive heart failure is a very serious problem that occurs when the heart can no longer effectively do its job of pumping blood. Hawthorn, as Donald Brown, N.D., has said, makes the heart a more efficient pump.

Hawthorn has been shown in studies to help the heart work more efficiently in at least five ways. It increases the contractions of the heart muscle; it reduces peripheral vascular resistance by dilating the blood vessels; it improves left ventrical ejection fraction; it improves blood flow to the heart; and it acts as a powerful antioxidant. No wonder hawthorn is considered such a wonderful heart herb. Hawthorn also acts as a mild diuretic.

A number of studies have proven hawthorn to be a remedy for stage I and II congestive heart failure. In fact, well over a dozen studies have come to the same conclusion.

Researchers gave 600mg a day of hawthorn extract or a placebo to people with stage II congestive heart failure. When they tested them on a stationary bike eight weeks later, the hawthorn group had statistically significant improvement in stamina and endurance. They also had significantly reduced blood pressure and heart rate and they pumped blood at a lower pressure. Overall, they also suffered fewer symptoms and less shortness of breath (*Phytomedicine* 1994).

Three years later, researchers gave 160mg a day of hawthorn extract or a placebo to 136 people with stage II congestive heart failure in a double-blind study. The heart performance significantly improved in the hawthorn group while it worsened in the placebo group. The hawthorn group also experienced a superior quality of life (*Fortschr Med* 1996).

In the same year, people with either stage I or stage II congestive heart failure were given 900mg of hawthorn leaf and flower extract. Their symptoms decreased by 66%. Those with stage I congestive heart failure were largely symptom free. People in this study with high blood pressure had their blood pressure reduced and their heart rate drop from 89 beats per minute to 79. There was also a significant reduction in arrhythmias, once again showing the versatility of this great heart herb (Loew *et al*, 1996).

In 1994, researchers found 900mg a day of hawthorn extract to be at least as good as the ACE inhibitor captopril in an eight-week double-blind study of 132 people with stage II congestive heart failure (*Munch Med Wschr*).

Recently, a number of studies on hawthorn and congestive heart failure have been published. One three-month double-blind study gave either 240mg hawthorn leaf and flower extract or a placebo to thirty-nine people with stage II congestive heart failure who were not on other medications. Exercise tolerance on a stationary bike went up by 11% in the hawthorn group while going down 17% in the placebo group, just shy of being statistically significant. People on hawthorn reported feeling better than those on placebo. There were no side effects (*Phytomedicine* 2001).

Another recently released study found that people with stage II congestive heart failure did significantly better when given 30 drops of hawthorn three times a day than when given a placebo (*Phytomedicine* 2003).

And a review of double-blind, placebo-controlled studies on hawthorn leaf with flower extract for chronic heart failure, with or without medication, found that hawthorn increased exercise tolerance, relieved symptoms of heart disease and improved heart function (*American Journal of Medicine* 2003).

But the most exciting hawthorn study of all was published recently in the *American Heart Journal* (2002). This one is exciting because, while all previous studies were on stage II congestive heart failure, this double-blind, placebo-controlled study looked at 209 people with the more severe stage III congestive heart failure. After sixteen weeks, the group given 900mg of standardized hawthorn leaf and flower twice a day had a statistically significant improvement compared to the placebo group. People also reported significantly greater improvement in their heart failure symptoms than did people in the placebo group. Plus, the hawthorn did all this while producing only half as many adverse events as the placebo, testifying to both the efficacy and the safety of hawthorn. While we have long known that doses up to 900mg of hawthorn are effective for stage I or II congestive heart failure, we now know that a higher dose of 1,800mg is effective for the more severe stage III.

Traditionally hawthorn has also been used to remove food stagnation, indigestion, gas, abdominal distention, diarrhea, hernia, and stomach pain.

Hawthorn can be taken standardized for 1.8% vitexin–4'-rhamnoside in a dose of 160–900mg divided into two or three doses. Hawthorn is also sometimes standardized for 18.75% proanthocyanidin content. The recent stage III study suggests that the dose for more severe congestive heart failure should be 900mg twice a day. If using the dried berries, fruits or leaves, take at least 1.5–3.5 grams three times a day. If you opt for a liquid hawthorn, then take 4–5ml of the tincture three times a day or 1–2ml of the extract three times a day. Hawthorn teas made as infusions from the dried herb are also very effective.

The safety of hawthorn as found in the stage III study has been consistently reported. Every major work on herb safety reports the complete safety of hawthorn, including during pregnancy and lactation. Long term use of hawthorn is also perfectly safe and without side effects (*J Am Coll Toxicol* 1994, *Fortschr Med* 1992).

A major follow-up study of 3,664 people with stage I or II congestive heart failure found that hawthorn was well tolerated and produced adverse reactions in only 0.7% of cases. The same study found that of 1,476 people taking only hawthorn, physicians rated the treatment as very good or good for over 90% of them (*Z Phytother* 1998). This study, yet again, confirms both the efficacy and gentleness of hawthorn.

Hawthorn has no contraindications or side effects. Although it has been reported that hawthorn may potentiate the effects of heart medications like digoxin and digitalis, this caution is based on speculation and is not backed up by any clinical studies (Donald Brown, N.D.; Egon Koch, D.M.V., in *HerbalGram* #59). In fact, a recent study has shown that there is no interaction between hawthorn and digoxin (*J Clin Pharmacol* 2003). The long term use of hawthorn is a safe, gentle and effective part of any program for a healthy heart.

Horehound (Marrubium vulgare)

Horehound has been used as far back as ancient Egyptian times. Horehound's main use is for respiratory problems, and it is used by itself or in combination with other herbs to treat respiratory complaints like asthma, bronchitis, whooping cough, pulmonary consumption, sore throats, and anywhere else where it is desirable to throw off excess mucous from the respiratory tract.

As well as being of tremendous value to the respiratory tract, horehound is also used for loss of appetite, dyspepsia, bloating and flatulence. This popular folk remedy was also used as a tonic herb to remove obstructions from the system, to treat chronic hepatitis, suppressed menstrual flow, tuberculosis, malaria, hysteria, leukemia, and malignancies. Many of these folk uses, however, are unconfirmed.

Take 4.5g of horehound a day. If making a tea, infuse 1–2g of the dried herb per cup, and drink three cups a day. The dose of the extract is 2–4ml three times a day.

There are no contraindications, side effects or drug interactions for horehound. It should not be used while pregnant, although it is not contraindicated for breast feeding.

Horsetail *(Equisetum arvense)*

Horsetail is not what it sounds like: it is, in fact, a herb. The name has to do, presumably, with the plant's appearance – it looks like a horse's tail. The primary uses of horsetail revolve around its wealth of mineral content and, especially, its silica content. Silica is very important to the body and, though richly available in the earth's crust, this inorganic form is not well used by the body. The best sources of usable silica are plants, and, of the plants, horsetail is by far the best.

Silica is crucial for hair, skin, bone, cartilage, ligaments, tendons, and all connective tissue in the body. These roles for silica explain horsetail's value in healing wounds, sprains, strains, breaks and peripheral vascular disorders, and building and repairing connective tissue and bone, as well as its role in healthy hair, skin and nails. It is also said to be of value in treating ulcers.

Horsetail also has a great affinity to the genitourinary system. It is a mild diuretic but, more importantly, its astringent properties make it a good herb for incontinence, for involuntary flow of urine in small drops, and for children who wet their beds. It is also used for inflamed prostate and benign prostatic hyperplasia, inflammation of the urinary tract, infections, stones, some forms of edema, for difficult or painful urination, and for slimming. Horsetail may also help where aluminum is a problem. Silica seems to stop the damaging effects of aluminum. This role may be another way horsetail helps bone, but it means that silica may also help in some kinds of senility.

Horsetail's use dates back to ancient Roman and Greek times, and it has been used by many First Nations people in North America, in India, Asia and Europe.

Though horsetail can be taken in pill form at a dose of 2g three times a day, this herb is best taken as a tincture or tea. As a tea, infuse or decoct 1/2–2 teaspoons (2–5g) of the dried herb per cup and drink three times a day. As a tincture, take 2–10ml three times a day. The dose of the extract is 2ml three times a day.

You should not use horsetail if you have a heart or kidney disorder, and you should not take it if you are on digitalis or cardiac glycosides, since, as a diuretic, it could increase their toxicity if potassium is lost. Powdered horsetail should not be given to children or used for a prolonged period of time; tinctures and teas can be. Horsetail is safe to use while pregnant and breast feeding.

Hyssop

(Hyssopus officinalis)

If you look at the ingredients in traditional herbal cough drops, you will often find hyssop listed. This is because hyssop is such a great herb to use for coughs. Hyssop has a long history of use as an expectorant herb to clear mucous congestion from the respiratory tract. This makes hyssop a popular treatment for colds, fevers, hoarseness, sore throats, coughs, pneumonia, bronchitis, and other infections where mucous has settled into the respiratory tract. It is frequently combined with other herbs for these purposes. A very good overall cough, congestion, asthma, and bronchitis formula is to combine hyssop, lobelia, elecampane, mullein, licorice, comfrey, coltsfoot, and wild cherry bark (see the Safety sections for comfrey and coltsfoot).

Over the years, hyssop has been used for numerous other purposes, such as stimulation of the circulation, intestinal catarrhs, for the prevention of frost bite, for eruptive diseases, kidney and liver problems, to remove discolouration from bruises, to expel intestinal worms, for digestive and menstrual problems, and eye pains.

Make a hyssop tea by infusing 1–3 teaspoons (5–15g) in a cup of water and drink it three times a day. You can also take it as a tincture at a dose of 1–4ml three times a day. Hyssop can also be widely found in sore throat lozenges and cough syrups.

 Hyssop is safe to use, but should not be used during pregnancy. There is no contraindication for breast-feeding women. There are no side effects, contraindications or drug interactions.

Kava Kava *(Piper methysticum)*

With a history steeped in magic and ceremony, kava kava's benefits are being confirmed, one by one, by modern science, but its mysteries remain unresolved. It calms without working like any of the traditional sedative drugs, and it kills pain by a method unlike any other painkiller. It seems to work in a unique way that science cannot quite capture.

Kava has an intriguing and colourful past. The herb is native to the Pacific Ocean islands of Micronesia, Melanesia and Polynesia. The use of kava was found everywhere in island life, from politics to religion, from magic to medicine, as well as work and life cycle events like births, deaths and marriages. The drinking of kava was surrounded by ceremony.

Traditionally, kava has been used as a medicinal herb for nerves, relaxation, insomnia, as a diuretic, for asthma, rheumatism, weight loss, syphilis, gonorrhoea, weakness and fatigue, colds, headaches, and digestive problems.

Much of the modern research on kava has focused on its anti-anxiety effects. Several studies have shown kava to help anxiety, nervousness and stress.

In 1996, researchers compared kava to a placebo in a double-blind study. They gave either 100mg of kava extract, standardized for 70mg of kavalactones, three times a day, or a placebo to 58 people with anxiety, for four weeks. The Hamilton Anxiety Scale revealed a significant reduction in anxiety symptoms in the kava group compared to the placebo group after only one week. The improvement continued to grow over the four weeks. There were no adverse reactions to the kava (*Phytomedicine*). The same results and the same lack of side effects were reported two years later (*Alt Ther* 1998), and a 1991 study also found a statistically significant reduction in the symptoms of anxiety,

> *The herb is native to the Pacific Ocean islands ... The use of kava was found everywhere in island life, from politics to religion, from magic to medicine, as well as work and life cycle events like births, deaths and marriages. The drinking of kava was surrounded by ceremony.*

including nervousness, heart palpitations, chest pain, headaches, dizziness, and stomach ache, without any side effects (*Arzneim Forsch*).

Kava has not only been compared to placebo. Several studies have shown kava to be as good as benzodiazepines, one of the major classes of anti-anxiety drugs. In a large and important study of 172 people, kava proved itself to be as good as the benzodiazepine drugs oxazepam and bromazepam. The double-blind study gave either 100mg dry kava extract, standardized for 70% kavalactones, three times a day, or one of the two benzodiazepine drugs for six weeks. The Hamilton Anxiety Scale showed that all three groups experienced a significant decrease in anxiety and that there was no significant difference between them, meaning that kava is as good as the drugs in easing anxiety. While there were fewer people in the bromazepam group who experienced no benefit at all, that same group had a higher rate of sedative side effects, and the researchers concluded that kava is comparable to either drug. Kava had fewer side effects than the drugs (*Z Allg Med* 1993).

Kava is also effective for the anxiety and depression experienced by menopausal and postmenopausal women. A double-blind, placebo-controlled study found that while anxiety scores changed hardly at all in the placebo group, they dropped from 18 or greater to 5 in the kava group. And while seven out of twenty women experienced improvements in depression when given a placebo, seventeen out of twenty in the kava group improved. The eight-week study used kava standardized for 70% kavalactones and gave 100mg three times a day for eight weeks. Surprisingly, the placebo caused side effects in six patients: two more than in the kava group (*Fortschritte der Therapie* 1991).

While these studies clearly show the anti-anxiety power of kava, that is not all this remarkable herb does. Kava also improves sleep quality without interfering with REM sleep (*TW Neurologie Psychiatrie* 1991): an important advantage over benzodiazepines, which do suppress REM sleep. There are powerful muscle-relaxing components in kava. Terry Willard, Ph.D., calls kava "the most powerful herbal muscle relaxant known." The muscle-relaxing properties combined with kava's pain-killing properties make it a good herb for back pain (combined with the anti-inflammatory bromelain and acupuncture it has been a life saver for Ted's back pain). It can also be used for headaches. Some components of kava have powerful antifungal properties against a wide range of fungi.

Perhaps the best thing about kava is that it not only works as well as drugs, but has advantages that recommend it. Unlike drugs, it produces no morning hangover when used for insomnia. Also, unlike with anti-anxiety drugs, people do not develop a tolerance to kava, so it does not lose effectiveness over time. The other intriguing thing about kava is that, while anti-anxiety drugs affect coordination and alertness, kava not only promotes relaxation without loss of coordination or alertness, it actually increases concentration and alertness. In one double-blind study, researchers gave either a placebo, a benzodiazepine, or 200mg of kava, standardized for 70% kavalactones, three times a day. While the drug inhibited recognition in a memory test, kava slightly improved it (*Neuropsychobiol* 1993). This ability of kava to relax while increasing concentration has been confirmed in many other studies (*Pharmacopsychiatry* 1994, *Phytother* 1994).

That's the good news. The bad news is that Kava kava is gone: it is now illegal in Canada and some other countries. Unfortunately, the safest and best treatment known for anxiety has been pulled from the shelves in a judgment that reeks of arbitrariness, double standards and bad science.

Several studies have shown kava to be as good as benzodiazepines, one of the major classes of anti-anxiety drugs.

According to an advisory posted on Health Canada's Web site, kava has been banned based on a safety assessment that concluded, not that kava is dangerous, but that there is insufficient evidence that it is safe.

Insufficient evidence? How about thousands of years of traditional use? Or over a dozen clinical studies and two meta-analyses which not only demonstrated kava's effectiveness, but consistently marvelled at its safety? How about at least eight toxicological studies on kava, not one of which showed any evidence of liver toxicity, including the most recent Duke University study (*CNS Spectrums* 2001)?

Health Canada and others have responded to a scare stirred up by a series of case reports claiming that some people who have used kava have suffered liver toxicity. There were twenty-eight cases in Germany and Switzerland. But regulatory decisions should be based on science, not panic. And according to all the current scientific data we have, the conclusion based on these reports is deeply flawed.

At least four separate analyses of the case reports have now concluded that there is no evidence that the liver damage was caused by the kava and that kava is a safe alternative for the treatment of anxiety. Many of the cases can be explained by pre-existent liver disease and simultaneous use of alcohol or drugs that are known to be liver toxins.

An American analysis of the reports by a toxicologist / pharmacologist at the University of Illinois, concluded that there was no clear evidence that the liver damage was caused by kava and that, when used properly, kava has no scientifically established potential for causing liver damage (Waller 2002). A German analysis said that connecting kava to the liver toxicity was not logical in the majority of cases and called the connection arbitrary (*German Pharmacists Journal* 2002).

And how about the double standard? Kava was pulled from the shelves on weak and arbitrary evidence that it causes liver toxicity. Aspirin and Tylenol cause liver toxicity. Studies have proven that hormone replacement therapy causes breast cancer and heart disease, but no one is calling for its removal from the shelves. And, most relevant to the present case, one review of the kava cases compared the risk of using kava to the risk of using the conventional alternative, benzodiazepines, and concluded that, based on the adverse events caused by each, switching people from kava to the drugs would increase, not decrease, the risk (*German Pharmacists Journal* 2002). So where's the science and the logic there? Or as another German reviewer put it, "In view of the current scientific knowledge, the hasty condemnation of Kava extracts appears neither logical nor justifiable. Professional judgment and correct risk / benefit analyses are lacking" (*German Pharmacists Journal* 2002).

Kava kava is a beautiful and magical herb, and it will be sorely missed.

Kava is often dosed according to kavalactones. For anxiety, take 45–70mg of kavalactones three times a day; for sleep, take 135–210mg of kavalactones in one dose an hour before bed.

There is evidence, however, that kavalactones do not work alone. One study found the whole plant to outperform isolated kavalactones. So it may be better to go for total kavalactones rather than a small dose of kava with a large percentage of kavalactones.

Although drinking large amounts of traditional kava beverages containing over 400mg of kavalactones for more than three months, can produce a scaly skin condition, this reaction has never occurred with standardized kava extracts used at the appropriate dose. When the skin condition does occur, it goes away when you stop drinking the kava beverage.

Most sources say not to use kava when pregnant or nursing. However, Brinker lists this caution as speculative, and Mills and Bone say that no adverse effect is expected during pregnancy or lactation despite the caution.

Some sources speculate that you should not use kava if you suffer depression. Some sources say not to use kava with the Parkinson's drug levadopa, though this caution is based only on one case report. Kava may potentiate anti-anxiety drugs and barbiturates.

It has also been suggested that kava could act synergistically with alcohol and increase the level of inebriation. However, one study found that kava did not act synergistically with alcohol (Herberg 1991), and another that it actually tended to counter alcohol's negative effect on concentration (Herberg 1993). Similarly, it has been claimed that motor reflexes may be effected when using kava so caution should be exercised when driving or using heavy machinery. However, once again, one study found no significant changes in driving performance with the use of kava kava (*Z Allg Med* 1991).

Since many of the liver toxicity case reports were marked by pre-existent liver disease and simultaneous use of alcohol or drugs that are known to be liver toxins, kava should not be used by anyone with a history of liver disease, who is on medication with liver toxic effects, or who frequently consumes alcohol.

Kelp   *(Laminaria species)*

Kelp is more like a food than a herb since it is considered a sea vegetable. It is highly valued for its abundance of minerals and is often used for its iodine content to activate an underactive thyroid. It is the herb we use the most in the clinic for underactive thyroid because it is safe, healthy and readily available. And since kelp has the ability to activate an underactive thyroid, it is often used in weight loss formulae. Its mineral content makes it valuable for stimulating hair growth, protecting bones, and for anyone who is chronically low in minerals. The Chinese have used kelp to help soften hard lumps and tumours, and here in the West, herbalists make use of kelp for much the same purpose. In fibrocysitic breast disease, kelp is used to reduce lumps. Kelp is rich in polysaccharides, which are known to have anti-cancer properties and to inhibit the growth of tumours. Kelp protects against breast cancer and may be one of the reasons for the low breast cancer rates in Japan, where it is frequently eaten. In Japan, kelp is often used to help individuals who have been exposed to radiation.

Dosing information for kelp is difficult to give, as it has traditionally been consumed as a food rather than as a supplement. Since you should not consume more than 2,000mcg of iodine, and since the average kelp supplement apparently contains 1,000mcg, use that as your guide.

At the proper dose, kelp is entirely safe. Excessive doses could provide too much iodine and interfere with thyroid function. Prolonged use can cause pimples to break out. Don't use kelp if you have hyperthyroidism. It is safe to use while pregnant or breast feeding. The drug lithium could enhance the possible hypothyroid action of excessive amounts of iodine. It is also possible that kelp could enhance the action of levothyroxine and thyroid replacement medications.

Khella *(Ammi visnaga)*

Though this little-known Egyptian herb is rarely discussed, it has been used since ancient times and deserves to be known, especially by three groups of people: those with asthma, angina and kidney stones.

It is hard to understand why khella is so seldom discussed for asthma because it is the perfect asthma herb. Khella has powerful antispasmodic action in the small bronchials. Though it has little effect during an attack, khella is effective for preventing attacks. German herbal authority Rudolf Fritz Weiss, M.D., calls khella the treatment of choice between attacks. Its antispasmodic effects are very long lasting and a single dose before bed can prevent night attacks. During the day, three doses will prevent attacks and help with the persistent lesser symptoms of asthma.

Khella is antispasmodic in the arteries that supply blood to the heart as well. Coupled with its ability to dilate the coronary arteries, khella is a good treatment for angina.

Kidney stones are another problem that benefit from khella's antispasmodic power. Its antispasmodic action in the ureter is good for relieving the excruciating pain of kidney stones and allowing them to pass more easily. Similarly, it can relieve pain from gallstones.

Khella's antispasmodic action also makes it useful for menstrual cramps. Interestingly, khella extract is also useful for repigmenting the skin of people with vitiligo, the condition that causes progressive white patches on the skin. Clinically, Linda has seen really good results using this herb as a part of a program for this problem. Herbalist Michael Tierra also says that ground khella seed has a long history of use as a contraceptive after intercourse. But this use is unconfirmed by current scientific research.

For angina, take 250–300mg of khella a day, standardized for 12% khelliln. For asthma, Murray and Werbach suggest the same dose. The dosage should be divided in three to prevent asthma attacks, or take just one of those doses at bedtime to get a good sleep by preventing night time attacks. Tierra suggests that a dose is 6–9g of the seed decocted or one-half to one teaspoon (2–5g) of extract.

Khella is very safe, even for long term use. Because it may increase sun sensitivity, as its effectiveness in vitiligo suggests, it may potentiate the effect of the sun sensitizing drug 8-methoxypsoralen.

Khella's antispasmodic action in the ureter is good for relieving the excruciating pain of kidney stones and allowing them to pass more easily. Similarly, it can relieve pain from gallstones.

Lavender *(Lavendula angustifolia)*

There are few things more spectacular than fields of purple lavender. Lavender is one of the most beautiful herbs and one of the most useful essential oils. It has been used since ancient times as an antiseptic. It is also antibacterial and antifungal. Although in different ways, lavender is used both as a herb and as an essential oil.

Lavender is a good herb for mood. A herbal tea made from lavender helps if you are having trouble sleeping. Germany's *Commission E* approves the internal use of lavender for restlessness, insomnia and nervous intestinal discomfort.

Though the herbal tea is perfectly safe to drink, the essential oil should not be used internally. Used properly, though, this highly useful essential oil is an effective sedative and antidepressant.

Despite its long traditional use, lavender has not been extensively researched. This is beginning to change. Recent studies have begun to confirm the many uses of lavender.

A recent review of the studies on lavender concluded that scenting a room with lavender essential oil can improve feelings of well being, sleep and alertness while decreasing aggression and anxiety (*Psychotherapy Research* 2002), a useful thing to keep in mind at home.

This remarkable ability of lavender to simultaneously promote relaxation and alertness has been noticed before. In a 1998 study, people given lavender had increased drowsiness, less depression and were more relaxed, but also performed math calculations quicker and more accurately (*Int J Neurosci*).

A very small but promising study looked at lavender's reputation as a sleeping herb. It found that inhaling lavender essential oil was as effective as tranquilizers in helping elderly people with insomnia to sleep (*Lancet* 1995).

Two more recent studies have also provided exciting confirmation of lavender's traditional uses. Many people with dementia manifest agitated behaviour. In a study of fifteen people with severe dementia and agitated behaviour, the common area of their long-stay facility was diffused with either lavender essential oil or water on different days. With the lavender,

60% did better than they did with the placebo (*International Journal of Geriatric Psychiatry* 2002).

In the most recent study, forty-five people suffering from depression were given either sixty drops of lavender tincture and a placebo, or 100mg of the antidepressant drug imipramine and a placebo, or sixty drops of lavender tincture and 100mg of imipramine. After four weeks, all three groups improved significantly, confirming lavender's power as an antidepressant. Interestingly, the group taking both imipramine and lavender experienced a significantly greater improvement than those taking either treatment alone, suggesting that people on imipramine for depression may be able to reduce their dose of the drug – and, therefore, its side effects – by adding lavender (*Progress in Neuro-Psychopharmacology and Biological Psychiatry* 2003).

Lavender essential oil may also promote hair growth, prevent scarring and promote healing. It is good for burns and scalds. It is also an excellent herb to use topically (using the essential oil) when trying to clear up acne, as it stops new breakouts and heals old ones while clearing up scars. It can also be used to heal the perineal after childbirth.

In ancient times, lavender was used as a wash, helping to purify both body and spirit. In Greece, Persia and Rome it was used to purify sick rooms and hospitals. Ancient writers referred to it as the broom of the brain because it was said to sweep away impurities. It was widely used for psychiatric problems and it is still used for these purposes today.

In ancient times, lavender was used as a wash, helping to purify both body and spirit. In Greece, Persia and Rome it was used to purify sick rooms and hospitals. Ancient writers referred to it as the broom of the brain because it was said to sweep away impurities. It was widely used for psychiatric problems and it is still used for these purposes today.

Inhaling lavender essential oil was as effective as tranquilizers in helping elderly people with insomnia to sleep.

When used internally, lavender can be taken as a tea or as a tincture. To make a tea, infuse one to two teaspoons (5–10g). As a tincture, take up to 2ml three times a day.

When used properly, lavender is perfectly safe. There are no known side effects, contraindications or interactions, though as noted, it may have an enhancing effect on imipramine.

Lavender is safe to take when pregnant or nursing, according to all the women's herbals and books on contraindications that we consulted. Brinker speculatively says that excessive internal use should be avoided during early pregnancy.

Lemon balm
(*Melissa officianalis*)

Giving off the lovely scent of lemon, this member of the mint family is a beautiful herb. We grow it in our garden, and we love to go out and gather some and infuse it into a tea. It tastes wonderful and seems to brighten everything up. It also makes a great ice tea in the summer.

In a world of daily tension and rush, lemon balm is one of nature's very best calming herbs. It is perfect for nervous tension and depression.

In fact, wherever the word "nervous" appears, lemon balm shows up. The *German Commission E* approves its use for "nervous sleeping disorders" and in *Herbal Medicine*, Weiss recommends it for "nervous stomach disorders."

Lemon balm has a gentle effect on insomnia, and this gentleness, along with its pleasant taste, makes it a perfect remedy for children. A recent study found a combination of valerian and lemon balm to be significantly better than a placebo in improving sleep (*Fitoterapia* 1999). And an earlier study found the same combination to be just as good as the drug halcion at helping people fall asleep and at improving the quality of their sleep. Actually, the herbs were better than the drug because the drug group (but not the herb group) felt hung over the next day and had trouble concentrating (*Therapiewoche* 1992).

As for stomach disorders, science has proven lemon balm's ability to relieve gas and spasming. So it is a good herb for gas, upset stomach, vomiting, and especially for indigestion that stems from anxiety or depression. We find it is especially helpful as part of a treatment plan for irritable bowel syndrome.

But lemon balm's magic doesn't stop with calming the stomach and mind, it is also a remarkable antiviral herb. James Duke, Ph.D., goes so far as to say that he would try lemon balm for any viral infection. Despite its versatility, lemon balm does have a specialty: the herpes virus. According to Duke, lemon balm contains at least four antiviral components that target herpes. It can be drunk as a tea, and then the dregs, or more tea, can be applied topically to sores. It has been used for mumps, shingles, genital herpes, chronic fatigue immune dysfunction syndrome (CFIDS or CFS) and more.

One type of herpes infection has received special attention with regard to lemon balm. A number of studies have found a lemon balm extract cream to effectively treat herpes and cold sores – a welcome relief to a lot of people. The drug most used for this condition has numerous side effects and, what's worse, a 1998 study found that it didn't even help.

Now the good news. Even though sores take 10 to 14 days to heal when left alone, when 115 people with herpes applied a cream containing lemon balm extract, 60% had their sores healed in only four days, 87% were better by the sixth day, and a full 96% had their sores healed by day eight (*Phytomedicine* 1994). In a second study, a lemon balm ointment was 2.5 times more effective than a placebo ointment on 116 people with herpes. Most recently, a 1999 study again found lemon balm extract cream to be effective (*Phytomedicine* 1999). Used regularly, the lemon balm cream can stop recurrent cold sores. In my clinic, I have applied lemon balm ointment to cold sores and seen them clear up very quickly.

And if that's not enough to convince you to include lemon balm in your arsenal, there's more. David Hoffmann praises it as a heart tonic that lowers blood pressure, and he and Michael Tierra mention its usefulness in treating fever. Rosemary Gladstar says it is excellent for headaches, and Duke also recommends it for migraine.

And one more interesting use: Duke says that injections of lemon balm decrease thyroid stimulating hormone and, so, help hyperthyroidism. He says that there is a good chance that it will work orally too. Ironically, he also recommends it as a top herb for hypothyroidism, since it normalizes thyroid levels whether they are too high or too low.

Lemon balm can be enjoyed as an infused tea two to three times a day. The herb can be used in pill form at a dose of 1.5–4.5g three times a day. The dose for extracts is 1.5–4.5ml; the dose for tinctures is 2–3 droppers full (approximately 80–120 drops) 3 to 4 times a day. If you are using the cream for cold sores, get a concentrated extract (70:1) and apply it twice a day.

Lemon balm is remarkably safe. It has no contraindications, side effects or drug interactions. Brinker says not to use it while pregnant, but all the other contraindication sources we consulted disagree. A survey of women's herbals and pregnancy books not only does not produce a contraindication for lemon balm, but presents an enthusiastic recommendation.

Licorice *(Glycyrrhiza glabra)*

Years ago, we went to Pioneer Village in Toronto and chewed on licorice stick for the first time. It seemed strange, but long before licorice was a candy, licorice root was a herb. It was sweet and delicious. So sweet that the glycyrrhizin in licorice root is fifty times sweeter than sucrose. That's why its botanical name is *glycyrrhiza glabra*, meaning sweet root.

Licorice is an ancient herb. It has been used for over 4,500 years in ancient cultures in such diverse places as Assyria, Egypt, India, China, Greece, and Rome. Today it is one of the most extensively researched herbs of all. Though it gets much less celebrity attention than the other major herbs, licorice is one of the most active and important herbs in the world. It is one of the most revered herbs in China where it appears in numerous formulae.

Just how active is it? Check this out. A look through the work of herb authority James Duke, Ph.D., reveals that licorice is tops in many categories: it contains the most antifungal compounds of any herb, more anti-depressant compounds than any other herb, and the most bacteria-killing compounds. On top of this, licorice root is powerfully anti-inflammatory, anti-ulcer, antiviral, antioxidant, expectorant, demulcent, antispasmodic, mildly laxative, immune supporting, adrenal gland supporting, hormone balancing, anti-cancer, and liver protecting. This amazing list just might make licorice one of the most versatile, valuable and underrated herbs in the world.

Probably the most important modern use of licorice is in the treatment of ulcers. Several head-to-head studies have shown licorice to be as or more effective than cimitidine (Tagamet), ranitidine (Zantac), or antacids (*Practitioner* 1975; *Practitioner* 1979; *Gut* 1982; *Lancet* 1982). Not only is licorice at least as effective as these drugs, it has several advantages over them. Because the acids that cimitidine and ranitidine block play a crucial role in digestion, these drugs can lead to digestive problems, nutritional deficiencies and also *candida* and, ironically, *H. pylori*, the bacteria that causes so many ulcers. Licorice does not inhibit acid: it actually heals the ulcer. Licorice improves both the quantity and the quality of the protective substances that line the intestine and improves blood supply to the intestinal lining. Test tube studies also suggest that licorice may be active against *H. pylori* (*Life Sci* 2002). Once the ulcer has been healed, licorice also seems to permit fewer relapses than the drugs (*Irish Med Journ*1985). Linda has used licorice to heal her own ulcer. It not only healed the ulcer quickly, but it also began to reduce the pain almost immediately.

Because of concern that the glycyrrhizin in licorice could cause high blood pressure, and because glycyrrhizin is not necessary for licorice's anti-ulcer effect, a special form of licorice known as deglycyrrhizinated licorice, or DGL, has become the most commonly used form of the herb for treating ulcers. Licorice root heals ulcers whatever the type: peptic, gastric, duodenal, and even mouth ulcers (canker sores).

Licorice is also a powerful anti-inflammatory herb. It is good for any inflammatory condition from rheumatoid arthritis, bursitis and tendinitis to allergies and asthma. Licorice has cortisol-like effects, which it accomplishes in a number of ways, including tricking the body. The glycyrrhizin in licorice root is similar in structure to cortisol and fools

[T]he most important modern use of licorice is in the treatment of ulcers. Several head-to-head studies have shown licorice to be as or more effective than cimitidine (Tagamet), ranitidine (Zantac), or antacids.

our bodies by passing itself off as this anti-inflammatory, antistress adrenal hormone. In addition to its own cortisol-like action, licorice also inhibits the breakdown of cortisol, allowing it to stick around and work longer. Licorice is able to boost the action of both the body's own and pharmaceutical corticosteroids. Amazingly, while enhancing the action of corticosteroid drugs, licorice is able to simultaneously counteract their negative effects (*Endocrinol Jpn* 1967). All of these cortisol effects make licorice a very good adrenal tonic. Since the adrenal glands are the body's major centre for dealing with stress, licorice is an excellent herb not only for inflammation, but also to support the body's efforts to deal with stress.

It also helps the body deal with infection. Licorice supports the immune system. It induces interferon and other immune system components and has antiviral, antibacterial and antioxidant properties against a host of invaders, including herpes, *staph*, *strep*, *candida*, and the common cold. It is also effective against malaria (*Antimicrob Agents Chemother* 1994).

But perhaps the greatest anticipation is over the promise that licorice is showing for the treatment of HIV / AIDS. Michael Murray, N.D., says that a number of studies have shown licorice's ability to improve immunity in people with HIV / AIDS. In one study, when sixteen people with HIV were given glycyrrhizin for three to seven years, none of them had their immune system worsen and none of them progressed to AIDS. In the control group that did not receive glycyrrhizin, their helper- and total T-cells and antibodies went down and two of the sixteen developed AIDS (*Int Conf AIDS* 1993). In another study, ten people with HIV were given glycyrrhizin for one to two years and ten people were not. None of the people given glycyrrhizin developed AIDS or AIDS-related symptoms, but, of the ten people not given glycyrrhizin, two progressed to AIDS and one developed AIDS-related complex (*AIDS Treatment News* 1990).

And now there's more excitement over licorice and a modern viral nightmare. Here in Toronto, as in other parts of the world, SARS has been a serious concern. Though so far researched only in test tubes and not in people, a recent study has found that the same licorice component, glycyrrhizin, which helps HIV / AIDS, powerfully inhibits the replication of the virus that causes SARS (*Lancet* 2003).

Other immune uses of licorice include colds and flus and all lung problems, including cough, sore throat, bronchitis, and tuberculosis. It is used for bladder infections, for bringing down fever, and for *candida* and chronic vaginal yeast infections. You can also make a tea of licorice and apply it to athlete's foot, add it to shampoos to fight dandruff (and maybe hair loss), and use it internally and externally for shingles. Daniel Mowrey, Ph.D., says that whole licorice root is one of those amazing tonic herbs that can work in both directions: it can boost immunity or suppress immunity as needed.

Another area in which licorice seems to work in both directions as needed is in conditions involving female hormones. Licorice root has the ability to bring estrogen and progesterone into balance. It can increase estrogen when it is low or decrease it when it is high, making it a good herb for both PMS and menopause.

Licorice is also a good liver herb. Traditional Chinese medicine considers licorice to be a liver tonic herb, and it is still used for liver damage. In Japan, glycyrrhizin has been used for decades as a treatment for hepatitis, and studies confirm that it helps (*Aliment Pharmacol Ther* 1998). Robert McCaleb says that research shows that glycyrrhizin improves liver function in up to 40% of people with hepatitis B and C – not bad when you consider the 45–50% track record of conventional treatment with interferon when the drug's side effects are factored in. Licorice has another important role for people with hepatitis: it is able to prevent the development of liver cancer in people with hepatitis C (*Cancer* 1997; *Oncology* 2002).

James Duke, Ph.D., says that licorice is also used in Japan for the treatment of cirrhosis, and Mowrey says that it is used in traditional Chinese medicine for jaundice. It is, Mowrey says, a very promising herb for hepatitis, cirrhosis and jaundice. Licorice also protects the liver from the damaging effects of Tylenol (Dehpour F, *et. al.*, 2000) as well as preventing gastric bleeding and ulcers caused by aspirin and corticosteroids.

Licorice may also have some benefits for the heart. A recent study found that it was not only able to reduce cholesterol and triglycerides, but also to reduce the dangerous oxidation of the bad LDL cholesterol that is a crucial step in the development of atherosclerosis (*Nutrition* 2002).

Licorice can also help benign prostate hyperplasia, and DGL is a good herb for heartburn. Topically, licorice creams are wonderful for skin conditions. Studies have shown that creams containing glycyrrhetinic acid are as good as or better than hydrocortisone creams for treating eczema and psoriasis. When people with eczema applied either a glycyrrhetinic acid cream or a cortisone cream, 93% of those using licorice improved compared to 83% of those using the drug (*Br J Clin Pract* 1958). Studies have also shown that glycyrrhetinic acid helps heal cold sores and genital herpes.

If you want to take licorice as a tea and enjoy its sweet flavour, make a decoction from 1–2g of the root and drink a cup two to three times a day. As an extract, take 2–4ml three times a day. If using the powdered root as a pill, take 1–2g three times a day. If the pill is a solid extract (4:1), take 250–500mg three times a day. If you are taking DGL to get rid of an ulcer, chew two to four 380mg (4:1) tablets between, or twenty minutes before, each meal. The tablets must be chewed so that they can mix with the saliva to be effective. If the ulcer is chronic and not acute, you may get by on just one to two pills each time.

At the proper dose, licorice is extremely safe. At higher doses over prolonged periods, the literature on licorice is full of warnings. The fear is that high doses or prolonged use can cause potassium loss and sodium and water retention, leading to high blood pressure. It is said that this problem can occur at high doses of over 10g a day for two to three weeks – which is not really a problem since it exceeds the recommended dose – or at doses of more than 3g for more than six weeks. The 3g a day dosage is within the recommended dose range and can be taken long term. The high blood pressure is not permanent, but goes away when you stop using the herb. The DGL form is free of this concern.

Although responsibly issued, this warning may have been overstated. Following a diet that is rich in potassium and low in sodium (which any healthy diet should be anyway) would likely eliminate the feared side effect, according to several experts. People whose diet is normally high in potassium and low in salt have been reported not to have this side effect, even those who already have high blood pressure (*Br Med J* 1969).

More importantly, the side effect doesn't seem to apply at all to people taking the whole licorice root. Almost all reports of high blood pressure have come from people consuming large amounts of highly concentrated licorice extracts or real licorice candy containing licorice extract, not the whole root. By the way, this is European licorice candy; most North American licorice candy doesn't actually contain any licorice. The whole root, which contains substances that balance the blood pressure-raising glycyrrhizin, does not have this effect. Taking the whole root as a pill, tea or stick has not resulted in this much-discussed side effect. Taking the proper dose of whole licorice root appears to be perfectly safe.

To be safe, people who already have high blood pressure, low potassium, severe kidney disorder, and possibly edema or congestive heart failure should probably choose a different herb.

There are also some strange contraindications for licorice. Some sources say not to use licorice if you have cirrhosis: an odd warning given its long tradition as a liver herb and its current use for cirrhosis in Japan. Some sources also contraindicate licorice for diabetics, although Brinker says that this warning is only speculative and that it is not because licorice aggravates diabetes, but because diabetics are more prone to low potassium and sodium retention. This is another warning that is probably overstated but may fit into that "caution" category. Herbalist Michael Tierra endorses licorice as a safe sweetener for diabetics, and licorice has been traditionally used to treat diabetes in Chinese medicine.

Licorice should be avoided by those with low bile production.

Pregnant women should not use licorice because it increases the risk of premature birth: though this warning, too, is based on large consumption of glycyrrhizin from licorice extract in European candy. Mills and Bone in their authoritative text say that up to 3g of the whole root is likely to be safe. A couple of sources also speculate on its avoidance while breast feeding, though many others, including the German Commission E and the American Botanical Council do not. Again, there is always more than one herb for any condition, so if you want to play it safe, choose another one.

As for drug interactions, licorice should not be used with potassium-depleting diuretics, digitalis or cortisone. Licorice may enhance the effect of laxatives. Prolonged use of high doses should be avoided if you are on the birth control pill because of the slight chance that the herb will counteract it. Similarly, it may be contraindicated during estrogen replacement therapy, though only one source mentions this contraindication. Licorice may enhance the action of MAO-inhibiting antidepressants.

The side effects that have turned up for licorice are usually from highly concentrated licorice extract as a flavouring. Many studies on this herb report no side effects at all.

Lobelia

According to herbal authors the Weiners, the Meskwaki tribe used lobelia to help cure quarrelling couples. They would slip a little in the couple's food to stop a divorce. It was also used by midwives to help ease tight muscles during childbirth.

Today, lobelia has many uses. Lobelia's powerful antispasmodic, expectorant properties make it ideal for treating upper respiratory problems like asthma, bronchitis, spasmodic coughs, whooping cough, pneumonia, and other upper respiratory problems. One of the ways that lobelia seems to work is by stimulating the adrenal glands to release hormones that cause the bronchial muscles to relax.

It is also of great benefit for any spasming in the neurological and muscular systems, like hysteria, epilepsy, convulsions, tetanus, febrile conditions, muscle spasms, and what traditional herbalists call "suspended animation," since it's one of the fastest acting antispasmodics. Lobelia is an effective herb to use when there has been food poisoning, since, at sufficient doses, it is an emetic and will induce vomiting. This aspect of lobelia makes it useful whenever you want to purge the system.

Often old-time herbalists would add a little bit of lobelia to almost every formula as a kind of catalyst to make the formula work better. Externally, lobelia can be applied to bruises, sprains, insect bites, tumours and cancers.

It is also helpful to use lobelia to quit smoking. The lobeline in lobelia has a chemical structure much like that of nicotine. It has similar physiological effects without the addictiveness. It satisfies the need for nicotine while you wean your body off it.

[T]he Meskwaki tribe used lobelia to help cure quarrelling couples. They would slip a little in the couple's food to stop a divorce.

If you are using the dried herb in pill form, take 200–600mg three times a day. If you prefer to make a tea, infuse about 1/4 teaspoon (1g) per cup and drink three cups a day. The dose of the tincture should not exceed 1ml three times a day. For the extract, take 0.2–0.6ml three times a day. For respiratory problems, like asthma, some suggest that a tincture made with vinegar instead of alcohol is better. Often a stimulant herb like peppermint is given before administering lobelia to help it work better.

Large doses of lobelia can cause nausea and vomiting; hence, this herb's dignified nickname: puke weed. This seemingly negative effect is actually a good thing. There have been no cases of serious side effects. Emetics like lobelia are valuable when purging is necessary, and its emetic quality assures the safety of lobelia. Although it has often been claimed that lobelia is a toxic herb, lobelia is safe either because it is not toxic at all or because it has a built in safety feature that causes you to vomit if you take too much of it.

Do not use lobelia if you have cardiovascular disease or if you suffer from nervous exhaustion, shock, paralysis, low vitality or indigestion. Lobelia should not be used if you are pregnant. Though virtually all herbals and women's herbals say that you cannot use lobelia if you are breast feeding, it is interesting to note that neither Brinker nor the American Herbal Products Association's *Botanical Safety Handbook* list breast feeding as a contraindication for lobelia.

Maitake mushroom *(Grifola frondosa)*

Of the three great medicinal mushrooms – shiitake, reishi and maitake – maitake is probably the least familiar. But maitake is finally emerging from the shadows: which is a pretty good trick if you're a mushroom. Maitake is a massive mushroom that does not resemble the common button mushroom at all. It can reach twenty inches (50 centimetres) in diameter and weigh over 100 pounds (45 kilograms). Its name means "dancing" mushroom, possibly because in ancient times people would dance with joy when they were lucky enough to find this delicious and medicinally valuable mushroom, since it was worth its weight in silver. Traditionally, this mushroom was considered so valuable that mushroom hunters would never divulge the location of their finds.

Mushrooms are not really plants at all. They belong to the kingdom of fungi, and, strangely, fungi are more closely related to animals than they are to plants. In his article in *HerbalGram* #54, Paul Stamets says that because they are more closely related to us, mushrooms can suffer from some of the same microorganisms that we do, meaning that we can benefit from the natural antibiotic defences they have developed. Stamets says that maitake mushrooms are antibacterial, antiviral and anti-candida.

> *Its name means "dancing" mushroom ... in ancient times people would dance with joy when they were lucky enough to find this delicious and medicinally valuable mushroom, since it was worth its weight in silver. Traditionally, this mushroom was considered so valuable that mushroom hunters would never divulge the location of their finds.*

But the real excitement over maitake mushrooms is in the realm of cancer research. Cancer expert Ralph Moss, Ph.D., says that a number of ingredients in this mushroom are showing anti-cancer effects in the laboratory. Many of these effects are due to its powerful ability to stimulate the immune system.

A lot of the research on maitake mushroom has been done on a component of it known as maitake fraction-D. In one exciting study (*J Orthomol Med* 1997), maitake fraction-D was given to 165 people with various kinds of advanced cancer. Amazingly, tumour regression, or a significant improvement of symptoms, was seen in 73% of those with breast cancer, 67% with lung cancer and 47% with liver cancer. It was also effective in people with prostate cancer. It was less effective in people with stomach cancer, bone cancer or leukemia. When the researchers tried adding the maitake fraction-D to chemotherapy, it enhanced the chemo while alleviating many of its side effects in all kinds of cancers. It also reduced pain.

A second study conducted recently also looked at the effect of maitake mushroom on people with a variety of advanced cancers. They gave a blend of maitake fraction-D and whole maitake powder to thirty-six people. There was cancer regression or significant symptom improvement in eleven out of sixteen people with breast cancer (68.8%), five out of eight with lung cancer (62.6%) and seven out of twelve with liver cancer (58.3%). Once again, when it was added to chemo, the chemo worked better, and, as previously found, it was less effective in leukemia and cancer of the stomach and brain (*Altern Med Rev* 2002). There was, however, one study that found an anti-cancer effect for a maitake extract on cancers including stomach and leukemia (Zhu *et al*, 1994).

The greatest excitement over maitake mushroom has been for prostate cancer. The maitake D-fraction was tested in a laboratory against hormone refractory prostate cancer (also known as androgen independent prostate cancer). When prostate cancer progresses to this stage, conventional therapy has been ineffective. But there was almost complete cell death when the cancer cells were treated with maitake D-fraction. When the D-fraction was combined with vitamin C, much smaller amounts worked almost as well. Amazingly, unlike chemotherapy and other methods that also damage the healthy cells around the cancer cells, maitake kills cancer cells without damaging the non-cancerous ones (*Mol Urol* 2000). It was also recently shown to increase the effectiveness of chemotherapy in test tubes in this difficult to treat cancer (*Journal of Alternative and Complementary Medicine* 2002).

Maitake mushrooms may hold promise not only for cancer, but perhaps also for AIDS. Research conducted at the National Cancer Institute in 1992 found that maitake mushroom had antiviral activity against HIV. In fact, Moss says that internal NCI documents reveal that it inhibited the growth of HIV at about the same rate as AZT. Too bad no one ever followed that up!

Maitake mushrooms may also help blood pressure, blood sugar, cholesterol, and stress.

 Maitake can be used as a supplement, as a tea or in cooking. The dose is 3–7 grams a day.

 Maitake mushroom is perfectly safe. There are no side effects, drug interactions or contraindications, including during pregnancy and breast feeding.

Marshmallow (*Althaea officinalis*)

This medicinal herb is not what it sounds like: it is not the puffy white marshmallow that people roast over fires. Rather, marshmallow root is a common herb that is used to heal wounds, burns, sore and chafed skin, to soothe sore throats and mouths, for dry cough, and gastrointestinal irritation. Its demulcent and emollient properties make it well suited to healing irritated surfaces, and it is, therefore, almost always included in formulae for ulcers, leaky gut, and for irritated mucous surfaces. Because it is such an effective wound-healing herb, it is well suited to healing gastroenteritis, peptic and duodenal ulcers, colitis, and enteritis. It is simply one of the best herbs to heal up an ulcerated digestive system. It is not surprising, then, that it has been used for over two thousand years in Europe. Its first recorded use, however, was in the ninth century BCE. It was widely used in Greek medicine. Its name Althea comes from the Greek *altho*, to cure.

In pill form, use either 5g of the leaf or 6g of the root. If you prefer a tea, either infuse 1–3 teaspoons (5-15g) of the leaf in a cup of water and drink three cups a day, or decoct 1–3g of the root in a cup of water and drink three cups a day. The *Commission E* recommends slightly lower doses of the tea. Tincture doses vary: herbalist David Hoffmann recommends 1–4ml three times a day, but others recommend the much higher dose of 5–10ml of the leaf two to three times a day, and 10–25ml of the root up to three times a day. Of the extract, take 1–2ml of the leaf two to three times a day or 2–5ml of the root up to three times a day.

 This very safe herb has no side effects or contraindications. It is perfectly safe to take while pregnant or breast feeding. There are no drug interactions, although marshmallow may delay the absorption of oral drugs that are taken at the same time. This possibility, however, is only speculative.

Milk thistle *(Silybum marianum)*

Milk thistle is a herb with both the weight of tradition and science behind it. It has been used for over two thousand years and is the subject of hundreds of studies, making it one of the most studied herbs of all.

Milk thistle is the most effective of the liver herbs and probably the best supported treatment of them all for liver toxicity (*Fitoterapia* 1995). All of this makes milk thistle one of the most important herbs for modern living. The liver is chiefly responsible for detoxifying our bodies of all of the chemicals and pollution that we are now exposed to on a daily basis. In today's world, keeping the liver healthy is a foundation stone of health, elevating milk thistle to a position of herbal prominence. Robert McCaleb calls the regular use of milk thistle a modern necessity.

Milk thistle is an important herb for the whole range of liver disease. It is used for hepatitis, cirrhosis, liver disease caused by alcohol, toxins or chemicals, and fatty liver. All but two of the many studies done on milk thistle have found it to be very effective in these conditions. Milk thistle may also be able to help with the new threat of hepatitis C. One review of the research on milk thistle concluded that the herb was effective for toxic and metabolic liver disease as well as acute and chronic hepatitis (*Economic and Medicinal Plant Research* 1988).

Robert McCaleb calls the regular use of milk thistle a modern necessity.

Milk thistle can also protect the liver from damage caused by pharmaceutical drugs, including acetaminophen (Tylenol), antidepressants and antipsychotics, cholesterol-lowering drugs, anticonvulsives and, possibly, anesthesia. It is a crucial herb for damage caused by alcoholism. Its long term use heals the damage, and those with cirrhosis live longer when they use milk thistle (*J Hepatol* 1989). Donald Brown, N.D., says that milk thistle is a key to any alcohol recovery program.

Milk thistle seems to be tailor-made for the liver, with a powerful and wide-ranging effect that protects and heals it in so many ways. The flavonoids found in milk thistle, known collectively as silymarin, are powerful antioxidants. But not only are they powerful antioxidants in their own right, they also greatly increase the amount of glutathione in the liver, as well as in the intestines and stomach. Glutathione is one of the body's most important antioxidants and most crucial detoxifiers. Silymarin also increases the activity of SOD, another of your body's important antioxidant enzymes (*Acta Physiol Hung* 1991).

Milk thistle protects the liver from harm from toxins, chemicals and drugs by preventing toxins from penetrating into the liver cells. It is even effective against the extremely poisonous death cap mushroom.

Perhaps most amazingly of all, milk thistle not only protects the liver from damage, it cures it, because it has the incredible ability to actually regenerate the liver. Milk thistle increases the production of new, healthy liver cells to replace the old damaged ones (Sonnenbichler *et al*, 1986, 1989). While it stimulates cell growth, however, it does so only for healthy cells; milk thistle does not stimulate cancerous liver cells (*Biochem Pharm* 1986).

[M]ost amazingly of all, milk thistle not only protects the liver from damage, it cures it, because it has the incredible ability to actually regenerate the liver.

Milk thistle also aids the liver by increasing the production and flow of bile and by stopping liver-damaging inflammation. This last ability allows milk thistle to prevent the fibrosis caused by inflammation from alcohol abuse and hepatitis (*Zeits Allegemeinmed* 1998).

Because milk thistle makes the liver work better, it is also a valuable herb for the many conditions that are not thought of as liver disease, but which are at least partly caused by a liver no longer able to work at full capacity. This long list of conditions includes any female hormonal condition because the liver is crucial for breaking down estrogen. It also includes digestion, constipation, mood disorders, and skin conditions like psoriasis and acne.

Recent research is also suggesting new uses for this valuable herb. It may help with allergies (*British Journal of Clinical Pharmacology* 1987). It might also help colitis and ulcers. Research shows that milk thistle could help with gallstones.

Milk thistle may also turn out to be an anti-cancer herb. Laboratory research conducted in test tubes, but not yet on people, shows that milk thistle can inhibit ovarian and breast cancer cells (*Eur J Cancer* 1996). A component of milk thistle, called silibinin, has been shown to be a strong fighter of prostate cancer cells in test tubes. When prostate cancer cells were treated either with a chemotherapy drug, silibinin or both, the silibinin boosted the chemo drug's ability to inhibit the growth of the cancer cells and powerfully increased apoptosis (*Clin Cancer Res* 2002). Apoptosis, unlike chemotherapy, is a very safe way of killing cancer cells without harming the non-cancerous cells around them.

This remarkable liver herb may turn out to be an effective kidney herb too. Research has found that milk thistle is also able to repair and regenerate kidney cells, increasing kidney cell replication by 25%–30% (Sonnenbichler, *et al* 1998).

Milk thistle is most often taken in pill form as a standardized extract. It should be standardized for 70%–80% silymarin and taken in doses of 140mg of silymarin two to three times a day. Notice that that's 140mg of silymarin, not of milk thistle: if the herb is standardized for 70% silymarin, you need to take 200mg of milk thistle to get 140mg of silymarin. If you are using a milk thistle tincture, take 1–2ml three times a day. As a powdered seed or as a tea made from the powdered seed, the *German Commission E* recommends 12–15g a day. Silymarin is poorly soluble in water, however, so teas made from this herb are not really recommended.

Milk thistle is extremely safe for everybody. With the exception of an occasionally mild laxative effect, milk thistle has no side effects. Large studies have found mild side effects in only 1% of people using milk thistle. One study found that of 998 people, tolerance was good or excellent in 98% (*Allg Med* 1998). Another study that monitored over 3,000 people found adverse events in only 1%: most of them were mild gastrointestinal complaints. There are no contraindications for milk thistle and no drug interactions.

Milk thistle has a long history of use for encouraging the flow of breast milk and is perfectly safe to use while breast feeding. Milk thistle is also perfectly safe for pregnant women. Brinker has recently speculated that it should be avoided during pregnancy, theoretically due to its actions, but also says that this contraindication is not consistent with the research. Milk thistle has actually been recommended for some uses during pregnancy. None of the women's herbals we consulted contraindicated milk thistle for pregnancy and all of the other authoritative texts on contraindications, including those of the *German Commission E*, the American Botanical Council and the American Herbal Products Association, endorse the use of milk thistle by pregnant women.

Motherwort (*Leonurus cardiaca*)

Motherwort is a wonderful herb that has many uses, although it is mainly used in three areas. Since it promotes blood circulation, motherwort is used for various heart problems, such as atherosclerosis, to dissolve blood clots, for angina, palpitations, anxiety, and heart neuralgia. The word *"cardiaca,"* in motherwort's botanical name, means heart.

Its second main use is for female problems. Motherwort was used as a folk remedy for female problems, which is where the "mother" in motherwort comes from. It is used for suppressed or absent menstruation, painful periods and, in combination with other herbs, for menopause and other female disorders. It is often combined with other female herbs like dong quai, cramp bark, chastetree berry, and the cohoshes. According to Michael Tierra, in ancient times, motherwort's ability to promote menstruation made it valuable to Chinese courtesans who used motherwort to prevent pregnancy and protect themselves from venereal disease.

The third main use of motherwort is to treat various nervous problems, such as hysteria, convulsions, insomnia, and other neurotic conditions.

Historically, motherwort has also been used for worms, typhoid fever, disturbed sleep, gastrointestinal stress, as a douche for vaginitis, rheumatism, goiter, high blood pressure, epilepsy, and to improve mood and fainting.

First Nations people of North America were well acquainted with motherwort and used it extensively much as it is used today: for female problems. In the Middle Ages, motherwort was used for nervousness and emotional excitement. It was also used to protect individuals from evil spirits.

Today, it is still widely used for blood pressure issues and for thyroid hyperfunction. Motherwort is an antispasmodic, carminative, nervine, emmenagogue, cardiac tonic, and diuretic.

In pill form, take 4.5g a day. To drink motherwort as a tea, infuse 1 teaspoon (5g) per cup of water and drink three cups a day. Take 2–4ml of the tincture three times a day (though the *German Commission E* recommends a much higher dose of 22.5ml, presumably in divided doses).

Motherwort is a very safe herb with no side effects, contraindications or drug interactions. Motherwort should not be used during pregnancy because it is an emmenagogue, and it could potentially bring on a miscarriage, though Brinker says that this contraindication is only speculative, and that it only applies to excessive doses in early pregnancy.

First Nations people of North America were well acquainted with motherwort and used it extensively much as it is used today: for female problems. In the Middle Ages, motherwort was used for nervousness and emotional excitement. It was also used to protect individuals from evil spirits.

Muíra puama *(Ptychopetalum olacoides, Liriosma ovata)*

Some herbalists believe that muira puama is one of the best herbs for treating impotence. This is not surprising as it has been used in Brazil for many years, where it is known as "potency wood." Muira puama is also wonderful for lack of libido in males and as a mild aphrodisiac in both men and women. A 1990 study confirmed muira puama's benefits. Muira puama was given to 262 men with either erectile dysfunction or poor libido. Within two weeks, 51% of the men with erectile dysfunction benefited, as did 61% of those with loss of libido (Waynberg, 1990).

But that's not all this herb does. Muira puama is also used to prevent other sexual problems and to treat diarrhea.

A recent study also showed it to be useful for memory problems caused by age or stroke. The study showed that it enhanced cognitive and physical performance, and so is thought to hold promise for Alzheimer's patients (Elisabetsky 2000).

There is not a lot of information available on dosage Try 10 to 30 drops (about 1ml) of the tincture or extract two or three times a day, or one hour before you're going to need it. The study mentioned above used an extract at a dose of 1–1.5 grams a day. You can also make a standard decoction and drink three to four cups a day.

Muira puama seems to be perfectly safe. There are no side effects, contraindications or drug interactions. It is safe to take while pregnant and breast feeding.

Muira puama has been used in Brazil for many years, where it is known as "potency wood."

Mullein

(Verbascum thapsus)

Mullein has been used since ancient times. In the Middle Ages, mullein was a popular skin and lung treatment. Later, it was used in Europe, the United Kingdom and the U.S. for tuberculosis. And then, in the nineteenth century, it was also used for inflammatory disorders of the ear, genitourinary tract, and for respiratory problems.

This herb is an expectorant, antispasmodic, astringent, and demulcent that is often used today in the treatment of lung and bronchial congestions, including spasmodic coughs, sore throats, irritated throats, bronchitis, and pneumonia. It is often smoked for lung and bronchial congestion and coughs. Mullein is also used to treat mumps, swollen glands, cramps, diarrhea, for lymphatic congestion, and earaches. We have been particularly impressed with mullein for earaches. We have used this herb in scores of people with earaches and have seen it work remarkably quickly. For earaches, mullein can be used alone, or it is often combined with garlic, calendula and St. John's wort and extracted in olive oil. Drops of the oil are then placed in each ear.

> *We have been particularly impressed with mullein for earaches. We have used this herb in scores of people with earaches and have seen it work remarkably quickly . . . [I]t is often combined with garlic, calendula and St. John's wort and extracted in olive oil.*

Take 3–4g of mullein three times a day. To make a mullein tea, infuse 1–2 teaspoons (5–10g) in a cup of water and drink three cups a day (the *Commission E* recommends a smaller serving of 2g twice daily). You could also use a tincture at a dose of 1–4ml (or even a little more) three to four times a day, or an extract at a dose of 1.5–2ml twice a day.

The flowers are macerated in olive oil and used for treating earaches. If you are using the traditional combination described above, strain the oil through a cloth and place five drops into each ear three times a day.

Mullein may also be smoked for treating lung and bronchial congestion. For lung, throat and bronchial problems, mullein is usually combined with other respiratory strengthening herbs like wild cherry, licorice, elecampane, comfrey, and coltsfoot (see information on Safety for comfrey and coltsfoot).

The root of this plant also has uses and can be decocted into a tea to relieve lymphatic congestion, diarrhea and cramps. For treating mumps and swollen glands, mullein is often used in a poultice.

Mullein is perfectly safe, including during pregnancy and breast feeding. There are no side effects, contraindications or drug interactions.

Myrrh, ARABIAN SOMALIAN

(Commiphora myrrha, Commiphora molmol)

Myrrh has been around and in use by many ancient cultures for thousands of years. It was used by the ancient Egyptians for embalming. It was considered so valuable to the ancient Egyptians that we were amazed to see on a trip to Luxor, Egypt, a huge part of an ancient wall of the graceful and unusually beautiful temple of Hatshepsut dedicated to a relief of myrrh trees being brought to Egypt. During Christ's time, it was one of the most precious commodities available. It was offered, along with frankincense and gold, as one of the "treasures" given as a gift to the infant Jesus (Matthew 2:11). Many cultures still use it as incense, and it is said to have purifying, calming and spiritual properties.

Myrrh is a herb with many uses. It is a fantastic antiseptic herb that can be applied externally to heal and disinfect wounds, bedsores, and hemorrhoids. Internally, it can be used for infections in the mouth and throat, such as gingivitis, mouth ulcers (canker sores), thrush, pyorrhoea, pharyngitis, and tonsillitis. Clinically, we have seen it quickly heal mouth, throat and tooth aches, often with just one dose. It is also used for sinusitis, nasal congestion from the common cold, and it is a good antimicrobial.

And that is not all. Myrrh can be used to treat indigestion, gas, painful or suppressed menstruation, arthritis, and bronchial congestion. Combined with other herbal antivirals and antibiotics, it can be used to fight off infections and inflammation.

Myrrh is best taken as a tincture. Take 1–4ml three times a day. To use topically in the mouth, put 5–10 drops of tincture in a glass of water and gargle or rinse with it three times a day. The resin, however, turns rubbery and sticks to the glass so don't use your favourite crystal. Myrrh can also be a valuable ingredient in toothpaste.

Myrrh is safe and has no side effects or interactions with drugs. It should, however, be avoided during pregnancy. Myrrh is fine if you are breast feeding. Herbalist Michael Tierra suggests that it should not be taken for more than a couple of weeks at a time unless it is balanced with demulcent herbs, because resins can be hard on the kidneys. For the same reason, the American Herbal Products Association's *Botanical Safety Handbook* says that doses over 2–4g could irritate the kidneys. That is why other sources say not to exceed 1g of the resin three times a day if you are taking the pill form. Myrrh is contraindicated when there is heavy uterine bleeding and arterial agitation. Brinker alone adds fever and acute internal inflammation: odd warnings given the traditional uses of this herb.

Myrrh, INDIAN (GUGULIPID)   *(Commiphora mukul)*

From the Ayurvedic tradition of India comes the resin of a type of myrrh tree known as *Commiphora mukul*. The standardized extract of this herb is known as gugulipid: a funny name, but a very serious cholesterol fighter.

Gugulipid works as well as cholesterol-lowering drugs, but without their significant side effects. One study found that gugulipid significantly lowered cholesterol and triglycerides in 70% of 205 people. Cholesterol went down 23.6% and triglycerides 22.6% (*J Assoc Phys India* 1989). Another study found similar results with cholesterol lowered by 25% and triglycerides by 30% (*Journal of Molecular and Cellular Cardiology* 1978). Overall, gugulipid can lower total cholesterol from 14–27%, the bad LDL cholesterol by 25–35%, triglycerides by 22–30%, and raise the good HDL cholesterol by 16–20%, according to Michael Murray, N.D. Raising the good HDL cholesterol is at least as important as lowering the bad – and more commonly discussed – LDL cholesterol.

Indian myrrh may also be beneficial for the heart in other ways. It acts as an antioxidant, preventing free-radical damage to LDL cholesterol and, so, protects against atherosclerosis (*Phytother Res* 1993) and inhibits platelet aggregation (*Planta Med* 1979). It may also aid in weight loss.

One surprising benefit of this cholesterol star is its effect on acne. When it was compared to tetracycline, Indian myrrh edged out the drug, with 68% of people improving compared to 65.2% on the drug. People with oily skin did far better on the herb (*J Dermatol* 1994). A second study found that gugulipid brought about excellent results in 30% of people with acne, good results in 47% and moderate results in the remaining 23% (*Ind J Dermatol Venereol Leprol* 1990).

One study found that gugulipid significantly lowered cholesterol and triglycerides in 70% of people . . .

One surprising benefit of this cholesterol star is its effect on acne. When it was compared to tetracycline, Indian myrrh edged out the drug, with 68% of people improving compared to 65.2% on the drug.

Take 500mg, standardized for 25mg of guggulsterones, three times a day.

This herb is extremely safe. It may cause a rash and should not be used by women who are pregnant or who are experiencing excessive uterine bleeding. There are no known drug interactions, though one source mentions reduced absorption of propranolol and diltiazem when taken with *comiphora mukul*.

Nettle

(Urtica dioica, Urtica urens)

In the wild, nettle is a herb that knows how to take care of itself. It protects itself and stings you if you don't pick it carefully. Perhaps that's because if everyone knew how valuable nettle truly was, there would be none left. Perspective is a funny thing: what is to one person a bothersome weed is to another a valuable herb. And nettle is one of the most useful plants we have.

Nettle is revered as a tonic herb. Herbalist Michael Tierra says that nettle is a tonic for the whole body, and especially for the lungs, stomach and urinary tract. It strengthens weak kidneys and is also used for urinary infections and stones. Herbalist Rosemary Gladstar also praises it as a tonic for the reproductive system.

For women, there are few tonics better, according to Gladstar. It is a great help for menopause, water retention, PMS, and excessive menstruation. It restores energy after childbirth and enriches and increases breast milk.

Part of nettle's value comes from its abundant store of easily absorbable nutrients. It is a treasure house of calcium, magnesium, silica, iron, potassium, zinc, chromium, and vitamins C and K. It is also very rich in chlorophyll.

Nettle is one of the best herbs for allergies and hay fever. Dr. Andrew Weil says that he knows of nothing as dramatic as the allergy relief offered by freeze-dried nettle leaves. In one double-blind, placebo-controlled study, freeze-dried nettle leaves significantly relieved the symptoms of allergies and hay fever in 70% of sufferers (_Planta Medica_ 1990).

Recent research is also pointing to nettle as an arthritis herb. Forty people with acute osteoarthritis were given either 200mg of diclofenac or 50mg of the same drug plus 50 grams of stewed nettle leaf. Diclofenac is a nonsteroidal anti-inflammatory drug (NSAID) commonly used for arthritis in doses of

> _Dr. Andrew Weil says that he knows of nothing as dramatic as the allergy relief offered by freeze-dried nettle leaves._

150–200mg; however, 50mg is not an effective dose, as previous studies on the drug have shown it not to work at 75mg. Nonetheless, both groups in this study improved by 70% (*Phytomed* 1997). Since the 50mg of diclofenac given to one group could not be responsible for the remarkable improvement, there are two possible answers: either the nettle leaf was responsible for the improvement or the nettle leaf enhanced the effect of the anti-inflammatory drug. An earlier study found that people with osteoarthritis could reduce their dose of NSAIDs by 50% with nettle leaf (*Therapiewoche* 1996). Given the common side effects of NSAIDs like aspirin, a 50% reduction in dose could be important. In 1996, another study found nettle leaf extract to be as effective as NSAIDs in rheumatic complaints (*Therapiewoche* 1996).

The leaf of the stinging nettle has many other uses. Duke recommends it for bronchitis, asthma and hay fever, and he says that its antibacterial activity makes it good for plaque and gingivitis when added to toothpaste or mouthwash. Hoffmann calls nettle a specific for childhood eczema and suggests it for nosebleeds and haemorrhages. Tierra also recommends it for bleeding, including uterine bleeding and endometriosis. He adds that it is perfect for anemia and that, applied to the scalp, it may help stimulate hair growth. Nettle leaf is also good for kidney stones, cystitis, nephritis, hemmorrhoids, diarrhea, dysentery, acne, and osteoporosis.

Not only the leaf of the nettle plant, but also the root has uses. Research is finding nettle root offers good relief for the urinary symptoms of benign prostate hyperplasia (BPH), the enlarged prostate that affects so many men. One study compared nettle root extract to a placebo and found the root to be better than the placebo for all urinary symptoms (*Urologe B* 1987). Urinary frequency was significantly reduced by nettle root extract in another placebo-controlled study, and a huge study of 4,051 men with BPH found a 50% reduction in night-time urination (*Allg Med* 1984). In an even larger study of urinary frequency and flow, 78% of 4,396 men improved after three months and 91% improved after six (Friesen A, 1988).

According to herbal authors the Weiners, in the second and third centuries BCE, nettle was used for an unusual purpose: as an antidote for hemlock. Too bad Socrates wasn't able to get any when he was forced to drink the poison while in prison in Ancient Greece! Nettle was also used as a counterpoison for henbane and as a cure for snakebite and scorpion sting.

For nettle leaf, use 2–5g of the dried leaf three times a day in pill form or as an infusion. As an extract, take 2–5ml three times a day, and take 7–14ml a day of the tincture. For the nettle root, use 4–6g of the dried root. If you are making a decoction, use 1.5g three to four times a day. The dose is 1.5ml three to four times a day of the extract and 5–7.5ml three to four times a day of the tincture. For BPH, the dose that has been used is 600–1,200mg of 5:1 extract a day, which is equal to 3–6g of the dried root.

Nettle is very safe, including during pregnancy and breast feeding. Brinker says to avoid excessive internal use during pregnancy, but no other contraindication text or women's herbal that we consulted gives this warning. Rosemary Gladstar lists it as a favourite herb that is highly recommended for pregnant women. Tori Hudson, N.D., calls it "one of the best herbs to use in pregnancy" and Aviva Jill Romm calls it "Second to none . . . a pregnancy herb par excellence . . . ." The only contraindication is if you have edema that is caused by a heart disorder or kidney insufficiency. There are no side effects for the leaf and only occasional mild gastrointestinal upset for the root. There are no negative drug interactions.

A Lot of Herbs For a Lot of Time

- The first Chinese herbal was written around 4,000 years ago
- India's Ayurvedic system of healing is also about 4,000 years old. The 5th century BCE *Sushruta Samhita* mentions around 760 herbal medicines
- The First Nations healers of North America used at least 2,582 plants medicinally
- Samoan herbalists can identify and use one hundred to two hundred species
- Throughout history, only 1% of plants have been used as foods, but an amazing 15% have been used as herbal medicines

Oregano
(Origanum vulgare)

This popular and delicious cooking herb has a history of use in respiratory and digestive conditions. It has also been used as an antiseptic for the mouth and throat as well as for cuts and wounds.

Recently, another use for this herb has emerged that has been newly documented. Oregano oil has proved to be a remarkable antifungal, anti-candida remedy. In fact, a recent study found oregano oil to be more than a hundred times more powerful against *candida* than caprylic acid, another popular natural remedy for *candida*. It is also being used for cold sores and to prevent colds and flus.

And, of course, oregano is a remarkable antioxidant herb that can be used anywhere an antioxidant is needed, such as to maintain health and for problems like arthritis and glaucoma.

Oregano can be made into a tea by infusing 1–2 teaspoons (5–10g) per cup of water. Drink three cups a day. Of course, the most delicious way to take oregano is as a seasoning. Add it generously to your food: especially Greek salads!

Of the oil, take it by the drop. If the oil is enteric-coated in a capsule, take 0.2–0.4ml twice a day between meals. If you are applying the oil topically for athlete's foot or other fungal infection, make sure that it has been diluted by at least 50% and apply it twice a day.

Oregano leaf is very safe. There are no side effects, contraindications or drug interactions. It is safe to use during pregnancy and breast feeding, though Brinker says to avoid excessive use during pregnancy.

Do not use the oil if you are pregnant. And don't apply it to hypersensitive, diseased or damaged skin. If you are applying it to mucous membranes, make sure it is no more than a 1% concentration. The oil is very strong. Don't apply it topically to children under two.

parsley (*Petroselinum sativum, Petroselinum crispum*)

Pretty much everyone knows parsley. It is often used decoratively with food. But this herb is not just a garnish on your plate to be thrown away. It is a wonderful source of minerals and vitamins and is high in chlorophyll and, therefore, useful for detoxifying. And it tastes wonderful in the Middle Eastern dish tabouli. Parsley has many herbal properties, including being a diuretic, carminative, emmenagogue, antispasmodic, expectorant, sedative, antirheumatic, antiseptic, and it can also be used to bring on menstruation.

But its main use is for the urinary tract. Parsley is used to soothe urinary tract inflammations, infections, and to get rid of excess water in the system, while the root is particularly suited to dissolving and expelling stones and gravel from the urinary tract system and from the gallbladder. All the parts of parsley can also be used to aid digestion and for bronchial and lung problems. It is useful for gas and indigestion. The seed of parsley can be used to treat rheumatic complaints. And, if you've eaten garlic and can't get rid of the smell on your breath, try chewing on parsley: its natural deodorant properties can help to remove smells. Parsley can also be used to stop unwanted breast milk from coming.

In pill form, take 6g a day of the crushed herb and root. Herbalist David Hoffmann says that you can also drink parsley as a tea by infusing 2 teaspoons (10g) of the dried herb per cup of water three times a day; the *German Commission E* gives the lower dose of 2g per cup three times a day. You can take 2–4ml of the tincture three times a day or 2ml of the extract three times a day.

Like all food herbs, parsley is very safe. But don't use it while you are pregnant. And though it is perfectly safe to use while breast feeding, avoid using it because parsley will dry up your breast milk. There are no side effects or drug interactions for parsley, and the only contraindication is for people with kidney inflammation. Occasional allergies are possible.

Passionflower *(Passiflora incarnata)*

Someday passionflower could be a herbal superstar, when more people realize what it can do. Right now this is a herb that does not get nearly enough attention. Passionflower is a gentle, effective sedative that does not produce a morning hangover or have a drug-like effect. Herbalist David Hoffmann says it is one of the best herbs for stubborn, chronic insomnia. Since passionflower is also a great herb for anxiety, it is the perfect herb to use if your sleeplessness is caused by nervousness or anxiety. A number of prominent herbalists have similarly noted that passionflower is an ideal herb to use if your insomnia is caused by worry or nightmares or if you can't sleep because you can't turn off your thoughts. It is also a useful herb if pain is keeping you awake at night.

Passionflower is a very gentle herb, making it perfect for children and the elderly. It is one of the relaxing herbs that is excellent for children who are hyperactive or who suffer from anxiety or nervous disorders.

An exciting study recently put passionflower's anti-anxiety powers to the test. It pitted the herb head to head with the benzodiazepine drug oxazepam in a double-blind study. Benzodiazepines are the drugs of choice for treating anxiety, but the passionflower worked just as well. In fact, passionflower got the nod because the drug caused significantly more problems in terms of impairment of job performance (*J Clin Pharm Ther* 2001). Clinically, we have found that passionflower is one of the best herbs for people suffering from frequent or occasional anxiety and even panic attacks.

Passionflower's anti-anxiety properties may make it a valuable herb in another innovative way. Researchers have now found that the combination of passionflower and the drug clonidine is more effective than the drug alone in helping people withdraw from opiates like morphine and codeine (*Journal of Clinical*

> *Benzodiazepines are the drugs of choice for treating anxiety, but the passionflower worked just as well. In fact, passionflower got the nod because the drug caused significantly more problems in terms of impairment of job performance.*

Pharmacy and Therapeutics 2001). Passionflower is also helpful in withdrawal from the anti-anxiety benzodiazepine drugs (*Eur J Herb Med* 1997).

Passionflower has other uses too. Since it is a strong antispasmodic, it is also a good herb for epilepsy and Parkinson's disease. Its antispasmodic properties also explain this herb's ability to help hysteria, cramps, menstrual cramping, PMS, and asthma. Passionflower also helps people suffering from neuralgia and shingles.

Passionflower makes a pleasant, relaxing tea. Infuse a teaspoon (5g) of dried herb per cup and sip it 30–45 minutes before you go to bed to help you sleep, or three to four times throughout the day to help you relax. As a tincture, use 5–10ml and, as an extract, use 2ml in the same way as the tea. If you are using the dried herb in a pill form, the dose is 2g three to four times a day: a single dose can be taken for insomnia.

Passionflower is a very safe and gentle herb: there are no side effects, contraindications or drug interactions. Brinker speculates that passionflower should be avoided during pregnancy, but a survey of several other authorities produced no such contraindication. However, some sources point out that since no data has yet proven passionflower to be safe during pregnancy and lactation, its use should, for now, be avoided.

Pau d'arco (*Tabebuia impetiginosa [formerly avellanedae], Tabebuia ipe*)

Pau d'arco has more traditional support than scientific, but this magical herb is pregnant with promise. Like so many amazing South American herbs, pau d'arco goes by many names, including Lapacho, Taheebo and Ipe Roxo.

Pau d'arco has been used for at least a thousand years by the traditional healers of Brazil. Its list of uses is epic: skin diseases, boils, colitis, dysentery, diarrhea, constipation, fever, sore throat, respiratory problems, snake bite, syphilis, wounds, ulcers, arthritis, cystitis, prostatitis, and cancer. Herbalist Michael Tierra says it is also useful for diabetes, anemia, hemorrhage, Parkinson's, arteriosclerosis, and ring worm.

Pau d'arco has wide antibacterial, antiviral, antiparasitic and antifungal properties. It has strong anticandida properties, and is a good herb for other yeast and fungal problems as well. Pau d'arco is effective against herpes types I and II and some strains of flu.

Pau d'arco has a reputation as a cancer-fighting herb and traditionally it was widely used for cancer. Cancer expert Ralph Moss, Ph.D., says that lapachol, one of its major active ingredients, has definite anti-cancer activity. It is probably not, he says, the only ingredient acting in this way. Studies, possibly marred by isolating single active ingredients, and by politics, have been confusing, disappointing and inconclusive. Unfortunately, the major cancer study did not use the whole herb, as traditional South American healers have. As Moss has pointed out, it is probably not a single active ingredient doing the work.

Pau d'arco has also been shown to have anti-inflammatory and immune-stimulating properties. In his book on pau d'arco, Kenneth Jones says that this herb increases the invader-devouring phagocytic action of immune cells by 40%.

The best way to prepare pau d'arco is to bring three cups of water to a boil. Then let it cool down a little and simmer 2 tablespoons of the dried inner bark for twenty minutes. Some say that contact with aluminum and plastic should be avoided. Drink 3–6 cups a day. Some recommend more for serious conditions. Pau d'arco can also be taken as a liquid extract at a dose of 3–7ml a day, and sometimes more for cancer. A similar recommendation of 15–30 drops 2 to 8 times a day is also given. Standardized extracts should be taken at a dose of 1.5–2g of lapachol a day. If you are using an unstandardized powdered herb, take 900mg three times a day.

Pau d'arco is very safe. Moss says that the bark of the yellow flowering pau d'arcos (*Tabebuia umbellata, pedicellata, argentea, aurea*) should be avoided, as should *Tabebuia neochrysantha*. *Tabebuia aurea* is traditionally used to induce abortions, so this variety should be avoided by pregnant women. Accurately identified pau d'arco, sold by reputable companies, is entirely safe and without side effects when used at the proper dose. It is more effective and safer to stick to the whole inner bark instead of isolated active ingredients. There are no reports of toxicity with the whole bark decoction. Pau d'arco is safe for long term use.

Brinker says that pau d'arco should be avoided during pregnancy, but lists this warning as only speculative and based on animal studies. The relevance of animal studies to humans is always questionable. The American Herbal Products Association's *Botanical Safety Handbook* does not include pau d'arco on its list of herbs to be avoided during pregnancy and classifies it as a herb that is safe when used appropriately. Other sources say to use pau d'arco with caution during pregnancy.

Because of its immune-stimulating properties, it is possible that pau d'arco should not be used with immunosuppressive drugs. It is also possible that it should not be used with anticoagulants because at high doses it antagonizes vitamin K-like warfarin. However, it should be noted that Terry Willard, Ph.D., says that there are also several vitamin K-like substances in the whole plant.

Peppermint *(Mentha piperita)*

Peppermint has been in use for a very long time. It gets its name Mintha from Greek mythology: Hades, who loved the nymph Minthe, metamorphosized her into a peppermint plant after the jealous Persephone crushed her. The herb was also used by the ancient Egyptians and later in Iceland.

This is one herb that actually tastes good. This may account for peppermint's being one of the most familiar herbs. However, it is much more than a pleasant-tasting tea: peppermint has many valuable herbal uses. It is one of the best herbs for colic and gas and for the bloating caused by gas. For these problems, it can be used as a tea or, perhaps even stronger, in the form of peppermint oil. It stimulates the production and flow of bile and digestive juices as well. Several double-blind studies have found peppermint to

Seventy-nine percent of people who took the peppermint oil had improvements in abdominal pain and gas.

be a great herb for indigestion. It can also help people with Crohn's and colitis.

Peppermint is an effective herb for irritable bowel syndrome. Again, the tea is good, but the enteric-coated peppermint capsule may be better. Peppermint oil eases the intestinal cramping, reduces gas, and soothes the irritation. It also fights *candida*, an important factor when fighting irritable bowel syndrome.

Several studies have looked at peppermint oil as a remedy for irritable bowel syndrome. Most, though not all, have found it to be effective. One double-blind study found that the herb was significantly better than a placebo. Seventy-nine percent of people who took the peppermint oil had improvements in abdominal pain and gas (*J Gastroenterol* 1997). Peppermint oil has also been shown to benefit older children suffering from irritable bowel syndrome. In a double-blind study of forty-two 8- to 17-year-old children suffering from this condition, enteric-coated peppermint oil, at a dose of 0.1–.2ml three times a day did reduce pain (although it did not help every symptom). On a severity of symptom scale, 76% improved compared with only 19% in the placebo group (*J Pediatr* 2001).

Recently, the *American Journal of Gastroenterology* (1998) published a meta-analysis of five studies on peppermint oil. The three that used enteric-coated peppermint oil were all effective, while neither of the two that used regular capsules were effective. Overall, however, the reduction in symptoms was significantly better than a placebo.

Even though research has suggested that the enteric-coated peppermint oil works better, a 1999 study challenges that conclusion. This double-blind study gave either enteric-coated or nonenteric-coated capsules containing peppermint and caraway oil. Both groups had significant drops in pain intensity, though the frequency of pain improved more in the enteric-coated group. Overall, the improved severity of the illness was similar in both groups with 81% improvement in the enteric-coated group and 82.8% in the other. Both were well tolerated, but the enteric-coated capsule was slightly better tolerated (*Pharmazie* 1999).

Most excitingly, a double-blind study found enteric-coated peppermint and caraway oil to be slightly more effective than the drug cisapride. Improvements in pain intensity and frequency were almost the same in both groups with a slight edge given to the herbs. Pressure, fullness and gas improved more in the herb group. Physicians rated the number of people in the herb group who improved much or very much as 78.6% compared to 70.9% in the drug group (*Arzneim-Forsch Drug Res* 1999). We have found that when you treat the other issues surrounding irritable bowel syndrome, such as food allergy, *candida*, and other parasites and stress, using enteric-coated peppermint oil capsules mixed with other herbs and fibre is very effective.

Peppermint is a wonderful herb for nausea and vomiting. It helps relieve the nausea of pregnancy and motion sickness. It may also help with postoperative nausea (*J Adv Nurs* 1997).

Applied topically, peppermint oil is a good painkiller and is as good as acetaminophen (Tylenol) at relieving tension headaches.

Peppermint oil is antiviral, antibacterial and antifungal, including being powerfully anticandida. It also contains antioxidants. And James Duke, Ph.D., says that peppermint fights the bacteria that causes gingivitis and tooth decay. Herbal authority Rudolf Fritz Weiss, M.D., also endorses peppermint for pancreatic disease.

Peppermint tea is also great for fighting colds, flus and fevers. Its diaphoretic properties encourage sweating, which helps to stimulate the immune system and "burn" the cold right out of you. For this purpose, it is often combined with other diaphoretic herbs like yarrow or elderberry.

As a tea, infuse 2g two to five times a day. Some simply say to make a standard infusion and drink it as often as you want. If you are taking the dried leaf in a pill form, try 3–6 grams a day. As a tincture, take 2–3ml three times a day. The dose for the peppermint oil capsules is 0.2–0.4ml three times a day.

Peppermint is a very safe herb to use. Though Brinker speculates that excessive amounts should be avoided in early pregnancy, all other sources consider it to be perfectly safe to use while pregnant or breast feeding. Peppermint has no drug interactions. It is free of side effects with the exception that the oil may cause a burning sensation in some people.

Peppermint oil should not be applied to the face or used by small children, and it should not be used by people with obstruction of the bile duct, gallbladder inflammation or severe liver damage.

Some sources say not to use peppermint oil if you suffer from chronic heartburn; however, herb expert James Duke, Ph.D., strongly recommends it for this use. He says that Andrew Weil, M.D., agrees, as does traditional use. Similarly, some sources say not to use peppermint oil without consulting a health care practitioner if you have gallstones. However, several authorities, like Michael Murray, N.D., Rudolf Fritz Weiss, Ph.D., James Duke, Ph.D., and others recommend peppermint oil for the treatment of gallstones, and some studies support this recommendation. See the section on artichoke for a fuller discussion of this warning. Brinker speculates that peppermint oil should be avoided by people with hiatus hernias.

Pygeum　　　　　　　　　　　　　　(Pygeum africanum)

Pygeum was originally used in Africa to treat urinary disorders. Today this herb is of special importance to men. It is used to both prevent and to treat benign prostate hyerplasia (BPH), prostatis, urinary tract infections, male infertility, and impotence.

Studies have confirmed pygeum's importance in men's health. When numerous clinical trials were looked at involving over 600 patients with BPH, pygeum was shown to be effective, especially in early cases. In one particular study, 30 patients with BPH were given 100mg of pygeum for 75 days. The patients showed significant improvement on objective parameters, such as increased urine flow rate and a drop in leftover urine volume (*Rev Bras Med* 1984). When a review of eighteen studies – including 1,562 men – on pygeum and BPH was undertaken, the herb was shown to bring about a significant improvement. Men taking pygeum were more than twice as likely to report improvement in their overall symptoms (*Am J Med* 2000).

In cases of infertility, pygeum may improve those whose infertility originates from reduced prostatic secretions. Pygeum has been shown to increase prostatic secretions and improve seminal fluid (*Urol Int* 1984; *Arch Int Urol* 1988; *Ann Urol* 1986). Among men with BPH or prostatitis, pygeum can improve the ability to achieve an erection (*Arch Ital Urol Nefrol Androl* 1991).

The dosage of a lipophilic extract of pygeum should be standardized to contain 14% triterpene, including beta-sitosterol and 0.5 percent n-docosanol, and taken at 100–200mg per day in divided dosages; 100mg can be taken in one dose. You can also take a standard decoction and drink three cups a day. Pygeum is often found mixed with other herbs like saw palmetto and stinging nettle for men's prostate health.

Pygeum is very safe. There are almost never any side effects, except for the very occasional and mild gastrointestinal upset. There are no drug interactions. We were unable to find any information on pregnancy and breast feeding (but that's not a problem, as enlarged prostates are not generally a problem for women).

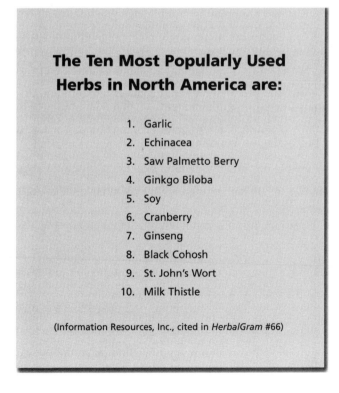

The Ten Most Popularly Used Herbs in North America are:

1. Garlic
2. Echinacea
3. Saw Palmetto Berry
4. Ginkgo Biloba
5. Soy
6. Cranberry
7. Ginseng
8. Black Cohosh
9. St. John's Wort
10. Milk Thistle

(Information Resources, Inc., cited in *HerbalGram* #66)

Raspberry leaf ⟨Rubus idaeus⟩

When most people think of raspberry, they think of a delicious fruit; yet raspberry has a lot more to offer. It is the leaves of this common plant that are most used in herbalism to treat various problems, especially disorders of a female nature.

Raspberry is used in pregnancy to help prevent miscarriage, and is often combined with other herbs for this purpose. It is also used to ease delivery, to tone the entire female system, to stop postpartum bleeding, heavy or frequent bleeding, and to aid in postpartum problems. Many women report that, if they consume raspberry leaf tea throughout the pregnancy or in the last three months, their labour is virtually pain free. Raspberry is also used for other female concerns, like menstrual irregularities, to bring on ovulation, to encourage breast milk, and for leucorrhea. It seems that raspberry works by toning and relaxing the uterus.

Raspberry can also be used for fevers, to treat children's and adults' thrush, and to cleanse the system. It will remove canker from the mucous membrane and can be used as a gargle for sore throat and mouth. It can also be used for diarrhea, dysentery and nausea.

Various species of raspberry have also shown antifungal activity and antiviral activity against a wide variety of viruses. Raspberry has also been found to be a diuretic, have blood sugar controlling properties, and to stimulate immunity.

And before men skip this page, herbalist Rosemary Gladstar says that raspberry leaf's best kept secret is that it has the same nourishing reproductive tonic effect on men as it does on women.

 Raspberry leaf makes a very pleasant-tasting cup of tea. Infuse 1–2 teaspoons (5–10g) in a cup of water and drink it freely. For pregnancy, drink two to three cups a day, and even more, if needed, during labour. As a tincture, take 2–4ml three times a day.

Raspberry leaf is very safe. There are no risks or side effects and it is, of course, safe to use during pregnancy and breast feeding. Although no other sources we could find list any drug interactions, one reliable source says that the tannins in raspberry leaf could interfere with the absorption of atropine, codeine, ephedrine / pseudoephedrine, theophylline / aminophylline. It also lists Cardec DM and Lotil / Lonox, presumably for the same reason.

Red clover   (*Trifolium pratense*)

That beautiful pink weed growing in your yard may be more valuable than you think. It may really be a lucky clover. Red clover has a colourful history in herbalism. And recently that pretty little weed is enjoying a blossoming of scientific research too.

Red clover has a long history of use as an alterative and expectorant. Canadian herbalist Terry Willard says that red clover is one of the strongest alteratives known. Alteratives, also known as blood purifiers, gently improve body function by aiding detoxification, elimination and digestion. Because of this, he recommends red clover as part of an arthritis formula.

Alteratives are also good for skin diseases, and red clover has a long history as a skin herb. In fact, herbalist Rosemary Gladstar recommends using red clover for all skin conditions. Herbalist Michael Tierra specifically names it for acne, psoriasis and eczema, and another herbalist, David Hoffmann, argues that red clover is one of the best herbs for children with these skin problems.

Red clover has also been traditionally used for respiratory conditions. According to Gladstar, it is one of the best respiratory tonics. Red clover is an expectorant and antispasmodic, making it very useful for coughs, colds, asthma, whooping cough, bronchitis and tuberculosis.

Though there are no studies on red clover and cancer, there is a history of use here too. In fact, red clover is one of the ingredients in the famous Hoxsey cancer formula. In his book on cancer, John Boik points out that red clover does contain the isoflavone genestein and reminds us that genestein is a promising anticancer agent. Old time herbalists used red clover topically for breast cancer and reported success.

Red clover is also used for detoxification and canker sores and it may help relieve menstrual cramping. It is rich in calcium and iron and has mild blood thinning properties. Red clover may also raise the good HDL cholesterol levels.

Recently, red clover has shown some promise for menopause.

Red clover contains isoflavones not unlike the anticancer, phytoestrogenic isoflavones found in soy. Strangely, unlike soy, early research was unable to find any real benefit to red clover for hot flashes. Recently, though, the trend has changed, and research on red clover has begun to find all kinds of benefits for women's health.

When thirty women were given 80mg of red clover isoflavones for three months in a double-blind study, the frequency of their hot flashes went down by 44%, while the frequency in the placebo group was unchanged (*Maturitas* 2002). However, a recent study has again questioned clover by showing mixed results. Although this study found no significant difference between red clover and a placebo at reducing the number of hot flashes, it did find that the red clover reduced the number of hot flashes faster than the placebo (*JAMA* 2003).

Red clover may help women who suffer breast pain prior to their periods. This cyclical breast pain is called cyclic mastalgia. In a small study, eighteen women suffering from cyclic mastalgia were given either 40mg or 80mg of isoflavones from red clover or a placebo for three months. Pain was improved in the placebo group by 13%, but it improved in the 40mg isoflavone group by 44% and the 80mg group by 31%. The improvement in the 40mg group was statistically significant (*The Breast* 2001).

There may be yet another benefit for women. One of the things that happens with age and menopause is that arteries begin to lose elasticity, which increases the risk of heart disease. When seventeen women were given either isoflavones from red clover or a placebo in a double-blind study (*J Clin Endocrinol Metab* 1999), elasticity improved by a significant 28% more in the red clover group, showing that red clover may not only help hot flashes, but one of the important cardiovascular risk factors that comes with menopause: good news in the wake of the recent HRT disaster.

You can take red clover as a tea by infusing 2-3 teaspoons of the dried herb and drinking it three times a day. If you are using the tincture, take 2-4ml three times a day. As a pill, take 2-4 grams a day. If the pill you are using is standardized for 40mg of isoflavones, take 1-2 a day.

 Red clover is a very safe herb with no side effects. However, it should not be used by women who are pregnant or breast feeding. It should also not be used if you are taking estrogen.

It is often said that people with blood clotting disorders or who are on blood thinning drugs should not use red clover because of the blood thinning properties of the coumarin found in this herb. But, according to Brinker, this warning is based on a myth: the coumarin in red clover has no blood thinning properties.

Red yeast rice
(Monascus purpureus)

This unusual cholesterol fighter is made by fermenting rice with red yeast and then killing off the yeast. It has been a traditional food and medicine in China for centuries, where it is used to promote blood circulation. Like the cholesterol drug lovastatin, red yeast rice blocks the production of cholesterol by inhibiting the action of an enzyme known as HMG-CoA reductase.

The many studies on red yeast rice have been impressive. In one, it lowered total cholesterol by 23%, LDL cholesterol by 31%, and triglycerides by 34%, while raising the beneficial HDL cholesterol by 20% (*Curr Ther Res* 1997). In another study, it lowered cholesterol by 26% compared to 7% by the placebo, LDL by 33% compared to 8% by the placebo, and triglycerides by 20% compared to 2% by the placebo (*Am J Clin Nutr* 1999).

There are probably a number of things in this nutrient that are working to improve cholesterol because the amount of HMG-CoA reductase inhibitors in it is not sufficient to explain its anticholesterol power.

 The studies have used 1.2–2.4mg. You might try 2.4mg a day in divided doses.

Red yeast rice is very safe. No serious side effects have been reported. Until more is known about how this supplement works, it may be best to avoid it if you have liver or kidney disease since, in part, it acts like lovastatin: however, unlike lovastatin, no harm to the liver or kidneys has been found in the studies. Again, until more is known, you should follow the same drug-related contraindications as for lovastatin. Its safety during pregnancy and breast feeding is not yet established, so, for now, red yeast rice should probably not be used. Since HMG-CoA inhibitors also inhibit the important nutrient Coenzyme Q-10, you should supplement CoQ10 while using red yeast rice just in case it has this effect too.

Reishi mushroom *(Ganoderma lucidum)*

Reishi mushroom is also called *ling zhi*, which means "spirit plant." Other Chinese names for this plant include plant of immortality, ten thousand year mushroom, and the herb of spiritual potency – all names that speak of its great value. This beautiful mushroom has been prized in traditional Chinese and Japanese medicine for four thousand years. It was considered a herb of the first rank and perhaps even, according to Terry Willard, Ph.D., the most valued herb of all. Considered an elixir of life, this overall tonic was believed to increase longevity and to treat a large number of conditions. Reishi was especially used for hepatitis, nephritis, arthritis, high blood pressure, asthma, bronchitis, ulcers, and insomnia.

Like the other mushrooms, shiitake and maitake, reishi mushroom is a great herb for the immune system. It has antioxidant, antibacterial, antiviral and anti-tumour properties. Reishi is a valuable herb for chronic fatigue immune dysfunction syndrome (CFIDS or CFS) and AIDS. It is also an exciting herb for cancer. It seems to fight cancer in a number of ways, including boosting the immune system, possessing anti-tumour properties, and encouraging cell differentiation.

Reishi is also a good herb for the heart. Reishi fights heart disease in many ways, including lowering cholesterol and blood pressure, preventing blood clots, dilating the arteries, and improving blood flow to the heart. It is also a good herb for arrhythmias and eases the chest pain of angina. It has been shown to be very helpful for people with heart attacks or angina (*J Tradit Chin Med* 1982). In one interesting study, people with high blood pressure who did not respond to ACE inhibitors had either reishi or a placebo added to the drug. Blood pressure fell significantly in the reishi group compared to the placebo group.

Respiratory illnesses also succumb to reishi. Numerous studies have found this mushroom to be very effective in bronchitis, asthma and sinus problems. For example, in 1970, over 2,000 patients with bronchitis were given reishi. In only two weeks, 60 to 90% of the patients were better or improved, especially the elderly patients and those with bronchial asthma (Chang and But, 1986). It is also good for allergies and has been used for pneumonia.

Reishi is also good for ulcers and has liver protecting and detoxifying properties; it has been shown to help hepatitis. A clinical report form China (Lui, 1994), shows that when reishi was given to 70,000 patients with hepatitis, 90% were cured. It is also a kidney tonic and may help moderate blood sugar levels.

This mysterious mushroom also seems to have profound psychological effects. It seems to have the remarkable ability to calm the nerves while revitalizing them at the same time. It is good for insomnia, anxiety and nervous conditions. Willard even says it is good for paranoia. Reishi has been used for the symptom cluster of fatigue, irritability, headache, dizziness, sleep disturbance, muscle ache, anxiety, and intolerance of loud noise known as neurasthenia. Herbalist Christopher Hobbs, who has written extensively on medicinal mushrooms, says that in his experience, reishi is an effective calming herb for people with nervousness, anxiety and sleeplessness who have weak adrenals or neurasthenia.

One more unexpected use of reishi: it is an excellent herb for altitude sickness, helping climbers in one study at heights up to 5,000 metres.

Reishi mushroom is also called ling zhi, which means 'spirit plant.' Other Chinese names for this plant include plant of immortality, ten thousand year mushroom, and the herb of spiritual potency – all names that speak of its great value ...

Considered an elixir of life, this overall tonic was believed to increase longevity ...

An active ingredient in reishi, called the triterpenes, has been found to have anti-allergy effects while other compounds of reishi have also demonstrated anti-allergy properties. Reishi seems to have the ability to stop the release of histamine, thereby stopping allergy reactions before they start. Reishi can even be used as an antidote for poisonous mushrooms and as a lotion to protect against the sun's harmful UV rays. There are six types of reishi – blue, red, yellow, white, black and purple – and all of them offer unique benefits to human health.

Like so many of the traditional herbs, the long list of powers is not merely the stuff of myth, but of a tradition that is now being proven by science.

As a decoction, drink three cups of reishi a day. As a pill, take 3g three times a day. As a tincture, one authoritative source says to take 10ml three times a day, while another herbalist gives the much smaller dose of 40 drops (about 2ml) three times a day.

Like all of the mushrooms, reishi is very safe. There are no serious side effects and it is safe to use while pregnant or breast feeding. Reishi is not contraindicated for anyone except, possibly, those on immune-suppressing drugs because of organ transplants, since it can enhance immunity: though this warning is only speculative. There may be some drug interactions. Because of its calming effect, reishi may increase the sedative effects of reserpine and chlorpromazine, increase the sleeping time brought about by barbitol and pentobarbitol, and inhibit stimulation by amphetamines. It is possible that it could strengthen anticoagulants and cholesterol drugs because of its own antiplatelet and anticholesterol activity.

Rhodiola rosea
(Rhodiola rosea)

Rhodiola rosea is a herb you've probably never seen in a herb book before. Though it has a long tradition of use in Russia, Scandinavia and Asia and has been extensively studied, it still remains virtually unknown in North America and Europe. Rhodiola is beginning to creep onto the shelves of health food stores, however, and perhaps soon this surprising herb will get the attention it deserves.

Like ginseng, Rhodiola rosea is an adaptogenic herb: a herb that is extremely safe, that increases resistance to a wide range of things that stress the body, and that balances the body whether the system needs bringing up or bringing down.

Rhodiola rosea improves mood, energy and mental clarity. It is used to combat fatigue and stress, both mental and physical, and has the amazing ability to increase mental and physical energy while calming you at the same time.

Rhodiola rosea seems to be able to increase learning, thinking and memory. Several studies have shown its ability to improve fatigue, weakness, work capacity, distractedness, insomnia, poor appetite, irritability, and headache. In one study, when people started taking the herb several days before beginning intense intellectual work, they improved the amount and quality of their work and suffered less fatigue. In a double-blind study comparing Rhodiola rosea to a placebo during final exams, students on Rhodiola had significantly improved final grades, mental fatigue, and general well-being (*Phytomed* 2000).

In another study, Rhodiola rosea showed its ability to help both the mental and the physical. In this study, the herb not only decreased mental fatigue and anxiety, but also increased work capacity, coordination, and general well-being (*Eksp Klin Farmakol* 2000).

A number of studies have shown Rhodiola rosea's power to increase physical work capacity, confirming its claim as an effective herb for mental and physical performance. In one study, Rhodiola was compared to eleuthero (formerly known as Siberian ginseng) and a stimulating drug. While eleuthero and the drug both increased work capacity by 6% compared to the placebo, the Rhodiola rosea topped them both with a 9% increase. Those on Rhodiola also had shorter recovery time. When athletes were given Rhodiola rosea before ski races and biathlons, their shooting accuracy, coordination, strength, endurance, and recovery time all improved.

Rhodiola rosea is also a strong antioxidant herb and may have anti-cancer properties. It is able to increase the effect of some anti-cancer drugs while decreasing their toxicity.

This versatile herb may also have sexual and reproductive benefits for both men and women. In one study, when thirty-five men who suffered from either erectile dysfunction, premature ejaculation or both were given 150–200mg of Rhodiola rosea for three months, twenty-six of them responded. And when forty women who suffered from amenorrhoea (the absence of periods) were given Rhodiola, twenty-five of them had their normal cycle restored, and eleven of them became pregnant.

Rhodiola also helps depression and helps protect the heart.

The dosage of Rhodiola rosea is based on its rosavin content: 3.6–6.14mg of rosavin seems to be a good amount. You can take 300–600mg of Rhodiola rosea standardized for 1% rosavin, 180–300mg standardized for 2% rosavin, or 100–170mg standardized for 3.6%. Rhodiola should be taken on an empty stomach, half an hour before breakfast and lunch.

Rhodiola rosea is a very safe herb. There are no side effects. If it overly activates or causes agitation, lower the dose and then increase it gradually. Rhodiola should not be used by people with bipolar disorder, since its antidepressant effect could trigger mania. There are no drug interactions with this herb, although it could have additive effects with other stimulants. Rhodiola's safety during pregnancy and breast feeding is unknown.

Rhubarb   (Rheum palmatum)

This plant is not just for pies and tarts; rhubarb is used for constipation, worms, dysentery, diarrhea, dysmenorrhoea, and amenorrhoea.

In large doses, it is used for constipation and is often combined with ginger, or anise, or peppermint and licorice to prevent cramping pains. Rhubarb is effective as a laxative because it first clears the bowels, then it checks them through its astringent properties to help stop diarrhea. It is often combined with other anthelmintic herbs to clear out intestinal worms. For diarrhea, take smaller dosages of rhubarb powder, in water, three times a day. It is often roasted or boiled for this purpose, which helps to take away its purgative properties and primarily leave its astringent properties. In one double-blind study, 90% of people who had upper digestive tract bleeding were cured when they used an alcohol tincture of rhubarb. In smaller dosages, rhubarb aids the digestion, toning the stomach and small intestines. When it is chewed, it encourages salivation.

Since rhubarb promotes blood circulation to the pelvic cavity, it is used for dysmenorrhoea and amenorrhoea. It also has antibiotic properties. Rhubarb is a strong alterative and it is often used in formulae to rid the body of toxic matter. Some species of rhubarb are part of a formula for cleansing, called Essiac, that is used in cancer therapies.

In pill form, the dose of rhubarb is 1–5g of the root a day. The same amount, which equals approximately 1/4–1 teaspoon (1–5g), can be used as a decoction: some say once a day and some say morning and night. Don't be surprised if traditional Chinese herbalists recommend much higher doses: up to 12g a day. You can also use a tincture at a dose of 1–2ml three times a day.

Rhubarb should not be used while you are pregnant or breast feeding. It should also not be given to children under twelve. If you have an inflammatory condition of the intestines, such as irritable bowel syndrome, Crohn's, colitis or appendicitis, or if you suffer from intestinal obstruction or abdominal pain of unknown origin, you should not use this herb. Avoid it with hemorrhoids and be careful if you have a history of kidney stones.

Overuse of rhubarb can cause potassium loss because of its laxative effect, which can increase the toxicity of cardiac glycosides. Limit use of this laxative herb to eight to ten days. If you are on diuretics or corticosteroids, rhubarb can enhance the potassium loss caused by these drugs. The laxative effect may also reduce the absorption of oral drugs, though this is only speculative. Rhubarb can improve the ACE inhibitor captopril in reducing the progression of chronic kidney failure (*Chin Med* 1996).

Rooibos *(Aspalathus linearis)*

Rooibos is a herb that is gaining in popularity every year. It was originally collected on South Africa's west cape by indigenous people. Since then, it has been grown in many other countries and is being exported all over the world. Why is this herb so popular? Because it makes a pleasant tasting non-bitter tea containing a number of different kinds of antioxidants, which have been shown in test tubes and in preliminary live animal studies to help protect against heart disease, cancer, stroke, and age-related brain oxidation. This does not mean they will work the same way in humans and, in our opinion, testing on animals is unethical. To see if these claims are accurate, further ethical research on humans needs to be done.

Traditionally, rooibos has been used for infant colic and is still used by physicians in South Africa for this purpose. Other unsupported but traditional claims for rooibos include help with digestive upset for adults, as a sleep aid, and for allergies, diaper rash, and eczema.

Rooibos is said to be high in many other nutrients. But so far the only nutrients that it seems to have a significant amount of are copper and fluoride. Some athletes, however, use rooibos to replace lost fluid throughout the day and find that it does provide measurable amounts of several minerals and electrolytes (*HerbalGram* #59). Rooibos does not have caffeine, and this makes it an attractive drink to many people who do not want caffeine's negative effects. It is also low in tannins, which can interfere with the absorption of iron.

In general, unfermented rooibos seems to have higher amounts of polyphenol antioxidants than fermented rooibos, and it seems to demonstrate higher antioxidant and antimutagenic abilities in the preliminary tests that have been done.

 Very few sources list this herb yet, so information on dosage and safety is scarce. Try infusing 1–4 teaspoons (5–20g) in a cup of water three times a day.

 Rooibos is very safe and is free of side effects. There are no contraindications or drug interactions. Although rooibos is considered safe to use in infants, because it has not been studied in humans, there is no information available on its safety during pregnancy and breast feeding.

Rosemary (*Rosmarinus officinalis*)

Usually used as a cooking herb, rosemary has a lot to offer for health. A cup of rosemary tea is as effective in relieving a headache as an aspirin. In India, it is even used for migraine headaches. Rosemary is also a tonic and stimulant that is said to be good for memory, and was used by the ancient Greeks and Chinese for this purpose. In *Hamlet*, Shakespeare has Ophelia say, "There's rosemary, that's for remembrance" (4.5.174-175). And James Duke, Ph.D., says that it just might be true, even in Alzheimer's cases. Rosemary is loaded in antioxidants and it has several compounds in it that prevent acetylcholine from breaking down. Acetylcholine is the neurotransmitter whose deficiency is linked to Alzheimer's.

Rosemary is also useful for nervousness. This herb has benefits not only *in* the head, but *on* the head as well, where it is said to strengthen and stimulate hair and to be beneficial for premature balding when used as a cold tea rinse or essential oil.

A cup of rosemary tea is as effective in relieving a headache as an aspirin.

Rosemary also has value as a cardiovascular herb. It has been used to help circulation, to lower blood pressure, and to decrease capillary permeability and fragility.

Rosemary is a carminative and is excellent for the stomach and intestines, where it soothes spasms, flatulence and digestive upset, making it ideal for those who suffer from irritable bowel syndrome. It is also active against *candida*.

This valuable herb is also used for rheumatism, for hepatic and bilary problems, for wound healing, and as an antiseptic.

You can take rosemary as a pill at a dose of 4–6g a day. You can drink rosemary as a tea by infusing 1–2 teaspoons (5–10g) of the dried herb per cup and drinking it three or more times a day. Or drink a cup for a headache instead of taking an aspirin. As a tincture, no one seems to agree on the dose. Herbalist David Hoffmann says 1–2ml three times a day. Other reliable sources say 2–5ml three times a day. And the *German Commission E* says 10ml three times a day. *Commission E* gives an extract dose of 2ml three times a day.

Rosemary is very safe. There are no side effects. It is interesting to note that every modern text on herbs we consulted, including the authoritative contraindication texts, said not to take rosemary during pregnancy, but not one traditional women's herbal we consulted agreed. It's probably best to play it safe. It is okay, though, to use rosemary while you are breast feeding. There are no other contraindications for this herb. With the exception of one warning that an alcoholic extract of rosemary could interact with the chemotherapy drugs doxorubicin and vinblastine (*Eur J Canc* 1999), there are no other drug interactions for rosemary.

What Are The Best Herbs To Take When Travelling Or To Keep Around As Part Of A Herbal Medicine Kit?

Although this will largely depend on where you are and what problems you are likely to face, a good kit will contain enough possible herbs to cover a wide variety of problems.

For example:

- echinacea for immunity and infections
- ginger for nausea and digestion
- goldenseal root for immunity, infections and traveller's diarrhea
- garlic for infection of all sorts and immunity
- slippery elm for digestion and sore throat
- tea tree oil as a topical antiseptic
- bromelain for inflammation and pain
- white willow bark for pain
- valerian for sleep, anxiety and as an antispasmodic
- wormwood for parasites.

Sage   *(Salvia officinalis)*

Sage has quite a reputation. In ancient times, sage was renowned for promoting longevity. It was even used in the Middle Ages in tonics to promote longevity. In the seventeenth century, according to the Weiners, the writer John Evelyn claimed that sage could make a man immortal.

Sage is renowned for its antispasmodic, astringent, carminative, and antiseptic properties. It is especially useful as an astringent for slowing down or drying up fluids. This makes it a great herb for excessive perspiration, night sweats and hot flashes, menopausal hot flashes, excessive menstrual bleeding, vaginal discharge, unwanted breast milk, diarrhea, and dysentery.

Traditionally, sage has also been used as a gargle for sore throats and cough. It is antibacterial and antiviral. Herbalist David Hoffmann calls sage a classic herb for inflammation of the mouth, throat and tonsil. It can be used internally and as a mouthwash or gargle for laryngitis, tonsillitis, mouth ulcers, and inflamed and bleeding gums.

Sage is also a very good herb for indigestion and upper respiratory infections, and herbalist Michael Tierra uses sage in combination with rosemary, peppermint and wood betony for headaches. Research has found sage to be antifungal, including against *candida*.

As the name suggests, sage has been used for at least two thousand years for improving memory. Recently, in a small but exciting study, its ancient reputation got put to the modern, scientific test. Thirty people in the clutches of mild to moderate Alzheimer's disease were given either sixty drops per day of sage extract or a placebo for four months. The ones on the sage improved significantly. The Alzheimer's scores increased by 22% in the placebo group, but went down 26% in the sage group (*Journal of Clinical Pharmacy and Therapeutics* 2003). James Duke, Ph.D., says that research has shown that sage can prevent the breakdown of acetylcholine, the neurotransmitter whose deficiency is linked to Alzheimer's.

Some believe sage possesses tranquilizing properties.

Sage is ... a great herb for excessive perspiration, night sweats and hot flashes.

Take 1–3 grams of the herb three times a day. As a tea, drink an infu-sion of sage three times a day or gargle it several times daily.

Sage should not be used during pregnancy and, since it dries up unwanted breast milk, it should not be used where breast feeding is desired. The contraindication for pregnancy may only apply to the alcohol extract, but the traditional wisdom and caution say to avoid it altogether; there are always alternative herbs. The alcohol extract is also contraindicated for long term use. There are no known drug interactions.

St. John's wort   (*Hypericum perforatum*)

St. John's wort is one of the most incredible herbs, and its story is equal-ly as impressive: full of soaring success, fame and controversy.

The story of St. John's wort begins in the early days – before the spectacular arrival of Prozac. The leading antidepressant drugs back then were the tricyclics, such as imipramine and amitriptyline. And the lead-ing antidepressant herb was St. John's wort. So the question is, which one was better, the herb or the drug? And the answer was, consistently, the herb. In one early double-blind study, 900mg of St. John's wort lowered depression by 56% compared to 45% by 75mg of the tricyclic antide-pressant imipramine. The herb's advantage was not only how well it worked, but that it worked so well with fewer and less severe side effects (*J Geriatr Psychiatry Neurol* 1994).

Several years later, St. John's wort was asked to prove itself against a higher dose of imipramine. But there was a wrinkle. Though the drug was allowed to perform at full dose, the herb was to perform at just over half its usual dose. This massive double-blind study matched only 500mg of St. John's wort against 150mg of imipramine in 324 mildly to moder-ately depressed people for six weeks. But the handicap didn't matter. The low dose of St. John's wort was just as good as the full dose of the drug. Levels of depression on the Hamilton Depression Scale dropped from 22.4 to 12 on the herb and from 22.1 to 12.75 on the drug.

Interestingly, anxiety scores were significantly better for St. John's wort. And again, St. John's wort was significantly safer. Thirty-nine percent of the herb group had side effects compared to a whopping 63% of the drug group. And while 16% of the drug group withdrew from the study, only 3% of the herb group did. So impressive was St. John's wort's performance, the researchers concluded that it should be considered for first-line treatment in mild to moderate depression (*BMJ* 2000).

These studies are typical of the herb's success. When twenty-three studies on 1,757 people with mild to moderate depression were put together, the herb was shown to be significantly better than a placebo and just as effective as drugs. In fact, when St. John's wort went up against the tricyclic drugs, it was successful even more often: 63.9% of the time versus 58.5% (Linde *et al*, 1996).

Recently, researchers again pooled the studies to compare overall evidence for the herb. This time they looked at thirty-four double-blind studies which included 3,000 people. The herb was consistently better than placebos and as good or better than drugs. And once again, the nod went to St. John's wort not only because of its success, but also because of its safety. The herb produces side effects in only 1-3% of people, compared to 20-50% on the drugs (*Phytomedicine* 2002).

The success of St. John's wort was spectacular. With the arrival of Prozac, though, a new challenger emerged. How would the herb fare against this best-selling star of the new class of antidepressant, the selective serotonin reuptake inhibitors (SSRI's).

The world champion, both in terms of fame and sales, is Prozac. And in 1999, St. John's wort went head to head with it for the first time (*Arzneim-Forsch Drug Res*). The study was double-blinded, lasted six weeks and included 149 people with mild to moderate depression. The dose of St. John's wort was smaller than the one usually given in the many previous trials: only 800mg. Still, according to the Hamilton Depression Scale, there was virtually no difference between the two treatments: 72.2% of the Prozac group responded and 71.4% of the St. John's wort group did.

The rematch between the herbal and the pharmaceutical champions came one year later (*International Clin Psychopharmacol* 2000). And this time they again threw in the now familiar wrinkle. St. John's wort was asked to perform at only 500mg: a far cry from its usual 900mg. But the big surprise was that, according to the Hamilton Depression Scale, the herb still matched Prozac. In fact, there was a slight advantage to the St.

John's wort, and significantly more people responded to it than to Prozac. What makes these results more impressive still is that the safety of St. John's wort was far better: a full 72% of the side effects reported in the study were in the Prozac group, and those side effects were much more serious than the ones that occurred in the St. John's wort group.

The authors concluded that for mild to moderate depression, the two are equal and that there is no advantage to Prozac. In fact, they went farther and concluded that for mild to moderate depression, based on efficacy and safety, St. John's wort should be regarded as a first treatment option, especially when the other choice is Prozac.

The SSRI class of antidepressant drugs have continued to challenge St. John's wort, but the herb has always responded to the challenge. A 2000 study compared St. John's wort to Prozac's popular cousin, Zoloft. Thirty people with mild to moderate depression participated in this double-blind study. The dose of the herb was the usual 900mg. And, once again, St. John's wort worked just as well as the drug (*Clinical Therapeutics*).

Prozac made another challenge in 2002 (*J Adv Ther*) and helped 58% versus St. John's wort's 50%. Doctor and patient ratings produced no difference in effectiveness. And again, recently(2002) St. John's wort met the SSRI challenge: in a double-blind study, the herb decreased depression by 50.2% compared to 41.6% by Zoloft. As usual, there were significantly more adverse effects in the drug group (*Canadian Family Physician* 2002).

In recent studies, St. John's wort brought about more improvement in more people than the SSRI Paxil while being safer (*British Medical Journal On Line Edition* 2005); and it also helped people with major depression significantly better than Prozac (*J Clin Psychopharmacol* 2005).

So the question of how the herb would match the new drugs was answered. The same as the old drugs: as good or better and significantly safer. The next question was how the herb would fare against severe depression. The answer here has been clouded with controversy.

In the first study, people with severe depression had similar improvement when they were given either imipramine or St. John's wort (*Pharmacopsychiatry* 1977). Then the controversy hit. The *Journal of the American Medical Association* (2001) published a study concluding that St. John's wort was ineffective in treating major depression. The study's lead author said that based on his findings, he would not recommend St. John's wort to any of his patients.

How could he possibly arrive at such a conclusion? The study showed only that the herb was ineffective against severe depression. Dozens of studies have shown it to be effective against mild to moderate depression. And whether we can even conclude from this study that St. John's wort is useless against severe depression is questionable.

The earlier study arrived at a very different result: it found St. John's wort to be as effective as drugs in the treatment of severe depression.

One difference between the two studies was the dose. The positive study used 1,800mg. So perhaps you simply need a higher dose for severe depression.

Also, significantly more people did respond to the St. John's wort than to the placebo – 27% versus 18.6%. The 27% is admittedly extremely disappointing, but the placebo was even more so. Usually in depression studies, the placebo works in 30-50% of people. This low placebo response suggests that something in the design of the study doomed the treatment to fail.

Expert Jerry Cott, Ph.D said in *HerbalGram* that there was a fundamental flaw in the study. The people's depression was so chronic and severe they did not respond to the placebo or to the herb because they were unlikely to have responded to any antidepressant.

The attack continued, though, with the reporting of a study in which St. John's wort did not help people with depression. The reports stated simply that St. John's wort doesn't work. But this study (*Journal of the American Medical Association* 2002) comparing the herb to, not only a placebo, but also to the antidepressant drug Zoloft, also found that the drug didn't work. Zoloft was included in the study because we know it works. Therefore, if the drug didn't work it's because the study didn't work. So, according to Jerry Cott, who was actually involved in the study's design, it's not St. John's wort that didn't work, it's the study that didn't work.

St. John's wort has uses beyond depression. It is used for wounds, ulcers and bites. The oil can be applied to burns. St. John's wort cream helps treat eczema(*Phytomedicine* 2003). St. John's wort also has antiviral and antibacterial properties and shows some early promise for cancer.

Recent studies have also suggested exciting new uses. St. John's wort also helps with childhood depression (*J Am Acad Child Adolesc Psychiatry* 2003), seasonal affective disorder (*J Geriatr Psychiatry Neurol* 1994, *Pharmacopsych* 1997, *Curr Med Res Opin* 1999), and perhaps even obsessive compulsive disorder (*Journal of Clinical Psychiatry* 2000). It improves the quality of deep sleep and helps people with hypersomnia who cannot stop sleeping. It also helps with anxiety.

And St. John's wort might be a valuable menopause herb as well. It eases menopausal symptoms in 76%-79% of women. It especially helps sweating and irritability. St. John's wort also helps menopausal women maintain satisfactory sex. Eighty-six percent of women will experience reduced libido during menopause. But in the study, 80% of women said their sexuality had been "substantially enhanced" by the herb (*Advances in Therapy* 1999).

Clinically, we have also seen St. John's wort improve men's interest in sex when depression is a factor.

St. John's wort is usually taken as an extract standardized for 0.3% hypericin. Though recent research has shown that hypericin is not the primary active ingredient, pointing instead to hyperforin, hypericin is still a good marker for a quality extract, and supplements are still usually standardized for 0.3%. The dose is 300mg three times daily. Some St. John's wort supplements are now standardized to 5% hyperforin as well. As a tea, St. John's wort may be taken as an infusion of 1-2 teaspoons of dried herb per cup of water, consumed three times daily. As a tincture, take 2-4ml three times a day, and as a fluid extract take 2ml twice a day. As a dried herb, take 2-5g a day. The successful study on severe depression doubled the usual dose and gave 600mg of standardized extract three times daily.

One of the interesting things that has emerged from recent studies is the effectiveness of the herb at much smaller doses than the 900mg always recommended. Remember, St. John's wort out dueled both imipramine and Prozac at only 500mg, suggesting that smaller doses may be just as effective against mild to moderate depression.

Aside from how well it works, St. John's wort has earned its place as the antidepressant of choice because it works safely. A review of 3,250 people on St. John's wort found side effects in only 2.43%. It also found no sedative effect or interaction with alcohol (Harrer *et al*, 1994; Woelk *et al* 1994). In Germany, in 3.8 million people using St. John's wort between 1991 and 1996, only thirty-two side effects were reported (Hippius 1998). In the U.K., no side effects had been reported to 1998. These figures are amazingly low. St. John's wort produces even fewer side effects in real life than it does in the studies, probably because in the studies, people think they are on a medication and expect side effects: a sort of inside-out placebo effect known as the *nocebo* effect! Perhaps the most telling statistic of all, though, was one produced by a 1999 study that compared the safety of St. John's wort with drugs from every major class of antidepressant. In placebo-controlled studies only 4.1% of people on the herb had side effects, while 19.8% experienced side effects on the drugs (Stevenson *et al*).

You often see articles claiming that St. John's wort can cause photosensitivity, an increased sensitivity of the skin to the sun. In the doses that a person would actually use, this warning is unnecessary. In order to experience severe photosensitivity, you would have to take thirty to fifty times the recommended dose (Ersnt *et al*, 1998).

There are no contraindications for St. John's wort. Though Brinker cautions against using it while pregnant, other major works on contraindications do not contraindicate it for pregnancy or breast feeding. There is very little data existing which suggests that use during pregnancy is a problem.

There has been one concern raised, though.

Some research has shown that St. John's wort may stimulate a detoxification system in the liver known as cytochrome P450. Cytochrome P450 detoxifies and breaks down a number of drugs. St. John's wort may also stimulate another system known as P-glycoprotein. Stimulating liver detoxification is a good thing, but it could become problematic if it reduces the amount of prescription drugs in the blood that a patient is relying on. Though not all studies have found that St. John's wort does stimulate this system – at least two found that it does not – the scale is tipping the other way, and the evidence is mounting that it does stimulate this system and could reduce levels of certain drugs in the blood. The evidence is strong for HIV protease inhibitor drugs like indinavir and for cyclosporine, an immune system suppressing drug used for organ transplants. There is also evidence for the immune suppressing drug tacrolimus and the anticancer drug imatinib (Gleevec). If you are on one of these drugs, you should not use St. John's wort. Other drugs that are broken down by cytochrome P450 and could also be a concern include calcium channel blockers, the birth control pill, cortisone, digoxin, warfarin and other anticoagulants, simvastatin, chlorzoxazone and benzodiazepenes.

Though this information is important, there may be a need to put it in perspective. Though the evidence is solid for cyclosporine, indinavir, tacrolimus and imatinib, the clinical relevance of this information for the other drugs has not yet been established. There is little clinical evidence of significant weakening of digoxin. Recent research shows that the asthma medication theophylline is not affected by St. John's wort despite always showing up on the list (*Journal of Clinical Pharmacology* 2004). There have been no reports of St. John's wort interacting with benzodiazepines. A similar case may be made for the birth control pill. Although it could reduce its effectiveness in theory, so many women use both that you would expect to have seen this interaction in practice. So we took a survey of some of North America's leading natural health practitioners, including Tori Hudson, Jane Gultinan, Terry Willard and Peter Laker. None have ever seen a woman become pregnant while using the pill with St. John's wort. There is a report that nine women in Sweden and the U.K. have become pregnant using the pill while on St. John's wort. But whether the St. John's was responsible is unknown. So while there is certainly a contraindication for St. John's wort with cyclosporine, indinavir, tacrolimus and imatinib there may be room for question in some of the other drugs. Though, in theory, drugs that are broken down by cytochrome P450 could be affected by St. John's wort, in fact a 2001 German review (*Phytomedicine* 2002)found only one interaction for every 300,000 treatments.

Sarsaparilla   (*Smilax medica*)

Sarsaparilla is a tonifying herb, a diaphoretic and powerful alterative herb that helps to clear heat from the body. And so Sarsaparilla has three main uses in traditional herbalism. Its first use is for skin diseases of an eruptive nature, such as psoriasis, rashes, acne, and eczema. For this purpose it is often combined with other herbs. Its second main use has historically been for the treatment of the venereal diseases gonorrhea and syphilis. Its third main use is for treating liver diseases such as jaundice and hepatitis. Sarsaparilla is also a powerful anti-inflammatory, making it useful in inflammatory conditions like gout, arthritis and rheumatic complaints.

Because of its ability to bind toxins, sarsaparilla deserves its reputation as a blood purifier, which is responsible for many of its uses. By removing the toxins from the gut, sarsaparilla stops them from overwhelming the liver and spilling into the blood, leading to inflammation and diseases like psoriasis, arthritis and gout. In a controlled study on 92 patients with psoriasis, sarsaparilla greatly improved symptoms in 62% of patients and totally cleared the disease in 18% of patients (*New Engl J Med* 1942).

Although unproven, herbalists have traditionally used sarsaparilla to increase sexual energy in men. Some list sarsaparilla as being a mild diuretic.

Sarsaparilla can be taken as a pill at a dose of 2–4 grams three times a day. You can also make a sarsaparilla tea by decocting 1–2 teaspoons (5–10g) of the dried root three times a day. If you prefer to use tinctures, take 1–4ml three times a day.

Sarsaparilla is a safe herb. Not all sources contraindicate it during pregnancy and breast feeding, but enough do to take this contraindication seriously. The *German Commission E* says that sarsaparilla can cause gastric irritation but the American Botanical Council. in their edition of *The Complete German Commission E Monographs*, says that this warning is wrong. The American Herbal Products Association's *Botanical Safety Handbook* isn't buying it either, saying that this claim is not substantiated anywhere else. *Botanical Safety Handbook* similarly says that the Commission's warning that sarsaparilla could interact with digitalis, bismuths and hypnotics is unsubstantiated. So, with the exception of pregnancy and breast feeding, at normal dosage there are no side effects, contraindications or drug interactions.

Saw palmetto berry   *(Serenoa repens)*

Saw palmetto berries are very good news for men. This herb is nature's answer to benign prostatic hyperplasia (BPH), the prostate disorder that affects so many men in the second half of their lives. Several studies have shown it to be more effective, faster acting and safer than the pharmaceutical drugs used for BPH. For BPH, saw palmetto is simply the best thing out there.

BPH causes men to have to urinate more frequently, to have to get up in the night more often to urinate, and to suffer a reduced force of their urine. It is believed that BPH occurs when testosterone builds up in the prostate and is converted into its more potent dihydrotestosterone (DHT) form.

Though it is no secret that saw palmetto works – it is probably one of the least contested herbs in the world; its efficacy and safety are rarely questioned – there are still many secrets and misconceptions about this herb.

The biggest secret is how it works. And though the answer is becoming clearer, it is still somewhat of a mystery. At first it was said that saw palmetto berry helped BPH by inhibiting the conversion of testosterone to DHT. Then researchers said that it did not lower DHT. Most recently, research has confirmed that it does lower DHT, but not everywhere; it lowers it selectively in prostate cells. Saw palmetto lowers prostatic DHT, but not as much as the BPH drug finasteride (Proscar) does. The drug

Several studies have shown it to be more effective, faster acting and safer than the pharmaceutical drugs.

lowers it by 80%, while the herb lowers it by 32% (*Urology* 2001) to 50% (*Prostate* 1998).

So why does the herb work better than the drug if it has smaller DHT reducing powers than the drug? Perhaps more is going on. Saw palmetto probably helps BPH through a combination of powers: it reduces DHT; it prevents DHT from binding to prostate cells; it is antiestrogenic, antispasmodic, and anti-inflammatory. All of these actions help treat BPH.

And this combination of actions is powerful. According to Michael Murray, N.D., the BPH drug finasteride takes six months to start working; saw palmetto takes four to six weeks. The drug will work on less than half of people after one year; the herb helps nearly 90%. The drug increases urine flow by 16% in a year; the herb increases it by 38% in three months.

Are there studies to prove all this? Absolutely. There are at least sixteen double-blind studies on saw palmetto. This remarkable herb can decrease night-time urination by 45%, urine left after urination by 42%, and increase flow rate by 50% (*Ann Urol* 1984).

Another study found that 83% of people found significant improvement with saw palmetto after forty-five days and 88% after ninety days with no serious side effects (*Curr Ther Res* 1994). Another recent three-year study also found it to be good or very good in 80% of cases (*Phytomedicine* 1996).

In 1996, saw palmetto berry went head to head with Finasteride, a leading prostate medication (*The Prostate*). The double-blind study lasted six months and included 1,098 people. Two-thirds improved in both groups, but saw palmetto produced fewer side effects, including erectile dysfunction. A year later, the herb was compared to the drug again (Bach *et al*). In this three-year study, saw palmetto improved symptoms more and was safer: 10.7% had to discontinue the drug because of side effects compared to only 1.8% on the herb.

In 1998, the *Journal of the American Medical Association* published a meta-analysis of studies on saw palmetto berry. It found the herb to be better than a placebo and to be as good as finasteride while producing a staggering 90% fewer adverse effects. While the drug caused erectile dysfunction in 4.9% of cases, the herb did so in only 1.1%.

Another advantage of saw palmetto berry over the drug is that finasteride changes PSA measures by 50% and so may mask prostate cancer. One of the enduring myths about saw palmetto berry is that it also affects PSA. But it doesn't. Several studies have now proven that the herb has no effect on PSA (*Prostate* 1999, *Urology* 2001).

Another claim that may be a myth about to fall is that saw palmetto does not actually shrink the enlarged prostate as finasteride does. A recent study found that a saw palmetto-nettle root combination actually shrank enlarged prostate tissue (*Urology Times* 1999).

The most recent challenge to saw palmetto berry came from a new class of drug called alpha-blockers. Alpha-blockers are now more commonly used for BPH than finasteride is. Saw palmetto berry may be better than finasteride, but how would the herb of choice stack up against the new drug of choice? New question; same answer. Saw palmetto berry works just as well as the alpha-blocker tamsulosin (Flomax). And once again saw palmetto berry was safer, causing significantly fewer incidents of sexual dysfunction than the drug (*European Urology* 2002). Clearly, the advantage still goes to saw palmetto berry.

Because the same hormone that is involved in BPH is also involved in thinning hair, not only in men but also in women, by inhibiting this hormone, saw palmetto berry may also help in cases of hormone-related thinning hair. One study that combined the herb with beta-sitosterol found that it did (*Journal of Alternative and Complementary Medicine* 2002).

Saw Palmetto berry, though rightly known as a herb for men, may help women with more than just thinning hair. According to Michael Murray, N.D., saw palmetto may be of value in conditions involving excessive male hormones in women, such as polycystic ovarian disease and excessive facial and bodily hair (hirsutism).

Saw palmetto berry should be taken as an extract that has been standardized to contain 85–95% fatty acids and sterols. The dose is 320mg a day standardized to 85–95% fatty acids and sterols. Another myth about this herb is that it needs to be taken in 160mg doses twice a day. Studies now add convenience to efficacy: go ahead and take saw palmetto all at once in one 320mg dose (*Phytotherapy Res* 1997, *Advanced Ther* 1999).

If the herb is not standardized, the traditional dose is about

1/2–1 teaspoon (2–5g) of the dried berries, decocted and consumed three times a day, although the tea may not work as well, since the active components may not be extracted in water. You could also try 2–4g of dried berries in pill form, 1–2ml of the tincture three times a day, or 1–2ml of the extract twice a day.

Saw palmetto berry is entirely safe. The studies are remarkably free of side effects. There are no contraindications or drug interactions.

The vast majority of authoritative texts say that you can use saw palmetto while pregnant and breast feeding. One book says the safety has not been established, though, and one women's herbal says not to use it. The American Botanical Council *Clinical Guide to Herbs* says that although this has not been confirmed by scientific studies, the potential hormonal activity of this herb means that it is not recommended during pregnancy or breast feeding. This possible disagreement is not a great concern, however, since saw palmetto berry is primarily a herb for men.

Schizandra *(Schizandra chinensis)*

Throughout history, schizandra has been used for its remarkable ability to increase energy and stamina. It has been used by the Swedish ski team for this purpose as well as by fighter pilots. Schizandra has a long history of use in Chinese folklore and has recently gained a great deal of attention in the West. It is considered a tonifying herb that is primarily used to give energy, much like ginseng. Schizandra strengthens tissues and eliminates secretions. It also has among its activities antifatigue, immune enhancing, and anti-inflammatory activity.

This herb has numerous uses, including treatment for asthma, chronic cough, night sweats, irritability, palpitations, dream disturbed sleep, insomnia, diarrhea, leukorrhoea, forgetfulness, to regulate blood sugar levels, for stress, hepatitis, neck and shoulder tension, to beautify the skin, for pain, digestion, as an expectorant, for frequent urination, weak kidneys, venereal disease, PMS, circulation, and for normalizing blood pressure. It works as an adaptogen that increases the body's resistance to stress, and it regulates gastric acidity, increases muscle endurance, and prevents liver damage. Yet, with all that this remarkable herb does, its effects are gentle.

Of the fruit, take 1.5–15g a day. If you are using schizandra in pill form, take 400–450mg of the powdered herb three times a day. The dose of the tincture is 1–4ml three times a day. The dose of the decoction is given as 1.5–9g.

Schizandra is very safe. Although very rare, abdominal upset, decreased appetite and skin rash are possible. Although no books contraindicate schizandra during pregnancy or breast feeding, in a recent update Brinker now says not to use it while you are pregnant. Some experts caution against the use of schizandra by those with epilepsy or by those with high inter-cranial pressure or severe hypertension.

Senna

(Senna alexandina; Cassia angustofolia; Cassia senna)

Senna is a herb with a single purpose: it is a powerful laxative suitable for occasional acute constipation. And it has been approved by many for this purpose. The *German Commission E* and the World Health Organization both approve its use for constipation. The *British Herbal Compendium* approves its use for constipation and any problem where soft stool is desired, such as in anal fissure or hemorrhoids. It is also used for other situations in which easy, soft stool is needed, such as after recto-anal operations, for clearing the bowels, before X-ray examinations, and before and after surgery of the abdomen. Traditionally, it is often used as a part of a cleansing program to detoxify the body.

The leaves are considered to have a stronger laxative effect than the pods.

Take 0.6–2 grams of the dried leaf a day. As a tea, you an infuse 0.5–3 grams a day. The dose of the extract is 0.6–2ml a day. Herbalist David Hoffmann says to take 2–7ml of the tincture three times a day, a somewhat higher dose recommendation. Never take senna for more than 8 to 10 days or at the most, according to some sources, one to two weeks.

Senna is a strong laxative that can cause gripping. For this reason it should be combined with a carminative herb like ginger. Senna should not be used by anyone with an intestinal obstruction or acute intestinal inflammation, including Crohn's, colitis, appendicitis, or by anyone with abdominal pain of unknown origin or anal prolapse. Children under twelve should not use senna.

All other concerns for senna apply only to its overuse: so don't overuse it! Overuse can cause loss of fluid, diarrhea and depleted potassium. Depleted potassium could increase the toxicity of antiarrhythmia drugs and cardiac glycosides. Senna may increase or decrease the activity of digoxin. It is speculated that the laxative action of senna might decrease absorption of oral drugs.

Should you take senna while you are pregnant or breast feeding? We don't know. Some sources say no. Some sources say yes, except in the first trimester. *Commission E* says not to use the leaf because we don't have sufficient knowledge. They say you can use the pod, but that during the first trimester you should only use it if nothing else works: that's usually good advice for this powerful herb anyway. Brinker says speculatively, no. However, he says that human studies have shown it to be safe at laxative doses. So, can you take senna while you are pregnant or breast feeding? Don't know. There are a lot of gentler ways to relieve constipation anyway.

Shepherd's purse (*Capsella bursa-pastoris*)

The use of shepherd's purse dates back at least 8,000 years. This little-discussed plant is one of the best herbs for stopping excessive bleeding and therefore has a special place as a woman's herb, though it can be used for any bleeding, including nosebleeds and cuts. It is an excellent herb for haemorrhaging and for excessive bleeding following childbirth. It is perfect for women who suffer from menorrhagia or metrorrhagia, or excessively heavy periods. It works well when taken several days or even weeks or months before the onset of menstruation. We usually find that it is most effective if used for the two weeks after ovulation, up to and including the actual period, every month for at least three months. And it combines very well with other astringent herbs and herbs that nourish and support the reproductive organs and iron levels to fully treat the problem. It is also effective for the heavy bleeding or internal bleeding of endometriosis.

Shepherd's purse is of great value for bruises, skin wounds and for varicose veins. It has also been used for inflammation, cystitis, diarrhea, blood in the urine (hematuria), arthritis, bleeding from the digestive tract and lungs, for hypertension, and as a diuretic.

As a loose herb, use 10–15 grams of shepherd's purse per day. As a tea, infuse between 1/2 a teaspoon and 2 teaspoons (2–10g) and drink 2–4 cups a day. The extract dose is 1–4ml three times a day. Shepherd's purse must be used fresh or as tinctures made from the fresh herb. If you are using shepherd's purse for menstrual problems, drink the infusion every two to three hours just before and during menstruation. Similarly, you can take 30 drops (1ml) of the tincture every half hour for bleeding and endometriosis, gradually reducing the dose as the symptoms improve.

Shepherd's purse has no known toxicity, even when it is used long term. It has no known side effects, contraindications or drug interactions. Shepherd's purse should not be used during pregnancy, although it is one of the best herbs to use for hemorrhaging during childbirth. It is safe to use while breast feeding. Use shepherd's purse with caution if there is a history of kidney stones. Excessive doses may cause heart palpitations.

shiitake mushroom (Lentinus edodes)

Our favourite way to use this natural immune booster is on the barbecue: skewered on a vegetarian shish kabob. Shiitake is not only the most important medicinal mushroom, it is also an important gourmet mushroom. Delicious!

Shiitake mushroom has traditionally been used in China and Japan to boost immunity; fight colds, measles, intestinal worms and arthritis; and to improve circulation, lower cholesterol, and treat heart disease. Today, it is also used to treat asthma, hepatitis B, ulcers, AIDS, and herpes. Lentinin, a component of shiitake mushroom, is one of the top-selling drugs for cancer in Japan.

Shiitake mushrooms contain very powerful immune-boosting substances that make it one of the most exciting remedies for any condition involving lowered immunity, and one of the most promising cancer fighters. But shiitake doesn't aggressively destroy tumours, bacteria and viruses the way antibiotics and chemotherapy do. It boosts the immune system and helps it to do its work the way it's supposed to. Shiitake is able to boost virtually the whole host of immune components.

Lentinin and LEM (Lentinus Edodes Mycelium extract) have both shown strong anti-tumour activity when used both orally and as an injection. When lentinin is added to chemotherapy, cancer patients live longer than when they get chemotherapy alone. This life-extending ability of shiitake mushroom has been shown in cases of stomach cancer, pancreatic cancer, colon-rectal cancer, and breast cancer.

In addition to its being anti-tumour,

This life-extending ability of shiitake mushroom has been shown in cases of stomach cancer, pancreatic cancer, colon-rectal cancer, and breast cancer.

When people suffering from CFS were given lentinin [a component of shiitake], their levels of natural killer cells returned to normal – a boost of more than 300% – and their fatigue and energy levels improved.

mushroom expert Paul Stamets says that shiitake is antibacterial, antiviral and immune enhancing; good for cholesterol, blood pressure and for moderating blood sugar; and is also a kidney and liver tonic as well as reducing stress and acting as a sexual potentiator (*HerbalGram* #54). Research has also proven shiitake to be effective against *candida* and against herpes I.

In his book on medicinal mushrooms, Christopher Hobbs says that the research suggests that LEM may be more effective than the AIDS drug AZT. Laboratory research has also suggested that lentinin can make AZT work better (*Advances in Applied Microbiology* 1993). When lentinin was combined with another AIDS drug, didanosine, it made that drug work better too, leading to greater improvement in immunity than the drug alone (*Journal of Medicine* 1995). In another study, when lentinin was given intravenously, it was beneficial for AIDS (*J Med* 1998). Thirty percent of people with HIV had their immunity improve within eight weeks when they were given lentinen (Abrams, Greco, Wong, *et. al.*, 1990).

Shiitake is also an important herb for chronic fatigue immune dysfunction syndrome (CFIDS or CFS). When people suffering from CFS were given lentinin, their levels of natural killer cells returned to normal – a boost of more than 300% – and their fatigue and energy levels improved (*Nat Immun Cell Growth Reg* 1987). CFS is a debilitating and increasingly common problem. Clinically, Linda has found shiitake to be helpful as part of a CFS program.

When shiitake is combined with laser surgery for treating genital warts, the results are much better than surgery alone (*CJIM* 1999), and it may also be useful for hepatitis B (*Alt Compl Ther* 1998). Shiitake mushroom also significantly lowers cholesterol levels, lowers blood pressure, and may prevent blood clots. In a totally different role, shiitake is also a kidney tonic that can help treat incontinence. It is a good herb against cold and flu and can be used by anyone for immune support.

If you are using the whole, dried mushroom in cooking, soups or as a decoction, use 6–16g a day. Of the fresh mushroom, use about 90g or, according to one source, 3–4 mushrooms a day. If you are using a tincture, take 2–4ml a day. One source lists 400mg–2g a day as the dose for shiitake capsules. If you are using LEM to treat a serious condition, take 1–2g two to three times a day. When the disease is more stabilized, decrease your dose to 0.5–1g a day.

 Shiitake, like most of the herbs that are also foods, is perfectly safe. There are no contraindications or drug interactions. Although one source says shiitake's safety during pregnancy and breast feeding has not been established, the American Herbal Products Association's *Botanical Safety Handbook* classifies shiitake mushroom as a herb that is safe when used appropriately and does not contraindicate it during pregnancy or breast feeding.

Skullcap *(Scutellaria lateriflora)*

Skullcap does not get nearly the respect it deserves, and it is entirely omitted from many of the major works on herbs. But when you turn to the herbals of the most respected traditional herbalists, skullcap always shows up – because they know how valuable this remarkable herb is.

Herbalist David Hoffmann honours skullcap by crowning it "perhaps the most widely relevant nervine." And Rosemary Gladstar calls skullcap one of the most versatile nervines. The great beauty of skullcap, according to herbalists Christopher Hobbs, David Hoffmann and others, is its ability to tonify the nervous system by nourishing, enriching, and reenergizing it at the same time as it calms it, making it a true nervous system tonic.

Gladstar says skullcap is good for any nervous system disorder, including stress, nervous exhaustion and insomnia. It is a good herb to take throughout the day to prepare you to ease into sleep at night. Skullcap is great for stress, tension and anxiety and has also been used for hysteria and depression. A recently released double-blind, placebo-controlled study has found skullcap to be an effective herb for anxiety (*Alternative Therapies* 2003). Hobbs says to turn to skullcap whenever nervousness comes out in spasms, tics, tremours or convulsions. This antispasmodic power also makes skullcap a good herb for epilepsy and Parkinson's. Clinically, Linda has also seen this herb help reduce tight muscles, allowing a crooked arm or leg to return to a more normal state.

Skullcap is also a good herb for hyperactive children and is useful for nervous headaches and PMS. In an unrelated use, skullcap is also a bitter that can aid digestion.

Herbalist Michael Tierra says that skullcap is one of the most effective herbs to help with withdrawal from drugs and alcohol. In addition to its ability to produce calmness, its detoxification properties help lessen the withdrawal symptoms.

Skullcap can be taken as an infusion at a dose of 1–2 teaspoons (5–10g) per cup three times a day. As a dried herb in pill form, take three grams up to three times a day. If you are using the tincture, use 2–4ml three times a day. For drug and alcohol withdrawal take 15 to 20 drops every hour or two.

Skullcap is a very safe herb. It has no side effects, contraindications or drug interactions. Some sources say not to take skullcap while pregnant because of limited information. However, the important *Botanical Safety Handbook* of the American Herbal Products Association does not contraindicated it in pregnancy and several reputable women's herbals agree, and at least one recommends skullcap as a nervine during pregnancy.

slippery elm *(Ulmus fulva, Ulmus rubra)*

Slippery elm is one of our favourites, and we always keep some of it around because it is so versatile. This is one of the most soothing of herbs. It is great for irritated and sore throats, dryness and coughs, and for ulcers. It soothes intestinal tract irritation and is useful for diarrhea and just about every kind of digestive problem, such as gastritis, colitis, Crohn's, IBS, gas, bloating, nausea, and haemorrhoids. It is sometimes mixed with other herbs for these purposes. In times of convalescence or wasting, it is an excellent nourishing food that stays down when nothing else will. It can even be used for morning sickness.

Externally, slippery elm can be mixed with a little hot water to form a poultice that is effective for ulcers and other wounds. It can also be made into a boulice for haemorrhoids and for vaginal irritation, and is often mixed with other herbs for these purposes.

Traditionally, slippery elm has also been used as part of a cancer program in a couple of herbal cancer remedies.

Decoct one part slippery elm to eight parts water (mixed well) for 10 to 15 minutes and drink half a cup three times daily. A simpler method that we often use is to mix about half a teaspoon (2g) of powdered bark into a cup of hot water and drink 2 to 3 times a day. Slippery elm lozenges are also available. Once you get used to the taste of sucking on a tree, they're actually not bad and kind of sweet. As a nourishing food, mix warm honey water with 4–6 tablespoons of slippery elm powder until it reaches the consistency you want. You can add cinnamon for flavour. Eat freely as needed.

Perfectly safe, even if you are pregnant or breast feeding. There are no side effects, contraindications or drug interactions. Because slippery elm is so mucilaginous, it is possible that it could interfere with the absorption of drugs taken at the same time.

Soy   (Glycine max)

One of nature's most powerful and versatile healers is a simple bean: the soy bean. Soy is excellent for the heart. Replacing animal foods with soy foods has been shown to improve cholesterol levels and lower the risk of coronary artery disease (*Arch Intern Med* 2001; *Am J Clin Nutr* 2002). Studies have consistently found soy to lower cholesterol: a meta-analysis of thirty-eight studies found soy diets to reduce cholesterol in 89% of the studies (*N Engl J Med* 1995).

Soy is also good for blood pressure. In a recent double-blind study, 40 people with mild to moderate high blood pressure were given either skim milk or soy milk for three months. There was a significantly greater decrease in blood pressure in the soy milk group (*J Nutr* 2002). Surprisingly, simply drinking 500ml of soy milk twice a day reduced blood pressure comparably to many blood pressure medications.

Soy is not only good for preventing heart disease, it is also great for preventing the other big killer: cancer. Population studies suggest that eating soy may be the reason for lower cancer rates in China and Japan. High levels of genestein, an important anti-cancer compound in soy, are associated with low incidence of breast and prostate cancer. Chinese and Japanese women have way fewer deaths from breast cancer than North American and European women. But when they move to North America, adopt a western diet and decrease their soy intake, their death rates from breast cancer climb to levels similar to ours. Japanese men who eat a lot of soy also have much lower mortality rates from prostate cancer. Risk of prostate cancer also goes down with an increased consumption of soy (*Br J Urol* 1996). Studies suggest that soy may protect against several other kinds of cancer, including colon cancer (*Nutr Cancer* 1994).

How does a simple soy bean fight cancer? There are many components in soy that help fight cancer, but the most important one seems to be the isoflavone genestein. Genestein takes cancer on in many ways. It induces apoptosis, a process in which cancer cells self-destruct without damaging the healthy cells around them. Genestein also inhibits the growth of the new capillaries that tumours need to grow. It also induces differentiation, a process that makes a cancer cell less aggressive. Since genestein is a phytoestrogen that is much weaker than your body's own estrogen, it also lowers estrogen by stealing receptor cites from your body's hormones. All of these actions make genestein a very promising anti-cancer agent.

Replacing animal foods with soy foods has been shown to improve cholesterol levels and lower the risk of coronary artery disease.

Surprisingly, simply drinking 500ml of soy milk twice a day reduced blood pressure comparably to many blood pressure medications.

One of the ways soy fights cancer is through its phytoestrogenic isoflavones. This mild estrogenic action also makes soy a big help during menopause. Only 3.6% of Japanese women, whose diet is rich in soy isoflavones, suffer from night sweats, compared to 30.9% of Canadian women, and only 19.6% of Japanese women have hot flashes, compared to a whopping 64.6% of Canadians.

When soy flour was given to fifty-eight menopausal women for three months, they had a 40% reduction in hot flashes (*Maturitis* 1995). In another study, women were given either 60 grams of soy protein, containing 76mg of isoflavones, or a placebo. The soy group had a 45% reduction in hot flashes compared to 30% in the placebo group – a significantly superior benefit (*Obstet Gynecol* 1998). Most recently, when a four-month study gave either 100mg soy isoflavones or a placebo, the women on the soy had a significant 40% decrease in menopausal symptoms (*Obstet Gynecol* 2002). Hot flashes were reduced by 61% versus only 21% in the placebo group in another recent study (*Menopause* 2002).

Soy is also turning out to be effective for another concern of menopause: osteoporosis. Studies are showing that soy isoflavones can stop bone loss and even reverse it (*Am J Clin Nutr* 1998; *Am J Clin Nutr* 2000). Soy isoflavones may stimulate bone-building cells (*Biochem Pharmacol* 2000), inhibit cells that break down bone (*J Cell Biochem* 1996), improve calcium absorption (*Biochem Pharmacol* 2000), and cause less urinary loss of calcium than animal protein (*J Clin Endocrinol Metab* 1988). And soy is not just for women. A new study comparing soy protein to milk protein has also suggested that soy protein may be good for men's bones (*J Nutr* 2002).

Now there's an additional benefit of soy for menopausal women: research is suggesting that it can help reverse the cognitive decline that is associated with menopause. In a recently released study, 60mg of soy isoflavones led to significant improvement in memory, logic, and attention compared to a placebo (*Pharmacology, Biochemistry & Behaviour* 2003).

For lowering cholesterol, use 30mg or more of soy protein, although some studies have found a benefit with as low as 20mg. For osteoporosis, take 90mg of soy isoflavones. For cancer, the limited dosage information seems to suggest 25–100mg of isoflavones for prevention and at least 100mg a day to treat it. For menopause, try 60–80mg of isoflavones a day. Some studies have found benefit with as low as 34mg and some sources recommend a much higher dose of 76–135mg of isoflavones.

To put all of these numbers into perspective, the amount of isoflavones that would be consumed in the average Asian diet is estimated to be 20–80mg a day, or even as much as 50–150mg, according to some sources. Of course, you can also get your soy by eating it in its various forms. Two to three ounces of soy would give you about 50–80mg of isoflavones.

 Soy is very safe. It can decrease the absorption of thyroid hormones if it is taken at the same time, so don't take any soy products within three hours of taking your thyroid hormones. Soy may also block the effects of tamoxifen on estrogen-dependent breast tumours.

Sugar cane wax extract (Saccharum officinarum)

This is the first time sugar cane has appeared as the protagonist when talking about health. Sugar cane wax extract is an amazing herb that not enough people have heard about. It is simply the best thing out there for cholesterol – natural or pharmaceutical. There are many choices in the fight against cholesterol. But if you knew that one of those choices had been studied head to head against virtually every kind of cholesterol-lowering drug and had been proven to be as good or better without the negative side effects, which would you choose?

Believe it or not, the cholesterol fighting champion is an extract from the wax of the sugar cane: the same sugar cane that seemed to have no redeeming qualities.

There have been at least 14 placebo-controlled, double-blind studies on sugar cane wax extract, and in every one of them total cholesterol , the bad LDL cholesterol, the ratio of bad LDL to beneficial HDL cholesterol, and the ratio of total to HDL cholesterol significantly improved. And what is more, sugar cane wax extract caused an equal or lesser number of side effects.

So it works. But does it work as well as pharmaceutical cholesterol lowerers? Actually, it works better. The drug of choice for high cholesterol is the statin class of drugs. Though these drugs effectively lower the bad LDL cholesterol, they have two major drawbacks. The first is that they do not effectively raise the beneficial HDL cholesterol – an even more important factor for preventing heart disease than lowering LDL cholesterol – and the second is that they negatively affect the liver.

In a head-to-head study against the statin drug lovastatin, sugar cane wax extract lowered LDL cholesterol just as well. But while lovastatin actually lowered the good HDL cholesterol, sugar cane wax extract raised it by 17%. And unlike lovastatin, sugar cane wax extract had no liver toxicity as well as fewer of the other side effects. In a second study of people with high cholesterol as well as additional coronary risk factors, sugar cane wax extract performed better than lovastatin with fewer side effects (*Curr Ther Res Clin Exp* 2000).

When sugar cane wax extract went up against the next statin drug, pravastatin, it produced a greater improvement in both LDL and HDL cholesterol with fewer side effects (*Curr Ther Res* 1997; *Int J Clin Pharmacol Res* 1999). Against simvastatin, sugar cane wax extract was at least as good with fewer side effects (*Can J Cardiol* 1997).

When compared to a second class of cholesterol drugs called fibrates, the nod went once again to the natural cholesterol fighter. While the drug more effectively lowered triglycerides, sugar cane wax extract was superior against total cholesterol, LDL cholesterol and HDL cholesterol. And once again, sugar cane wax extract was the choice for safety. Unlike the drug, sugar cane wax extract did not adversely affect the liver and produced fewer side effects.

Sugar cane wax extract has also been studied against the drug acipimox (*Int J Tissure React* 1999). Sugar cane wax extract was the clear winner, more effectively lowering total and LDL cholesterol and more effectively raising HDL. What's more, sugar cane wax extract lowered Lp(a), the little-discussed but worst cholesterol of them all, by 32.6% (57.4% in those whose levels were too high to begin with). According to Michael Murray, N.D., elevated Lp(a) is a ten times greater risk factor for heart disease than elevated LDL cholesterol.

And finally, when sugar cane wax extract went up against the drug probucol, it proved superior in lowering total and LDL cholesterol as well as triglycerides (*Curr Ther Res Clin Exp* 1997).

Sugar cane wax extract has a number of other features to recommend it. It is

[Sugar cane wax extract has] been studied head to head against virtually every kind of cholesterol-lowering drug and had been proven to be as good or better without the negative side effects.

safe for people with high cholesterol who have liver disease. In fact, it may even improve the liver disease (*Curr Ther Res Clin Exp* 1996). In people with high blood pressure in addition to their cholesterol problems, sugar cane wax extract improves total, LDL, and HDL cholesterol while significantly lowering blood pressure (*Curr Ther Res*).

Sugar cane wax extract is also effective and safe in diabetics with high cholesterol (*Diabetes Care* 1995). In 1999, sugar cane wax extract was compared to lovastatin in type II diabetics with high cholesterol (*Int J Clin Pharmacol Res*). Sugar cane wax extract produced a greater decrease in total and LDL cholesterol. While lovastatin caused an unfortunate decrease in HDL, sugar cane wax extract increased it. Sugar cane wax extract also decreased blood pressure compared to the drug. Lovastatin had a negative effect on liver enzymes; sugar cane wax extract once again did not. Side effects were fewer with sugar cane wax extract, and all those who were forced to withdraw from the study were on lovastatin.

But the news gets better. Sugar cane wax extract's heart benefits don't stop with cholesterol. It acts as an antioxidant, preventing LDL cholesterol from oxidizing. Oxidation of LDL cholesterol is a necessary step in the development of atherosclerosis.

Sugar cane wax extract has also been shown in several studies to significantly inhibit platelet aggregation without effecting coagulation. Sugar cane wax extract compares favourably to aspirin and may even have some advantages while additionally producing fewer side effects (*Pharmacol Res* 1997). The combination of sugar cane wax extract and Aspirin is also effective.

Sugar cane wax extract also prevents and reverses atherosclerosis and blood clots. It improves angina (*Int J Clin Pharmacol Ther* 1996) and is good for intermittent claudication (*Angiology* 1999; *Angiology* 2001). In the most recent study on sugar cane wax extract, the herb was compared to lovastatin in people with intermittent claudication. Pain-free walking distance improved 34% in the sugar cane wax extract group but not at all in the lovastatin group. While both treatments lowered total and LDL cholesterol, sugar cane wax extract also lowered fibrinogen by 6% and raised HDL by 32% while lovastatin helped neither of these heart disease risks (*Angiology* 2003).

The starting dose for sugar cane wax extract is 10mg with dinner. If it has not worked after two months, increase the dose to 20mg. Typically, sugar cane wax extract should lower LDL cholesterol by 20–25% within six months at 10mg and by 25–30% at 20mg, Michael Murray, N.D., says HDL should go up by 15–25% after two months.

Sugar cane wax extract is very safe, producing side effects even less frequently than placebo. In a study that followed 27,879 people for an average of 2.7 years, only 0.31% suffered side effects and only twenty-two had to stop using sugar cane wax extract. It works synergistically with the antiplatelet aggregation properties of Aspirin, but has no adverse drug interactions. Murray says that because cholesterol is needed for fetal development, sugar cane wax extract should not be used while pregnant. He also cautions that the effects on breast feeding and on children are currently unknown.

Most Asked Questions and Answers

Can multiple herbs be used together?
Yes. Herbs may be used alone or in combination to tolerance or to specific needs.

Can herbs be used with drugs?
Yes, few herbs have drug herb interactions. See interactions throughout this book.

Can I get off of drugs and on herbs instead?
Working with a practitioner, using established tapering patterns, many people can come off of their drugs.

Why use a herb over a drug?
Usually herbs are safer, with less side effects than drugs and have wider actions against more conditions. So often one herb can be used to treat more than one problem at a time. Herbs are also rich in nutrients and are often less expensive too.

Tea tree oil   *(Melaleuca alternifolia)*

Possessing some of the widest ranging antimicrobial properties of any plant, tea tree oil makes an excellent disinfectant and has a reserved place of honour in any first aid kit.

Tea tree oil is a useful part of any acne program. It is an effective alternative to benzoyl peroxide that produces less stinging, burning, dryness, and redness (*Med J Aust* 1990).

In addition to being antiseptic, tea tree oil is antifungal. It works against athlete's foot, smelly feet, irritated feet and is as effective as conventional treatment against fungus-infected toenails (*Fam Pract* 1994).

Tea tree oil is a useful part of any acne program. It is an effective alternative to benzoyl peroxide that produces less stinging, burning, dryness, and redness improved.

It also kills *candida* and *Trichomonas vaginalis* (*Essential Oils Data Search* 1985; *Obstet Gynecol* 1962) and has been reported to reduce the symptoms of acute bladder infection very quickly. Recently, tea tree oil was found to be active even against antibiotic-resistant strains of bacteria. It is also effective for diaper rash and jock itch when combined with calendula cream.

Keep tea tree oil around and use it whenever you need to disinfect a cut or any kind of wound.

Just apply the undiluted oil directly to the area of skin or nail that needs it at least twice a day. For acne, apply a 5–15% solution three to four times a day.

Tea tree is extremely safe topically, but should not be taken internally. As a powerful essential oil, it may occasionally cause mild contact dermatitis. However, it is one of the very safest essential oils and usually causes little irritation even when used for long periods. There are no drug interactions.

Triphala

Triphala is an herbal combination from India's Ayurvedic herbal tradition composed of three fruits: *Terminalia chebula*, *Emblica officianalis*, and *Terminalia belerica*. It is a gentle laxative that unlike many other laxatives is safe to use long term. It is not habit forming and has no adverse effects. In fact, it is considered to be as safe as food. Clinically, Linda has found it to be one of the most effective laxatives that there is.

Triphala is not just for constipation, however. Interestingly, because it is actually a bowel tonic, triphala can also be used for the opposite problem: diarrhea. It is a tonic for cleansing and tuning up the digestive system. Triphala doesn't only cleanse the digestive system, but is a good blood and liver tonic and detoxifier as well. It is considered a rejuvenator for the whole body.

Traditionally, triphala has also been used to strengthen the eyes, and is used for cataracts and glaucoma. It can also be used as a daily eyewash to get rid of redness and soreness.

Triphala has been used to eliminate parasites, and recent research has discovered that it also possesses strong antioxidant activity (*International Journal of Pharmacognosy* 1997).

For improving general health, triphala can be used for up to a year at a low dose of 1–2g twice a day. It can be used this way on and off throughout life. As an occasional laxative, triphala can be used at a higher dose of 10–15g for shorter periods. If you want to try triphala as an eyewash, steep one teaspoon (5g) of the powder in one cup of boiled water. Let it cool and strain it. Using an eyecup, bathe the eye two to three times a day.

Triphala is very safe, even long term. It is not habit forming, so avoids the problem with many other laxatives. There are no side effects. We were unable to find information specifically on pregnancy and breast feeding.

Though the research on turmeric is still in the early stage, research is generating enormous excitement.

In India, turmeric has a very long history of use as an anti-inflammatory and anti-arthritis herb. In acute inflammation, curcumin, an important component of turmeric, is as effective as cortisone or the nonsteroidal anti-inflammatory drug, phenylbutazone; in chronic inflammation it is half as effective but safer.

When people suffering from rheumatoid arthritis were given either curcumin or the powerful nonsteroidal anti-inflammatory drug phenylbutazone, there was significant improvement in both groups, and the curcumin worked as well, or almost as well, as the drug (*Indian J Med Res* 1980). When the two went head to head again – this time for treating postoperative inflammation – the herb was as good or better (*Int J Clin Pharmacol* 1986). Turmeric is also safer than the nonsteroidal anti-inflammatory drugs when it comes to causing gastric ulcers.

Turmeric is not only a valuable anti-inflammatory. It has also shown potential value with the big three: cancer, heart disease and AIDS. In fact, turmeric is one of the most promising anticancer herbs of all. Cancer expert John Boik notes that turmeric is showing potential not only for the prevention, but even for the treatment of cancer. It is looking good in virtually any form of cancer. Cancer expert John Boik reports that several test tube studies show that curcumin inhibits, and even decreases, the proliferation of a variety of cancer cells. And test tube studies are showing promise against prostate, breast, skin, colon, stomach and liver cancers (*Carcinogenesis* 2000; *Clin Cancer Res* 2001; *Anticancer Res* 2001; *Mol Urol* 2000; *Prostate Cancer Prostatic Dis* 2000; *Prostate* 2001; *J Invest Dermatol* 1998).

Turmeric seems to battle cancer on many fronts. Among the many important ways it fights cancer, turmeric inhibits angiogenesis (*Mol Med* 1998) and induces apoptosis (*Clin Immunol* 1999). Angiogenesis is the formation of new blood vessels that supply nutrients to tumours and allow them to grow. Inhibiting this supply line starves the tumour. Apoptosis is a very safe way of killing cancer cells without harming the healthy noncancerous cells around them. Turmeric also induces this action. Turmeric also helps because it's a powerful antioxidant.

An exciting recent study found curcumin to powerfully induce apoptosis in both hormone dependent and hormone independent prostate cancer cells. This finding is important because when prostate cancer becomes hormone independent, it is hard to treat. This makes curcumin an exciting possibility for the prevention and treatment of advanced prostate cancer (*Prostate Cancer Prostatic* Dis 2000).

From cancer to heart disease, turmeric again shows promise. Turmeric lowers cholesterol and triglycerides and protects cholesterol from free radical damage (*Indian J Physiol Pharmacol* 1992; *Age* 1995). It also prevents blood platelets from clumping together, protecting against atherosclerosis (*Thromb Res* 1985; *Arzneimforsch* 1986). A recent study also found that turmeric effectively reduced elevated fibrinogen levels (*Mech Ageing Dev* 2000). Elevated fibrinogen levels can cause atherosclerosis and are an important risk factor for heart disease.

Curcumin might also help people with HIV. Several studies suggest that curcumin can inhibit the replication of HIV in a number of ways. One study found that a large dose of curcumin raised CD4 counts in HIV positive people (*Int Conf AIDS* 1994), meaning it raised the level of important immune cells that are deficient in those with HIV.

Besides the big diseases, this valuable herb has other uses as well. Turmeric is used for digestive problems like gas and bloating. Eighty-seven percent of those with indigestion improved after one week on turmeric, compared to 53% of those who were given a placebo (*J Med Assoc Thai* 1989). Turmeric increases the output of bile, which can help a number of digestive problems. It protects the liver. And a couple of small recent studies raise the hope that curcumin can help Crohn's disease (*Digestive Diseases and Sciences* 2005) and turmeric can help irritable bowel syndrome (*J Alt Comp Med* 2004).

Herbalist Michael Tierra says that because turmeric promotes blood circulation and is an anti-inflammatory, it is a great herb for bruises and injuries. Used internally and externally, it heals wounds and relieves pain. Its topical use is also good for relieving the pain of arthritis and neuralgia. Tierra also notes that turmeric reduces fever, helps treat hepatitis, helps regulate menstrual cycles and helps PMS. James Duke, Ph.D., adds getting rid of worms to turmeric's resume.

As in Indian curries, the benefits of turmeric can be enjoyed by eating it: a healthy, inexpensive and delicious way of using turmeric. As a supplement, the dose of the powdered root is 1-4g a day. The dose of the infusion is 1.3g of the root twice a day. Take 1.5-3ml of extract or 10ml of tincture.

Some sources recommend a higher dose. Mills and Bone recommend an extract dose of 5-14ml a day divided into 4-5 doses. Michael Murray, N.D. suggests a standardized turmeric that delivers 200-400mg of curcumin three times a day for cancer and has suggested as high as 400-600mg of curcumin three times a day for inflammation. He also suggests taking it with bromelain on an empty stomach to increase absorption.

Turmeric is extremely safe. There are no side effects. It is safe during breast feeding but should not be used during pregnancy.

The texts also say to avoid turmeric in cases of bile duct obstruction and to use it with gallstones only after consulting a practitioner. The gallstone caution is the usual one for herbs that increase bile: see the section on artichoke for a full discussion. Tierra states that turmeric is an important aid in helping prevent and dissolve gallstones. Murray and Pizzorno and Robert McCaleb agree. Brinker lists this caution as speculative. High doses of turmeric may enhance the effect of blood thinners, and turmeric may enhance the effect of insulin.

Usnea

(Usnea longissima, Usnea barbata, Usnea florida, and other species)

Usnea is a lichen, a bizarre organism which is really two organisms, a fungus and an algae, living symbiotically as one. In addition to its immune system stimulating properties, usnea has very powerful antibacterial, antiviral and antifungal properties. Against some strains of bacteria, usnea is even more powerful than penicillin. It is especially effective against the *Streptococcus* bacteria that causes strep throat, *Staphylococcus* bacteria, and tuberculosis.

Usnea can also be used for other respiratory tract infections like bronchitis, pleurisy and pneumonia. It is also used for urinary tract infections.

It is an antifungal herb, effective against athlete's foot and *candida*. Usnea is also very effective against *Trichomonas vaginalis*, a sexually transmitted parasite that causes some urinary tract infections

Usnea can be taken in pill form at a dose of 100mg three times a day. Or you can take 3–4ml of the tincture three times a day. You can also gargle usnea to help with sore or strep throat by putting a dropper full in water and gargling several times a day. Lozenges are also available: take 100mg lozenges 3–6 times a day. Usnea can also be decocted as a tea or applied externally for fungal infections or infected cuts.

There are no side effects, contraindications or drug interactions for usnea. The alcohol extract could be irritating if not diluted in water. Though one source says that the safety of usnea while pregnant or breast feeding is not known, the American Herbal Products Association's *Botanical Safety Handbook* and the *German Commission E Monographs* both list it as safe.

Uva ursi
(Arctostaphylos uva-ursi)

If you are a woman and suffer from frequent urinary tract infections, uva ursi is one herb you should become familiar with. It is simply the best herb for getting rid if UTIs and keeping them from coming back (for men too). Uva ursi is also commonly known as bearberry. This little-discussed herb is considered by many traditional herbalists to be one of the most useful and effective herbs for urinary tract infections. It has a long tradition of use for urinary tract problems by First Nations healers.

Uva ursi is a urinary tract antiseptic as well as a diuretic and astringent herb. It is especially effective against *E. coli*, the bacteria that causes about 90% of all urinary tract infections, but is also effective against other bacteria that cause them. Uva ursi can be used both preventatively and to treat infections.

In one impressive double-blind study, 57 women who suffered recurrent urinary tract infections were given either a placebo or uva ursi for one year. Five of the twenty-seven women given the placebo had a recurrence of infection, but none of the thirty women given uva ursi did (*Curr Ther Res* 1993). This study shows that regular use is safe and effective for preventing urinary tract infections.

Herbalist Michael Tierra says that uva ursi is also good for treating blood in the urine. Clinically, Linda has found uva ursi to help flush out the system when stones are involved, as well as other problems that cause blood or inflammation of the urinary tract. For stones, she usually combines the herb with gravel root and marshmallow, although aloe and IP6 could be used as well.

> *[Uva ursi] is simply the best herb for getting rid if UTIs and keeping them from coming back.*

As a tea, infuse three grams and drink up to four cups a day. As a powdered herb in pill form, take 10–12 grams a day. Take either 3–5ml of the tincture three times a day or 3ml of the extract up to four times a day. If you are using a solid extract of uva ursi standardized for 10% arbutin as a pill, take 250–500mg a day.

Uva ursi can cause nausea and vomiting in sensitive individuals, and it should not be used while pregnant or breast feeding. It should not be given to children under 12.

There are no other cautions. Many sources say that you should not take uva ursi for more than a week, although the study discussed above found no problem with taking uva ursi for a year. Uva ursi only works in alkaline urine, so it should not be taken with substances that cause acidic urine.

valerian *(Valeriana officinalis)*

For cats it is a treat not unlike catnip; for us valerian is simply one of the best herbs for insomnia that there is. Many herbalists hail valerian as the most important sedative herb of them all. It is the herbal superstar of sleep, with dozens of studies hailing it as the conqueror of insomnia. Valerian first helps you fall asleep and then helps you sleep more restfully with less night-time awakening. Equally importantly, valerian does all this with none of the morning hangover effect that is so common with sleeping pills. The only problem with valerian is the smell, but try telling your cat that: felines go crazy over it. The smelliness problem, however, can be avoided by taking valerian in pill form.

All kinds of early studies demonstrated this herb's ability to ease people into sleep faster without a hangover effect the next day. One double-blind, placebo-controlled study significantly improved sleep in 89% of people, with 44% of them reporting perfect sleep. The herb helped people fall asleep faster and produced a better quality sleep (*Pharmacol Biochem Behav* 1989).

Recently, valerian has made its case against benzodiazepines, the most commonly used insomnia medications. The first head-to-head challenge came in the year 2000 when valerian went up against the drug oxazepam. Seventy-five insomniacs were given either 600mg of valerian extract or the drug thirty minutes before bed for four weeks. Sleep quality improved significantly in both groups and the herb was just as effective as the drug – more effective really since it beat the drug on side effects. Also of great interest, since benzodiazepines are currently the most popular drug for anxiety, was that valerian equaled the drug on anxiety scores (*Forsch Komplementarmed Klass Naturheilkd*). The rematch occurred two years later. In a six-week double-blind study of 202 insomniacs, the herb again came out on top with 82.2% of the valerian group reporting very good results compared to 73.4% in the drug group (*Eur J Med Res* 2002).

Traditional herbalists often like to blend herbs instead of using them singly, and several studies have put valerian to the test in combination with other relaxing herbs. Two especially promising combinations are valerian with hops or with lemon balm. The valerian-hops combination helps people fall asleep significantly faster and to wake up less often (*Eur J Med Res* 2000). This same combination has proven to be as effective as benzodiazepines for sleep disorders, without producing the withdrawal symptoms that the drug produced (*Wien Med Wochenschr* 1998). At least two other studies on this combination have found the same positive results.

Another excellent combination for insomnia is valerian-lemon balm. At least two studies have shown this combination to work (*Psychopharmacotherapy* 1996; *Fitoterapia* 1999) and a third found it to have benefits over the sleeping drug Halcion. While the herbal combination was as good as the drug at helping people fall asleep and at improving the quality of sleep, the herbs were better because the drug group (but not the herb group) felt hungover the next day and had trouble concentrating (*Therapiewoche* 1992).

Other good choices that we have seen work wonders clinically are valerian with St. John's wort, to further increase deep sleep; or with lemon verbena; or with skullcap, for those that can't stop repetitive thoughts; or with motherwort, for those who need an antispasmodic. It also combines well with passionflower, for those with anxiety; and with 5-HTP, for those with fibromyalgia or anxiety, depression, or insomnia.

Valerian's use for anxiety has been validated by a number of studies. It is also used for children with behavioural hyperactivity or learning disabilities. In one interesting study, 74.4% of children with disorders ranging from nervous restlessness to sleep disorders, anxiety, headaches, learning disorders, nail biting, and thumb sucking had good or very good results with valerian (*Medizinische Welt* 1975).

Like so many relaxing herbs, valerian also has antispasmodic properties. This makes it a good herb for muscle cramps, spasms and pain, as well as for epilepsy, colic, headaches, and menstrual pain.

Valerian may also be a useful herb for the heart. Daniel Mowrey, Ph.D., reports that valerian can lower blood pressure and help correct arrhythmias. James Duke, Ph.D., adds that it increases blood flow to the heart and improves its pumping ability.

Valerian as a tea tastes terrible. But if you do decide to take it as a tea, make an infusion of 1–2 teaspoons (5–10g) of the root per cup of water and drink it as necessary. Unlike most roots, valerian is infused and not decocted so as not to destroy the important volatile oils. The pot must be covered to prevent their escape. If you are using the tincture, 1–3ml can be taken three times daily for anxiety or as an antispasmodic, or as a single dose of 5ml 30–45 minutes before bed for insomnia. As a pill made from the dried root, use 1.5–2 grams either before bed or as needed. If the valerian is standardized as an extract, take 150–300mg standardized for 0.8% valeric acid, or 300–500mg standardized for 0.5% volatile oils 30–45 minutes before going to sleep. If you are using valerian for anxiety, you can take a morning dose of the standardized extract as well, according to Donald Brown, N.D.

One of the great benefits of valerian is its remarkable safety, even for long term use. There are no contraindications, side effects or drug interactions. Valerian is safe to use while pregnant or breast feeding. It should not be used, however, in children under the age of three. At proper doses, valerian does not lead to addiction or dependence. It does not impair reaction time, alertness or concentration, and should not impair ability to drive or operate machinery.

Many herbalists hail valerian as the most important sedative herb of them all. It is the herbal superstar of sleep, with dozens of studies hailing it as the conqueror of insomnia... Traditional herbalists often like to blend herbs instead of using them singly, and several studies have put valerian to the test in combination with other relaxing herbs. Two especially promising combinations are valerian with hops or with lemon balm.

wild cherry bark

(Prunus serotina)

Wild cherry bark is excellent both for calming the respiratory nerves and for digestive weakness. It is therefore used for coughs, including whooping cough, bronchitis, sore throat, asthma, ulcers, gastritis, diarrhea, dysentery, and colitis. It is especially useful in irritating coughs. For coughs, it is often combined with other herbs, such as, elecampane, crampbark, lobelia, comfrey, coltsfoot, licorice, horehound, and ginger (see Safety section for comfrey and coltsfoot).

The dose of wild cherry bark is 2–4g a day. It can be taken as a tea by infusing one teaspoon (5g) per cup of water three times a day or as needed. Herbalist Michael Tierra says that high heat weakens its cough relieving properties and suggests that wild cherry bark be infused in cool water overnight. Warm it slightly and drink it as often as needed. As a tincture, take 1–4ml three or four times a day.

There are no side effects, contraindications or drug interactions for wild cherry bark. However, you should not exceed the recommended dose or use it for prolonged periods of time. Most sources, including the women's herbals we consulted, do not contraindicate wild cherry bark during pregnancy; however, one source says that its safety is not yet established and Brinker speculatively says not to use it. So, perhaps for now, it should be avoided. No one says not to use it while breast feeding.

Herbs can be used to prevent disease as well as to treat them. And if more people used them regularly, we would be a lot healthier. Best general herbs that pretty much everyone can take to stay healthy (see potential interactions in book):
- Milk thistle: to detoxify pollution and chemicals and as an antioxidant that rebuilds and cleanses the liver, including damaged liver cells
- Gingko: a good general antioxidant for memory and circulation
- Any one of grape seed, pine bark, green tea, rosemary, sage, turmeric – good general antioxidants for good overall health

white willow bark   (Salix alba)

Money may not grow on trees, but Aspirin does. It grows on willow trees. White willow bark is a herbal painkiller. It contains substances that are transformed in the body to salicin and then to salicylic acid. Salicylic acid is the precursor of acetylsalicylic acid, or Aspirin. Like white willow bark, Aspirin kills pain; unlike Aspirin, white willow bark doesn't effect your stomach. In fact, side effects with white willow bark are very rare: it's a natural Aspirin without the side effects.

The painkilling prowess of white willow bark has been known for thousands of years. The ancient Greeks used it for gout and other inflammatory joint diseases. On our own continent, First Nations healers used it for fever, colds, asthma, and pain, including low back pain.

Today, nature's Aspirin is used much the same way. White willow bark is analgesic, anti-inflammatory and anti-fever. Herbalist David Hoffmann says to use it for arthritis, gout, headache, fever, and mild diarrhea. Herbalist Michael Tierra adds sciatic and neuralgic pains, and James Duke, Ph.D., says not to forget toothache. In Germany, the *Commission E* approves white willow bark for fever, rheumatic ailments and headaches.

Research has found the same results as tradition. When 78 people with osteoarthritis were given either 1,360mg of white willow bark, containing 240mg of salicin, or a placebo every day for four weeks, there was a statistically significant difference in favour of the herb (Schmid, 1998).

Modern research has confirmed not only the ancient use of white willow bark for arthritis, but for back pain too. Chrubasik reports data showing that white willow bark, containing 240mg of salicin, did a better job of pain killing than conventional treatment in people with low back pain. Then in 2000, Chrubasik studied 191 people with chronic low back pain that had been acting up usually for more than three months. The study was double-blinded, giving the patients either white willow bark or a placebo. The white willow bark extract contained 15% salicin, and they were given either 120 or 240mg salicin a day for one month. She wanted to see how many people would be free of pain without drugs for five days in the final week. The answer: 6% in the placebo group,

21% in the low dose willow group, and 39% in the high dose willow group. The 120mg group was significantly better than the placebo group after two weeks; the 240mg group took only one week to significantly pass the placebo. The difference in improvement became greater and greater over the next three weeks. Significantly more people on the placebo had to take drugs for their pain during all four weeks (*Am J Med*).

One interesting surprise emerged from this study: 240mg of salicin is the equivalent of 50mg of Aspirin, which is not enough to act as a painkiller. But it was enough in this study, suggesting that other things are working in white willow bark along with the salicin.

One to two teaspoons (5–10g) of white willow bark can be decocted for five to ten minutes and drunk three to four times a day as a tea. The dried bark can also be taken in pill form at a dose of 1–3g three times a day. As a tincture, take 5–8ml three times a day, and as an extract, take 1–2ml three times a day. White willow will often be standardized for salicin content. The *German Commission E* recommends 60–120mg of salicin but, as the recent studies show, 240mg of salicin a day may be a more effective dose.

Although the effects of white willow bark are similar to Aspirin, the safety, side effects and interactions are very different. First of all, white willow is free of Aspirin's damaging effect on the stomach. White willow bark also does not act as a blood thinner the way Aspirin does. Though it has a weak but significant effect on platelet aggregation, according to research done by Krivoy and Brook, this effect probably only matters for people with impaired platelet function. They say that there is no clinical evidence that people who use white willow bark for back pain are affecting platelet aggregation.

White willow bark is extremely safe. According to the *Commission E*, although theoretically white willow bark could have drug interactions similar to Aspirin's, there is actually no indication of this in the literature or the studies done to date.

There is no restriction for pregnant or nursing women, and there is no evidence that the herb should be contraindicated in small children with flu due to concerns about Aspirin and Reyes Syndrome.

wild indigo
(Baptisia tinctoria)

It may not taste good, but wild indigo is simply one of the best herbs there is for infections. The root of this little-discussed plant should come to mind whenever there is a severe infection. It is a potent anti-inflammatory that marshals the body's defences against infection. Wild indigo has antibiotic, antiviral, alterative, antiseptic, and strong anti-inflammatory actions. It is used for the most severe infections, including those with foul discharge and blood poisoning. Wild indigo is also used for infections of the ear, nose, mouth, and throat. It is used for swollen lymph glands as well as laryngitis and tonsillitis.

Other key uses of wild indigo include malignant ulcers, putrid ulcerations, diphtheria, tonsillitis, typhoid, dysentery, meningitis, leucorrhea, and ulceration of the cervix. Externally, it helps infected ulcers and sore nipples. According to Tierra, it combines well with bloodroot into an ointment and can be used for treating tumours, cancers, boils, and ulcers. Obtain experienced advice first.

We have personally seen wild indigo, combined with, myrrh, echinacea and goldenseal, heal surgical incisions that would not heal and were putrefying, even in diabetics, after antibiotics had failed. Wild indigo is also commonly combined with echinacea and thuja in a very well studied immunity formula known as Esberitox.

To take as a tea, herbalist David Hoffmann says to decoct 1/2–1 teaspoon (2–5g) of the root and drink three times daily. Another source gives the lower dose of 0.5–1g three times a day as a tea. Herbalist Michael Tierra suggests taking only one tablespoon of the tea every 3–4 hours. You can also take 1–2ml of the tincture three times daily.

There are no side effects when wild indigo is taken at the recommended dosage. It is speculated that wild indigo should not be used long term – more than two to three weeks – except under the supervision of a qualified practitioner. Brinker says that you should not use this herb if you have hyperemia, or excess blood in the vessels supplying a part of the body.

It is speculated that wild indigo should not be used by pregnant women. However, it should be noted that Esberitox has been established to be safe for pregnant women. Esberitox delivers 90mg of wild indigo per day. Use during breast feeding is fine.

wild yam
(*Dioscorea villosa*)

Yam has become a fairly controversial herb in the past few years due to the presence of diosgenin. Diosgenin can, in a laboratory, be turned into progesterone and testosterone. However, this conversion does not occur in the body. Because these hormonal precursors may have similar properties to the hormones, wild yam may still have similar effects.

Wild yam is an antispasmodic herb that is valuable in cases of colic, colitis and Crohn's, irritable bowel syndrome, and abdominal and menstrual cramps. It is also useful when suffering from gas. Gallstones and liver problems can also benefit from yam. It is a wonderful herb for clearing liver problems.

Wild yam is a very good anti-inflammatory and is excellent for rheumatism and rheumatoid arthritis. It also has some benefits for the heart. It has helped patients who have high blood pressure and atherosclerosis. Yam has been shown to lower triglycerides while raising the good HDL cholesterol.

As a herb for women, wild yam has been used for normalizing hormones and, in addition to menstrual cramps, it can be used for infertility, miscarriage, morning sickness, menopause, fibroids, and endometriosis.

Wild yam can be taken in pill form at a dose of 1g of the dried powdered root three times a day. To make a tea, decoct 1–2 teaspoons (5–10g) of the dried powdered root and drink it three times a day. As a tincture, take 2–4ml three times a day.

Wild yam is nontoxic and has no side effects even when used long term. Brinker says not to use wild yam if you have bile duct obstruction caused by impacted gallstones, bile duct inflammation, or bile duct or pancreatic cancer. He also says not to use it in jaundice caused by hemolytic anemia or other causes of excess bilirubin, acute or severe liver disease, liver cancer, or intestinal spasm. It must be noted, though, that intestinal spasm is one of the common traditional uses of wild yam.

As for pregnancy, two sources say that the safety of wild yam has not been established. However, neither Brinker nor the American Herbal Products Association's *Botanical Safety Handbook*, two very authoritative sources, say that this herb should be avoided during pregnancy. Furthermore, not only do none of our women's herbals contraindicate it during pregnancy, but several experts on women's herbs recommend it. Tori Hudson, N.D., and herbalist Rosemary Gladstar say to use it for morning sickness and for threatened miscarriage, and herbalist Amanda McQuade Crawford also recommends it for the latter.

Wormwood (*Artemisia absinthium and Artemisia annua*)

An aptly named herb, wormwood is primarily used to expel worms and parasites and to tone digestion. Its anti-inflammatory properties make it useful for treating inflammation in the digestive tract as well as to treat various aches and pains, much like white willow bark. It is a very powerful bitter and can therefore be used to stimulate the digestive process, including improving appetite. Wormwood is used for gastritis, jaundice, hepatitis, fevers, and liver problems.

A relative of wormwood, *Artemisia annua's* most exciting use is its ability to cure malaria. According to Terry Willard, Ph.D., *Artemisia annua* has been used for malaria for over 2,000 years. It destroys the membranes of parasites, causing them to starve to death. Herbalist Michael Tierra says that clinical studies using artemisinin, a compound found in *Artemisia annua*, have demonstrated 100% cure rate in 485 cases of tertian malaria and a 92.7% cure rate in 105 cases of subtertian cerebral malaria. The U.S. army is considering using *Artemisia annua* as a treatment for drug-resistant malaria: and research at the Walter Reed Army Research Institute has proven its effectiveness. It is being endorsed as a natural alternative to chloroquine to prevent malaria when travelling. When we went into malaria country last year – Thailand and Cambodia – we tried *Artemisia annua*, and we're still alive (although, to be honest, we hardly saw a mosquito).

In another study, the wormwood component artemisinin was given to 2,099 people with malaria. It reversed the symptoms in every one of them. Willard says that this discovery is especially important because the mosquitos in southeast Asia are becoming resistant to quinine and chloroquine. And the drugs often can produce side effects.

James Duke, Ph.D., says that there are components other than artemisinin that make *Artemisia annua* effective against malaria, so he recommends using the whole herb. Also, *Artemisia annua* helps to cool the body, making it a good herb to use when travelling to very hot countries where malaria is a factor.

Wormwood is such an effective pesticide that it has traditionally been used in gardens to get rid of unwanted visitors.

You should not exceed the recommended dose of wormwood, but the experts don't agree on exactly what that dose is. For the infusion, the low end is about 1.5g per cup two to three times a day; the mid range is 1/2–1 teaspoon (2–5g) three times a day; and the high end is 1–2 teaspoons (5–10g) three times a day. For the tincture, the low end is about 0.5–1ml (10–20 drops) fifteen minutes before each meal, and the high end is 1–4ml three times a day.

As for *Artemisia annua*, Terry Willard told us that to prevent malaria, he gives 300–600mg of *Artemisia annua* twice a day, starting three days before travelling and continuing until one week after returning home. Because of the bitter taste, he usually uses capsules. We used the tincture and it wasn't so bad. Willard recommends 20–40 drops two to three times a day for brave tincture users like us. If you are unlucky enough to actually have to treat malaria, he says to increase the dose to 3–9 grams – and even as high as 24 grams – a day.

Wormwood should not be used long term, although Brinker says that this applies only to the alcoholic extract (tincture) and not the tea or pill. Exceeding the recommended dose or taking wormwood long term (more than four weeks) could lead to side effects. Short term use of the tea or tincture (two to four weeks) produces no side effects. Actually, one study reports that less than 1ml of the tincture three times a day for a full nine months produced no side effects. But for now, to be sure, you should probably not use it for more than a month.

Wormwood has no contraindications or drug interactions and no side effects when used at the right dose for the right amount of time. It should not be used during pregnancy, and one authoritative source says not to use it while breast feeding (although several other good sources do not give the breast feeding warning).

These concerns do not seem to apply to *Artemisia annua*, which, in the American Herbal Products Association's *Botanical Safety Handbook*, receives only a "do not use during pregnancy" warning. Most other books do not include this herb.

If Herbs and Drugs are Used at the Same Time, are Interactions Possible?

Often the answer is yes. Sometimes interactions are possible. Though interactions are always thought of as negative, remember that interactions are often beneficial. Herbs may interact with drugs by reducing the drug's side effects. Herbs and vitamins might correct nutritional deficiencies caused by drugs. Herbs might also enhance the action of the drug. If the herb does enhance the action of the drug, have your doses monitored as they may need to be adjusted. Occasionally, the interaction is negative and needs to be avoided.

Yarrow *(Achillea millefolium)*

Yarrow has been used for hundreds of years by people all over the world. It is rumoured to have been used to help the Greek mythological figure Achilles heal his wounds. Rosemary Gladstar presents a version of the legend that says his mother dipped him in a bath of yarrow when he was born to protect him, but she held him by his heel while doing it. And, of course, that is the place where he was wounded: the only part of him not to be bathed in yarrow. More commonly, Achilles is said to have been dipped in the river Styx but many sources say the botanical name *"Achillea"* was given to this magical herb to commemorate Achilles' use of it to treat his wounds. And certainly it was used by the ancient Europeans to heal battle wounds. Yarrow was also used to heal battle wounds during World War I. In North America, it was used by the Aboriginal people to cure colds and flus and gastrointestinal problems.

Yarrow also has a strong association with witchcraft and oracles. It has this reputation for witchcraft because it was widely used by the wise women healers of Europe. It has associations with being a "flying herb," Gladstar says, and for "calling in the spirits" (don't try this without supervision by a qualified herbalist!). In China, it was traditionally used to help cast the circle for consulting the I Ching, an ancient book of wisdom.

Today, yarrow has a wide range of uses. It is commonly used as a herb for colds, flus and fevers because of its diaphoretic, or sweat-inducing, properties. For this use, it is often combined with elder flower and peppermint.

Yarrow can also lower blood pressure and stimulate digestion, as well as relieve gas and indigestion. It is used for cramp-like or bilious conditions of the digestive tract, to stimulate appetite, and for spasmodic complaints of the digestive tract.

The ability of yarrow to dry up excessive bleeding – which made it work for Achilles and others who were wounded – makes it a very useful herb for many kinds of hemorrhaging. It can be taken internally or crushed and applied externally for wounds that bleed badly. Topically, it is good for hemorrhoids. It can also be used for heavy menstrual bleeding, or menorrhagia, and it can be used for the opposite purpose, to bring on delayed or absent periods (amenorrhea). To lessen the profuse bleeding of menorrhagia, it should be taken for several days before menstruation begins. It can also prevent excessive bleeding following childbirth.

Yarrow has other uses as a herb for women. It is excellent for menstrual cramps and for aiding in labour and childbirth.

Take 4.5 grams of yarrow a day. Or drink it as a tea: infuse 1–2 teaspoons (5–10g) three times a day. If you are using the tea to treat a fever, drink it hourly. If you prefer tinctures and extracts, take 2–5ml of the tincture or 1–2ml of the extract three times a day.

Yarrow is a very safe herb. There are no side effects, contraindications or drug interactions. One – and only one – source says it may increase sensitivity to sunlight. It should not be used during pregnancy, but is fine while breast feeding (though that same single source says not to; all the other authoritative contraindication texts say it is fine). Gladstar even says that during pregnancy, it is only in the early stages that yarrow should not be used and that it has never been known to actually precipitate an abortion as feared. Still, the majority of the sources say not to risk it.

yohimbe bark   *(Pausinystalia yohimbe, Corynanthe yohimbe)*

Yohimbe bark comes from Africa, where it was used in tribal marriage rituals. And, interestingly, the herb is said to be an aphrodisiac for both men and women. It is still used for the same purpose today. Yohimbe is a powerful aphrodisiac that may benefit both men and women. It dilates blood vessels and, therefore, increases blood flow to the penis, helping in cases of erectile dysfunction, the inability to attain or maintain an erection. By dilating blood vessels of the skin and mucous membranes, it helps the blood to rise closer to the surface of the sex organs, so it can also help with lack of desire or to increase stimulation in women.

Although there have been some studies on yohimbe, it is not a well-studied herb. The active ingredient, yohimbine, is more well studied, and it is used in pharmaceutical drugs. It has been shown to be effective for impotence of vascular, diabetic and psychogenic origins. It improves the quality and the length of time of an erection. The *German Commission E's* unapproved monograph for yohimbe reports its unofficial use for sexual disorders, as an aphrodisiac, and for feebleness and exhaustion.

You can take an amount of yohimbe that contains 5–6mg of yohimbine three to four times a day. The traditional dose of the tincture is 5–10 drops three times a day. To make a tea, Rosemary Gladstar says to decoct one ounce of yohimbe bark in two cups of boiling water for no more than four minutes, then turn the heat down and let it simmer for twenty minutes more. Sip it slowly an hour before you need it.

Many herbalists and practitioners find this herb very difficult to work with. It is very powerful and stimulating and can cause a host of side effects that, though rare, include anxiety, nervous excitation, tremours, insomnia, dizziness, nausea and vomiting, increased blood pressure, and rapid heart rate.

Yohimbe should not be used by anyone who is suffering from schizophrenia, depression, bipolar depression, or anxiety. Don't use it if you have high blood pressure, angina, heart disease, or kidney disease. It is also speculated that you should not use yohimbe long term if you have liver disease, chronic inflammation of the sexual organs or prostate, or if you are elderly. It is also speculated that you should not give it to children (although we do not know why you would give it to children). You should probably not use it if you are pregnant or breast feeding.

Yohimbe may interact with tricylcic and monoamine oxidase inhibitor antidepressants, hypotensive drugs, phenothiazines, clonidine, alprazolam, naloxone, brimonidine, and sympathominetics (drugs like epinephrine that stimulate the sympathetic nervous system).

We could go into more detail about how yohimbe and these drugs negatively interact with each other, but the point is that you probably should avoid using this herb, and certainly shouldn't use it without supervision. There are safer alternatives available, like Muira puama and Ginkgo biloba.

COMMONLY USED ABBREVIATIONS

Abstr Gen Meet Am Soc Microbiol	Abstracts of the General Meeting of the American Society for Microbiology American Society for Microbiology General Meeting
Acta Nerv Super	Activitas Nervosa Superior
Acta Otalaryngol	Acta Oto-Laryngologica
Acta Physiol Hung	Acta Physiologica Hungarica
Acta Physiol Pharmacol Bulg	Acta Physiologica et Pharmacologica Bulgarica
Aliment Pharmacol Ther	Alimentary Pharmacology & Therapeutics
Atlern Ther Health Med	Alternative Therapies in Health and Medicine
Altern Med Rev	Alternative Medicine Review: a Journal of Clinical Therapeutic
Atlern Ther Health Med	Alternative Therapies in Health and Medicine
Altern Med Rev	Alternative Medicine Review: a Journal of Clinical Therapeutic
Am J Clin Nutr	The American Journal of Clinical Nutrition
Am J Med	American Journal of Medicine
Am J Epidemiol	American Journal of Epidemiology
Am J Chin Med	American Journal of Chinese Medicine
Am J Dis Child	American Journal of Diseases of Children
Am J Cardiol	The American Journal of Cardiology
Ann Ottalmol Clin Ocul	Annali di Ottalmologia e Clinica Oculista
Ann Ottal Clin Ocul	Annali di Ottalmologia e Clinica Oculista
Ann Trop Med Parasitol	Annals of Tropical Medicine and Parasitology
Ann Urol	Annales d'Urologie
Ann Pharmacother	The Annals of Pharmacotherapy
Anesth Analg	Anesthesia and Analgesia
Anticancer Res	Anticancer Research
Antimicrob Agents Chemother	Antimicrobial Agents and Chemotherapy
Arch Intern Med	Archives of Internal Medicine

Arch Ital Urol Nefrol Androl	ArchivioItaliano di Urologia, Nefrologia, Aandrologia
Organo Ufficiale dell'Associazione per laRricerca in Urologia	Urological, Nephrological, and Andrological Sciences
Arch Pediatr Adolesc Med	Archives of Pediatrics & Adolescent Medicine
Archives Neurology	Archives of Neurology
Arch Gynecol Obstet	Archives of Gynecology and Obstetrics
Arthritis Rheum	Arthritis and Rheumatism
Arzneimforsch	Arzneimittelforschung
Arzneim-Forsch Drug Res	Arzneimittel-Forschung Drug Research
Aviat Space Environ Med	Aviation, Space, and Environmental Medicine
Blood Coagulation Fibrinolysis	Blood Coagulation & Fibrinolysis: an International Journal in Haemostasis and Thrombosis
BMJ	BMJ (Clinical research ed.)
Biochem Pharm	Biochemical Pharmacology
Biomed Pharmacother	Biomedicine & Pharmacotherapy
Br Med J	British Medical Journal
Br J Clin Pract	The British Journal of Clinical Practice
Br J Clin Pract Suppl	British Journal of Clinical Practice Supplement
British J Clin Pharmacol	British Journal of Clinical Pharmacology
Br J Urol	British Journal of Urology
Boll Ocul	Bollettino di Oculistica
Bull Soc Opthalmol Fr	Bulletin des Sociétés d'Ophtalmologie de
Can J Cardiol	The Canadian Journal of Cardiology
Cancer Epidemiol Biomarkers Prev	Cancer Epidemiology, Biomarkers & Prevention: A Publication of the American Association for Cancer Research
Cardiovasc Drug Rev	Cardiovascular Drug Reviews
Chin Med	Chinese Medicine
CJIM	Chinese Journal of Integrative Medicine
Clin Physiol Biochem	Clinical Physiology and Biochemistry
Clin Drug Invest	Clinical Drug Investigation
Clin Cancer Res	Clinical Cancer Research: an Official Journal of the American Association for Cancer Research
Clin Immunol	Clinical Immunology
Curr Med Res Opin	Current Medical Research and Opinion

Curr Ther Res	Current Therapeutic Research, Clinical and Experimental
Curr Ther Res Clin Exp	Current Therapeutic Research, Clinical and Experimental
Deutsche Apotheker Zeitung	Deutsche Apotheker-Zeitung
Drugs Exp Clin Res	Drugs Under Experimental and Clinical Research
Eksp Klin Farmakol	Eksperimental'naia i Klinicheskaia Farmakologiia
Endocrinol Jpn	Endocrinologia Japonica
ESCOP	European Scientific Cooperative on Phytotherapy
Eur J Nutr	European Journal of Nutrition
Eur J Cancer Prev	European Journal of Cancer Prevention: the Official Journal of the
ECP	European Cancer Prevention Organisation
Eur J Clin Nutr	European Journal of Clinical Nutrition
Eur J Med Res	European Journal of Medical Research
Eur J Obstet Gynecol Reprod Biol	European Journal of Obstetrics, Gynecology, and Reproductive Biology
Eur J Cancer	European Journal of Cancer
Fam Pract	Family Practice
Fortschr Med	Fortschritte der Medizin
Forsch Komplementarmed Klass Naturheilkd	Forschende Komplementärmedizin und Klassische Naturheilkunde
High Alt Med Biol	High Altitude Medicine & Biology
Hong Kong Med J	Hong Kong Medical Journal Xianggang yi xue za zhi / Hong Kong Academy of Medicine
Hum Psychopharmacol	Human Psychopharmacology
IMAJ	The Israel Medical Association Journal
Ind J Dermatol Venereol Leprol	Indian Journal of Dermatology, Venereology and Leprology
Indian J Pharmacology	Indian Journal of Pharmacology
Indian J Physiol Pharmacol	Indian Journal of Physiology and Pharmacology
Ind Pediatr	Indian Pediatrics
Indian J Med Res	The Indian Journal of Medical Research
Indian J Opthalmol	Indian Journal of Ophthalmology
Indian J Exp Biol	Indian Journal of Experimental Biology
Infect Immun	Infection and Immunity

International Clin Psychopharmacol	International Clinical Psychopharmacology
Internat J Immunother	International Journal of Immunotherapy
Int Conf Aids	International Conference On Aids
Int J Clin Pharmacol	International Journal of Clinical Pharmacology, Therapy and Toxicology
Inter J Clin Pharmacol Ther	International Journal of Clinical Pharmacology and Therapeutics
Int J Clin Pharmacol Res	International Journal of Clinical Pharmacology Research
Int J Neurosci	The International Journal of Neuroscience
Int J Epidemiol	International Journal of Epidemiology
Int J Impot Res	International Journal of Impotence Research: Official Journal of the International Society for Impotence Research
Int J Cancer	International Journal of Cancer
Int J Tissure React	International Journal of Tissue Reactions
Inflamm Res	Inflammation research: official journal of the European Histamine Research Society
Irish Med Journ	Irish Medical Journal
J Adv Nurs	Journal of Advanced Nursing
J Assoc Physicians India	The Journal of the Association of Physicians of India
J Urol	The Journal of Urology
J Gen Med	The Journal of Gene Medicine
J Am Acad Dermatol	Journal of the American Academy of Dermatology
J Rheumatol	The Journal of Rheumatology
J Ethnopharmacol	Journal of Ethnopharmacology
J Women Health & Gender Based Med	Journal of Women's Health & Gender Based Medicine
J Dent Med	The Journal of Dental Medicine
J Periodontal Res	Journal of Periodontal Research
J Obstet Gynecol Br Common	The Journal of Obstetrics and Gynaecology of the British Commonwealth
J Med	Journal of Medicine
J Med Assoc Thai	Journal of the Medical Association of Thailand
J Mal Vasc	Journal des Maladies Vasculaires

J Alt Comp Med	Journal of Alternative and Complementary Medicine
J Altern Compliment Med	Journal of Alternative and Complementary Medicine
J Am Acad Child Adolesc Psychiatry	Journal of the American Academy of Child and Adolescent Psychiatry
J of Ag Food Chem	Journal of Agricultural and Food Chemistry
J Natl Cancer Inst	Journal of the National Cancer Institute
J Travel Med	Journal of Travel Medicine: Official Publication of the International Society of Travel Medicine and the Asia Pacific Travel Health Association.
J Psychiat Res	Journal of Psychiatric Research
J Drug Dev Clin Pract	Journal of Drug Development and Clinical Practice
J Sex Educ Ther	Journal of Sex Education and Therapy
J Sex Marital Therapy	Journal of Sex & Marital Therapy
J Ind Med Assoc	Journal of the Indian Medical Association
J Res Indian Med	The Journal of Research in Indian Medicine
J Fr Opthalmol	Journal Français d'Ophtalmologie
J Orthomolec Med	the Journal of Orthomolecular Medicine
J Nutr	The Journal of Nutrition
J Epidemiol	Journal of Epidemiology / Japan Epidemiological Association
J Am Coll Toxicol	Journal of the American College of Toxicology
J Clin Pharmacol	Journal of Clinical Pharmacology
J Clin Pharm Ther	Journal of Clinical Pharmacy and Therapeutics
J Clin Endocrinol Metab	The Journal of Clinical Endocrinology and Metabolism
J Clin Phychopharmacol	Journal of Clinical Psychopharmacology
J Hepatol	Journal of Hepatology
J International Med Res	The Journal of International Medical Research
J Dermatol	The Journal of Dermatology
J Invest Dermatol	The Journal of Investigative Dermatology
J Gastroenterol	Journal of Gastroenterology
J Geriatr Psychiatry Neurol	Journal of Geriatric Psychiatry and Neurology

J Pediatr	The Journal of Pediatrics
J Tradit Chin Med	Journal of Traditional Chinese Medicine Chung i tsa chih ying wen pan
JAMA	The Journal of the American Medical Association
Jpn J Canc Res	Japanese Journal of Cancer Research
Life Sci	Life Sciences
Mech Ageing Dev	Mechanisms of Ageing and Development
Med Welt	Die Medizinische Welt
Med Hypotheses	Medical Hypotheses
Med J Aust	The Medical Journal of Australia
Medizinische Welt	Die Medizinische Welt
Meth Find Exp Clin Pharmacol	Methods and Findings in Experimental and Clinical Pharmacology
Min Cardioangiol	Minerva Cardioangiologica
Min Ginecol	Minerva Ginecologica.
Min Angiol	Minerva Angiol
Mol Med	Molecular Medicine
Mol Urol	Molecular Urology
Munch Med Wschr	Münchener Medizinische Wochenschrift
Nat Immun Cell Growth Reg	Natural Immunity and Cell Growth Regulation
Neuropsychobiol	Neuropsychobiology
New Engl J Med	The New England Journal of Medicine
NY State J Med	New York State Journal of Medicine
Nutr Res	Nutrition Research
Nutr Cancer	Nutrition and Cancer
Obstet Gynecol	Obstetrics and Gynecology
Panminerva Med	Panminerva Medica
Pediatr Res	Pediatric Research
Pharmazie	Die Pharmazie
Phytomed	Phytomedicine
Phytother Res	Phytotherapy Research
Phytother	Phytotherapy
Planta Med	Planta Medica
Prev Med	Preventive Medicine
Psychopharmacol Bull	Psychopharmacology Bulletin
Prensa Medica Mexicana	La Prensa Médica Mexicana
Phlebologie	Phlébologie
Proc Soc Exp Biol Med	Proceedings of the Society for Experimental Biology and Medicine. Society for Experimental Biology and Medicine

Prostate	The Prostate
Prostate Cancer Prostatic Dis	Prostate Cancer and Prostatic Diseases
Pharmacol Res	Pharmacological Research: the Official Journal of the Italian
Pharmacological Society	Pharmacological Society
Pharmacol Biochem Behav	Pharmacology, Biochemistry, and Behavior
Pharmacopsych	Pharmacopsychiatry
Quad Clin Ostet Ginecol	Quaderni di Clinica Osterica e Ginecologica
Rev Bras Med	Revista Brasileira de Medicina
The FASEB Journal	The FASEB Journal: Official Publication of the Federation of American Societies for Experimental Biology
Therapiewoche	Die Therapiewoche
Thromb Haemostat	Thrombosis and Haemostasis
Thromb Res	Thrombosis Research
Tokai J Exp Clin Med	The Tokai Journal of Experimental and Clinical Medicine
Tohoku Journal of Experimental Medicine	The Tohoku Journal of Experimental Medicine
Urol Int	Urologia Internationalis
Urologe B	Der Urologe. Ausg. B
Vutr Boles	Vutreshni Bolesti
VASA	VASA. Zeitschrift für Gefässkrankheiten. Journal for Vascular Diseases.
Wien Med Wochenschr	Wiener Medizinische Wochenschrift
Z Allg Med	Zeitschrift für Allgemeinmedizin
Zeits Allegemeinmed	Zeitschrift für Allgemeinmedizin
Z Phytother	Zeitschrift für Phytotherapie: Offizielles Organ der Ges. f. Phytotherapie e.V.

SUGGESTED READING

HERBS

Blumenthal M, Busse WR, Goldberg A, Gruenwald J, Hall T, Riggins CW, Rister R (eds). Klein S, Rister RS (trans). *The Complete German Commission E Monographs: Therapeutic Guide to Herbal Medicine*. Austin, TX: American Botanical Council, 1998.

Blumenthal M, Goldberg A, Brinckmann J (eds). *Herbal Medicine: Expanded Commission E Monographs*. Austin, TX: American Botanical Council, 2000.

Blumenthal M, Hall T, Goldberg A, Kunz T, Dinda K (eds). *The ABC Clinical Guide to Herbs*. Austin, TX: American Botanical Council, 2003.

Boon, Heather, Michael Smith. *The Botanical Pharmacy*. Kingston, ON: Quarry Press, 2000.

Brinker, Francis, N.D. *Herb Contraindications & Drug Interactions*. Sandy, Oregon: Eclectic Medical Publications, 2001 (Updates made available on-line by the author up to April, 2004).

Brown, Donald. *Herbal Prescriptions for Health & Healing*. Roseville, CA: Prima Health, 2000.

Crawford, Amanda McQuade. *Herbal Remedies for Women*. Rocklin, CA: Prima Publishing, 1997.

Duke, James. *The Green Pharmacy*. New York, NY: St. Martin's Paperbacks, 1997.

Gladstar, Rosemary. *Herbal Healing for Women*. New York, London, Toronto, Sydney, Tokyo: A Fireside Book, 1993.

Hobbs, Christopher. *Ginseng: the Energy Herb*. Loveland, CO: Interweave Press, 1996.

Hobbs, Christopher. *Medicinal Mushrooms*. Santa Cruz, CA: Botanica Press, 1995.

Hobbs, Christopher. *Vitex: The Women's Herb*. Santa Cruz, CA: Botanica Press, 1996.

Hoffmann, David. *The Herbal Handbook: A User's Guide to Medical Herbalism*. Rochester, VT: Healing Arts Press, 1998.

Hoffmann, David. *The Complete Illustrated Holistic Herbal: A Safe and Practical Guide to Making and Using Herbal Remedies*. Shaftsbury Dorset, Rockport, MA: Element Books, 1996

Jones, Kenneth. *Cat's Claw: Healing Vine of Peru*. Seattle, WA: Sylvan Press, 1995.

Mabey, Richard. *The New Age Herbalist*. New York, NY: Collier Books, 1988.

McCaleb, Robert, Evelyn Leigh, Krista Morien. *The Encyclopedia of Popular Herbs*. Roseville, CA: Prima Health, 2000.

McGuffin, M., Hobbs, C., Upton, R., Goldberg, A. American *Herbal Products Association's Botanical Safety Handbook*. Boca Raton FL: CRC Press, 1997.

Mowrey, Daniel. *Guaranteed Potency Herbs: Next Generation Herbal Medicine*. New Cannan, CT: Keats Publishing, 1990.

Mills, S., Bone, K. *Principles and Practice of Phytotherapy*. Edinburgh, London, New York, Philadelphia, St. Louis, Sydney, Toronto: Churchill Livingstone, 2000.

Mowrey, Daniel. *Herbal Tonic Therapies: Remedies from Nature's Own Pharmacy to Strengthen & Support Each Vital Body System*. New Cannan, CT: Keats Publishing, 1993.

Murray, Michael. *The Healing Power of Herbs*, 2nd ed. Rocklin, CA: Prima Publishing, 1995.

Romm, Aaviva Jill. *The Natural Pregnancy Book: Herbs, Nutrition, and Other Holistic Choices*. Freedom, CA: The Crossing Press, 1997.

Tierra, Michael. *The Way of Herbs*. New York, NY: Pocket Books, 1998.

Vogel, Virgil J. *American Indian Medicine*. Norman, USA: University of Oklahoma Press, 1970.

Weiner, Michael, Janet Weiner. *Herbs That Heal*. Mill Valley, CA: Quantum Books, 1994.

Weiss, Rudolf Fritz. *Herbal Medicine*. Beaconsfield, England: Beaconsfield Publishers,1988.

Willard, Terry. Herbs: *Their Clinical Uses*. Calgary, AB: Wild Rose College of Natural Healing, 1996.

Willard, Terry. *Textbook of Advanced Herbology*. Calgary, AB: Wild Rose College of Natural Healing, 1992.

SUPPLEMENTS AND NATURAL HEALTH

Boik, John. *Cancer & Natural Medicine: A Textbook of Basic Science and Clinical Research*. Princeton, MN: Oregon Medical Press, 1996.

Boik, John. *Natural Compounds in Cancer Therapy: Promising Nontoxic Antitumor Agents from Plants & Other Natural Sources*. Princeton, MN: Oregon Medical Press, 2001

Hudson, Tori. *Women's Encyclopedia of Natural Medicine: Alternative Therapies and Integrative Medicine*. Los Angeles, CA: Keats, 1999.

Lininger, SW., Gaby, A., Austin, S., Brown, D., Wright, J., Duncan, A. *The Natural Pharmacy: Complete Home Reference to Natural Medicine*. Roseville, CA: Prima Publishing, 1999.

Moss, Ralph W. *Cancer Therapy: the Independent Consumer's Guide to Non-Toxic Treatment & Prevention*. Brooklyn, NY: Equinox Press, 1992.

Murray, Michael. *Encyclopedia of Nutritional Supplements*. Rocklin, CA: Prima Publishing, 1996.

Murray, Michael and Pizzorno, Joseph. *Encyclopedia of Natural Medicine*, 2nd ed. Rocklin, CA: Prima Publishing, 1998.

Murray, Michael and Pizzorno, Joseph. Eds. *Textbook of Natural Medicine*. Edinburgh, London, New York, Philadelphia, St. Louis, Sydney, Toronto: Churchill Livingstone, 1999.

Murray, Michael, Tim Birdsall, Joseph Pizzorno, Paul Reilly. *How to Prevent and Treat Cancer With Natural Medicine*. New York, NY: Riverhead Books, 2002.

INDEX

abdominal pain
    artichoke for, 7
    cayenne for, 32
    cinnamon for, 42
    dong quai for, 55
    hawthorn for, 105
    kava kava for, 110
abscesses
    arnica for, 6
    black walnut for, 18
    bromelain for, 19
    cat's claw for, 29
    chickweed for, 41
Achillea millefolium, 212–13
acne
    aloe vera for, 2
    burdock for, 21–22
    chastetree berry for, 39
    green tea for, 101
    Indian myrrh for, 140
    lavender for, 117
    milk thistle for, 133
    nettle for, 142
    red clover for, 155
    sarsaparilla for, 175
    tea tree oil for, 194
acquired immune deficiency syndrome.
    See AIDS
adaptogens
    ashwagandha, 9
    Asian ginseng, 84–85
    eleuthero, 63
    rhodiola rosea, 161
    schizandra, 179
aging
    alfalfa for, 1
    aloe vera for, 2
    fo ti for, 71
    ginkgo biloba for, 78
    grape seed extract for, 96
AIDS
    Asian ginseng for, 86
    astragalus for, 10
    cat's claw for, 31
    grape seed extract for, 96
    licorice for, 122
    maitake mushroom for, 129
    reishi mushroom for, 158

shiitake mushroom for, 183, 184
    turmeric for, 196
alfalfa, 1–2
allergies
    aloe vera for, 2
    butterbur for, 23
    dong quai for, 55
    garlic for, 74
    ginkgo biloba for, 82
    grape seed extract for, 96
    licorice for, 121
    milk thistle for, 133
    nettle for, 141
    reishi mushroom for, 159–60
    rooibos for, 164
Allium sativum, 73–75
aloe vera (*Aloe vera*), 2–3
Althaea officinalis, 130–31
altitude sickness
    ginkgo biloba for, 78, 82
    reishi mushroom for, 159
Alzheimer's disease
    ginkgo biloba for, 79, 80
    grape seed extract for, 96
    muira puama for, 136
    rosemary for, 165
    sage for, 167
amenorrhoea. *See* menstruation (absent)
Ammi visnaga, 114–15
anal fissures
    cascara sagrada for, 27
    senna for, 180
Ananas comosus, 19–20
andrographis (*Andrographis paniculata*), 3–5
anemia
    anise for, 5
    arnica for, 6
    Asian ginseng for, 87
    astragalus for, 10
    black walnut for, 18
    catnip for, 28
    dandelion for, 50
    dong quai for, 55
    nettle for, 142
    pau d'arco for, 148
Angelica sinensis, 54–56
angina

circulation improvement
    bilberry for, 13, 14
    butcher's broom for, 22
    cayenne for, 32
    ginger for, 77
    hyssop for, 108
    rosemary for, 165
    schizandra for, 179
    shiitake mushroom for, 183
cirrhosis
    dandelion for, 50
    gotu kola for, 94
    licorice for, 123, 125
    milk thistle for, 131–32
Citrux x paradisi, 97–98
cleavers, 43
clover, red. *See* red clover
cold sores
    lemon balm for, 119
    licorice for, 124
    oregano for, 142
colds
    andrographis for, 3–4
    anise for, 5
    Arabian Somalian myrrh for, 138
    Asian ginseng for, 85
    astragalus for, 10
    catnip for, 28
    cayenne for, 32
    chamomile for, 35
    echinacea for, 57–58
    elder for, 60, 62
    elecampane for, 62
    eleuthero for, 64
    garlic for, 74
    hyssop for, 108
    kava kava for, 109
    licorice for, 122
    oregano for, 142
    peppermint for, 151
    red clover for, 155
    shiitake mushroom for, 183–84
    yarrow for, 212
colic
    anise for, 5
    buckthorne for, 20
    catnip for, 28
    chamomile for, 35
    fennel for, 67
    fo ti for, 72
    ginger for, 77
    peppermint for, 149
    rooibos for, 164
    valerian for, 202
    wild yam for, 208

colitis
    buckthorne for, 21
    cascara sagrada for, 27
    cat's claw for, 31
    chamomile for, 35
    dandelion for, 50
    fennel for, 67
    goldenseal for, 92
    marshmallow for, 130
    milk thistle for, 133
    pau d'arco for, 147
    peppermint for, 150
    slippery elm for, 186
    wild cherry bark for, 204
    wild yam for, 208
colon cancer
    garlic for, 74
    green tea for, 99
    shiitake mushroom for, 183
    soy for, 188
    turmeric for, 196
coltsfoot, 43–44
comfrey, 44–46
Commiphora mukul, 139–40
Commiphora myrrha, 138–39
Commiphora molmol, 138–39
common cold. *See* colds
congestive heart failure.
    See heart failure
conjunctivitis
    eyebright for, 66
constipation
    alfalfa for, 1
    aloe vera for, 2
    artichoke for, 7
    black walnut for, 18
    buckthorne for, 20
    cascara sagrada for, 27
    cayenne for, 32
    dong quai for, 55
    fennel for, 67
    milk thistle for, 133
    pau d'arco for, 147
    rhubarb for, 162
    senna for, 180–81
    triphala for, 195
convulsions
    lobelia for, 126
    motherwort for, 135
    skullcap for, 185
Corynanthe yohimbe, 213–14
coughs
    andrographis for, 4
    anise for, 5
    black cohosh for, 17

Eupatorium purpureum, 98
Euphrasia officinalis, 66
exhaustion
    ashwagandha for, 9
    skullcap for, 185
    yohimbe bark for, 214
eyebright, 66
eye problems. *See names of individual problems*
eye inflammation
    black walnut for, 18
    eyebright for, 66
eye strain
    bilberry for, 12
    eyebright for, 66

fatigue
    andrographis for, 4
    Asian ginseng for, 87
    astragalus for, 10
    kava kava for, 109
    rhodiola rosea for, 161
female problems. *See names of individual problems*
fennel, 67–68
fenugreek, 68–69
fertility problems. *See* infertility
fever
    alfalfa for, 1
    andrographis for, 4
    ashwagandha for, 9
    astragalus for, 10
    burdock for, 21–22
    calendula for, 26
    cat's claw for, 29
    catnip for, 28
    cayenne for, 32
    chickweed for, 41
    cleavers for, 43
    elder for, 60
    feverfew for, 70
    ginger for, 77
    gotu kola for, 93
    hyssop for, 108
    lemon balm for, 119
    licorice for, 122
    lobelia for, 126
    North American ginseng for, 89
    pau d'arco for, 147
    peppermint for, 151
    raspberry leaf for, 154
    turmeric for, 197
    white willow bark for, 205
    wormwood for, 209
    yarrow for, 212

feverfew, 70–71
fibrocystic breast disease
    burdock for, 21–22
    chastetree berry for, 39
    kelp for, 114
fibroids
    burdock for, 21–22
    chastetree berry for, 39
    wild yam for, 208
fibromyalgia
    valerian for, 202
flatulence. *See* gas
flu
    anise for, 5
    Asian ginseng for, 85
    astragalus for, 10
    buckthorne for, 20
    cayenne for, 32
    chamomile for, 35
    echinacea for, 58
    elder for, 60–62
    eleuthero for, 64
    garlic for, 74
    licorice for, 122
    oregano for, 142
    pau d'arco for, 148
    peppermint for, 151
    shiitake mushroom for, 184
    yarrow for, 212
fo ti, 71–72
Foeniculum vulgare, 67–68
food poisoning
    goldenseal for, 91
    lobelia for, 126
forgetfulness. *See* memory improvement
fractures
    butcher's broom for, 22
    comfrey for, 44, 46
    gotu kola for, 94
    horsetail for, 107
frost bite
    cayenne for, 32
    hyssop for, 108
fungal infections. *See names of individual infections*

Galium aparine, 43
gallstones
    artichoke for, 8
    dandelion for, 50–51
    khella for, 115
    milk thistle for, 133
    parsley for, 145
    peppermint for, 152
    turmeric for, 198

peppermint for, 151
rhodiola rosea for, 161
rosemary for, 165
sage for, 167
skullcap for, 186
valerian for, 202
white willow bark for, 205
hearing problems
ginkgo biloba for, 78, 81
heart arrhythmias. *See* arrhythmias
heart attack prevention
cayenne for, 33
ginkgo biloba for, 78
green tea for, 100
reishi mushroom for, 159
heart disease
cinnamon for, 42
eleuthero for, 63
garlic for, 73, 74
grape seed extract for, 96
green tea for, 99, 100
red clover for, 156
reishi mushroom for, 158
shiitake mushroom for, 183
soy for, 188
turmeric for, 196–97
heart failure
Asian ginseng for, 86
goldenseal for, 92
hawthorn for, 103–105
heart pain
cinnamon for, 42
motherwort for, 134
heart palpitations
black cohosh for, 15
cramp bark for, 46
kava kava for, 110
motherwort for, 134
schizandra for, 179
heartburn
chamomile for, 35
licorice for, 123
peppermint for, 152
hematuria (blood in urine)
gravel root for, 98
shepherd's purse for, 182
uva ursi for, 200
hemorrhaging
cat's claw for, 29
cayenne for, 32
nettle for, 142
pau d'arco for, 148
shepherd's purse for, 181
yarrow for, 212
hemorrhoids

Arabian Somalian myrrh for, 138
buckthorne for, 20
butcher's broom for, 22
cascara sagrada for, 27
fo ti for, 72
nettle for, 142
senna for, 180
slippery elm for, 186
yarrow for, 212
hepatitis
andrographis for, 4
cleavers for, 43
dandelion for, 50
licorice for, 123
milk thistle for, 131
reishi mushroom for, 158–59
sarsaparilla for, 175
schizandra for, 179
shiitake mushroom for, 183–84
turmeric for, 197
wormwood for, 209
herbs. *See also names of individual herbs*
contraindications, x–xi
definitive terms, ix
dosages, x
drugs and, x–xi, 193, 211
infusions and decoctions, viii
medicine kit, 166
most popular, 153
pills and liquids, viii
standardization, ix
hernia
hawthorn for, 105
herpes
aloe vera for, 2
black walnut for, 18
buckthorne for, 20
echinacea for, 59
lemon balm for, 119
licorice for, 122, 124
oregano for, 142
pau d'arco for, 148
shiitake mushroom for, 183–84
high blood pressure (hypertension)
astragalus for, 10
cayenne for, 33
dandelion for, 50
dong quai for, 54, 55
eleuthero for, 64
fo ti for, 72
garlic for, 73
ginger for, 77
green tea for, 100
hawthorn for, 103
lemon balm for, 119

Asian ginseng for, 88
pregnancy. *See* childbirth; infertility;
  contraindications for individual herbs
premature ejaculation
  rhodiola rosea for, 162
premenstrual tension. *See* PMS

prostate cancer
  garlic for, 74
  green tea for, 99, 101
  maitake mushroom for, 129
  milk thistle for, 133
  soy for, 188
  turmeric for, 196, 197
prostate, enlarged. *See* benign prostatic
hyperplasia
Prunus serotina, 204
psoriasis
  aloe vera for, 2
  black walnut for, 18
  burdock for, 21–22
  calendula for, 26
  cayenne for, 32
  chickweed for, 41
  cleavers for, 43
  gotu kola for, 93
  licorice for, 123
  milk thistle for, 133
  red clover for, 155
  sarsaparilla for, 175
Ptychopetalum olacoides, 136
purple butterbur. *See* butterbur
Pygeum africanum, 152–53
pygeum, 152–53
pyrrolizidine alkaloids (PAs)
  in butterbur, 25
  in coltsfoot, 44
  in comfrey, 45
  in gravel root, 98

radiation therapy
  Asian ginseng and, 87
  astragalus and, 10
  kelp and, 114
rashes
  aloe vera for, 2
  calendula for, 26
  chickweed for, 41
  cleavers for, 43
  rooibos for, 164
  sarsaparilla for, 175
raspberry leaf, 154–55

rectal cancer
  green tea for, 99

red clover, 155–57
red ginseng. *See* Asian ginseng
red yeast rice, 157–58
reishi mushroom, 158–60
reproductive problems. *See names of
individual problems*
respiratory problems. *See names of individual problems*
Reynaud's disease
  bilberry for, 13
  ginkgo biloba for, 78
Rhamnus catharticus, 20–21
Rhamnus purshiana, 27
Rheum palmatum, 162–63
rheumatism
  arnica for, 6
  ashwagandha for, 9
  black cohosh for, 17
  burdock for, 21–22
  cat's claw for, 29
  cayenne for, 32, 33
  cramp bark for, 46
  dandelion for, 50
  elder for, 61
  eleuthero for, 63
  feverfew for, 70
  kava kava for, 109
  motherwort for, 135
  rosemary for, 165
  wild yam for, 208
rheumatoid arthritis
  black cohosh for, 17
  bromelain for, 19
  cat's claw for, 31
  cayenne for, 33
  devil's claw for, 51–52
  ginger for, 77
  licorice for, 121
  turmeric for, 196
  wild yam for, 208
rhodiola rosea (*Rhodiola rosea*), 160–62
rhubarb, 162–63
rice, red yeast. *See* red yeast rice
Roman chamomile. *See* chamomile
rooibos, 164–65
rosemary, 165–66
Rosmarinus officinalis, 165–66
Rubus idaeus, 154–55
Ruscus aculeatus, 22–23

Saccharum officinarum, 190–93
sage, 167–68

The Young Adult's Guide to Meditation

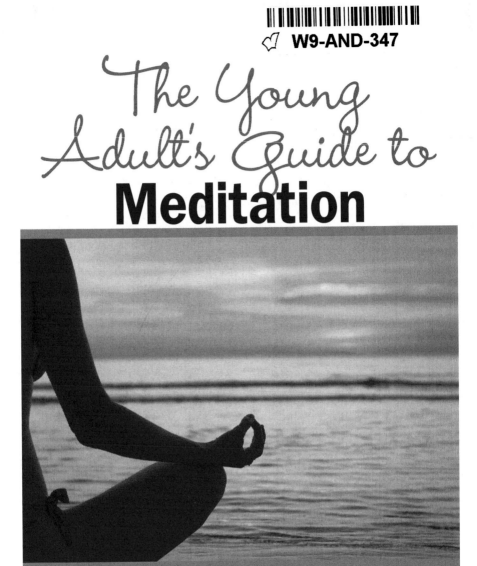

Easy Techniques that Reduce Stress and Relieve Anger, Anxiety & Depression

THE YOUNG ADULT'S GUIDE TO MEDITATION: EASY TECHNIQUES THAT REDUCE STRESS AND RELIEVE ANGER, ANXIETY & DEPRESSION

Copyright © 2016 Atlantic Publishing Group, Inc.
1405 SW 6th Avenue • Ocala, Florida 34471 • Phone 800-814-1132 • Fax 352-622-1875
Website: www.atlantic-pub.com • E-mail: sales@atlantic-pub.com
SAN Number: 268-1250

Library of Congress Cataloging-in-Publication Data
Names: Atlantic Publishing Group, issuing body.
Title: The young adult's guide to meditation : easy techniques that reduce
   stress and relieve anger, anxiety & depression.
Description: Ocala, Florida : Atlantic Publishing Group, Inc., [2015] |
   Includes bibliographical references and index.
Identifiers: LCCN 2015035966| ISBN 9781601389879 (alk. paper) | ISBN
   1601389876 (alk. paper)
Subjects: LCSH: Meditation--Juvenile literature. | Meditation--Therapeutic
   use--Juvenile literature. | Stress management for teenagers--Juvenile
   literature.
Classification: LCC BF637.M4 Y68 2015 | DDC 158.1/2--dc23 LC record available at http://lccn.loc.
gov/2015035966

Printed in the United States

YA 158.12 YOU
The young adult's guide to
meditation : easy
techniques that reduce
stress and relieve anger,

led Paper

35340636235490   Oct 16

Reduce. Reuse.
RECYCLE.

A decade ago, Atlantic Publishing signed the Green Press Initiative. These guidelines promote environmentally friendly practices, such as using recycled stock and vegetable-based inks, avoiding waste, choosing energy-efficient resources, and promoting a no-pulping policy. We now use 100-percent recycled stock on all our books. The results: in one year, switching to post-consumer recycled stock saved 24 mature trees, 5,000 gallons of water, the equivalent of the total energy used for one home in a year, and the equivalent of the greenhouse gases from one car driven for a year.

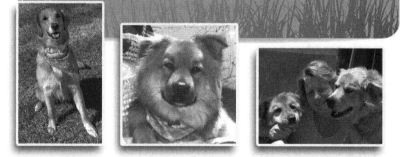

Over the years, we have adopted a number of dogs from rescues and shelters. First there was Bear and after he passed, Ginger and Scout. Now, we have Kira, another rescue. They have brought immense joy and love into not just into our lives, but into the lives of all who met them.

We want you to know a portion of the profits of this book will be donated in Bear, Ginger and Scout's memory to local animal shelters, parks, conservation organizations, and other individuals and nonprofit organizations in need of assistance.

– Douglas & Sherri Brown,
President & Vice-President of Atlantic Publishing

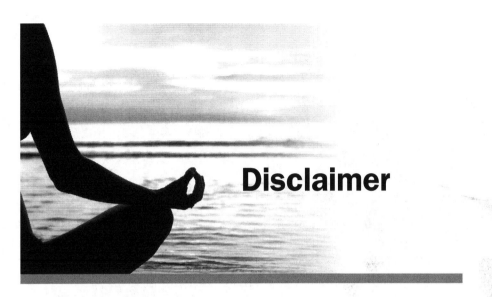

Disclaimer

This publication does not offer medical advice. Any content presented in this publication is for informational purposes only, and is not intended to cover all possible uses, directions, precautions, drug interactions, or adverse effects. This content should not be used during a medical emergency or for the diagnosis or treatment of any medical condition. Please consult your doctor or other qualified health care provider if you have any questions about a medical condition, or before taking any drug, changing your diet or commencing or discontinuing any course of treatment. Do not ignore or delay obtaining professional medical advice because of information presented herein. Call 911 or your doctor for all medical emergencies.

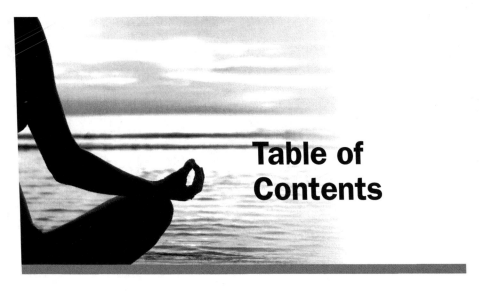

Table of Contents

CHAPTER 4
Preparing the Body for Core Meditation 67

CHAPTER 5
Beginning Core Meditation with Concentration 89

CHAPTER 6
Continuing Core Meditation with Mindfulness 109

CHAPTER 7
Finishing Core Meditation with Lovingkindness 129

CHAPTER 8
Divine Meditation 145

CHAPTER 9
Meditation in Everyday Life **159**

Conclusion **173**

Appendix A
Nine Grassroots Solutions for Consciousness Elevation....**175**

Appendix B
The Seven Natural Laws of Nature **179**

Appendix C
The Twelve Laws of Karma **181**

Introduction

ow do you really feel about life? Are you stressed or frustrated? Maybe standardized tests, schoolwork, or difficult friendships are getting you down. If you are reading this book, then there is a possibility that something in your life is not working and you have come to the point where you have had enough and finally want to do something about it by learning meditation. Meditation is the devotional exercise of training the mind to connect with the body. This connection creates a higher consciousness that results in some life benefit. Think back to when you were a child. When a child enters this world, it enters with the pure loving light of creation, free of judgments and attachments. It understands nothing of the conflicts of this world. However, as the child gradually encounters the successes, failures, joys and miseries that accompany modern life, the light of pure creation slowly dims within the child. Over time, it develops a *type of mindset* based on those experiences, which then determines the physical, intellectual, emotional and spiritual and quality of its life. Once fully grown and subjected to the various influences that formed the mindset, the individual then incorrectly comes to associate suffering as part of the

process of growing up. He or she never questions whether this suffering was intended, or whether there may be something very wrong with this widely accepted belief.

Whatever mindset you have developed in life (optimism, pessimism, fear, determination, confidence, anxiety, self-loathing, etc.) your ego was the source that created it. Through the development of your mindset, you perceive your sense of self in relation to the world around you. The ego drive is the impulse that satisfies what your sense of self thinks it needs. It comes through in our thoughts, our actions, our emotions and even our bodies. For example, when you defend your own beliefs, behave in certain ways toward others, or compete against others, your ego drive is working to protect the self it created. Over the past few centuries, the ego drive has

been useful in shaping life to meet many of society's physical and emotional needs. However, it also has been the source of physical and emotional stresses. Worse, it has removed our connection to something more satisfying than what the ego-driven material world has to offer. While the ego-driven material world continually strives to come up with solutions to the sense of lacking it creates, these solutions usually end up proving useless as a remedy.

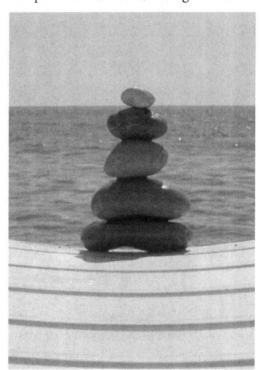

If you are like most people, your ego drive created some type of mental or emotional issues that you are either consciously or unconsciously aware of, and it ultimately has lead to your own suffering. If you can begin to

understand that a mindset was programmed into you as you aged, you can begin to understand that it is capable of being changed and that none of it has its origin in the spiritual dimension. This book will help you shed your past mental and emotional conditioning so that you can begin to achieve whatever intention you set for yourself as you move forward in your life. People turn to meditation because scientific and historical research shows that meditating at least 10 minutes a day can dramatically alter the way the body responds to stress. It can correct bad habits, support physical healing and improve task performance in everyday activities. Having an intention plays an important role in helping you continue a meditative practice once you have started. This book can help you find and explore a specific intention if you do not already have one. No single reason for meditation exists, but the most common reasons for why people meditate include a desire to reduce the stress in their life; a desire for physical, emotional, or spiritual healing; a desire to improve their relationships; and a desire to improve their life's work. Meditation will teach you that the way to achieve what you want out of meditation (and out of life) is to release yourself from the egocentric experiences that may have negatively formed your mindset and changed your consciousness.

This book has been divided into nine chapters arranged in a chronological way to help you understand how to begin your meditative practice and deepen it further by adding new techniques. Starting with an explanation regarding the history and science of meditation, this book will move toward getting you started by helping you further identify and explore a specific intention for continued meditative practice. From there it moves toward defining the three core meditations, including an overview of the techniques and exercises that correspond to each core meditation. Once you understand what you will need to begin your regular meditative practice, chapters 5,6 and 7 will each include exercises for putting together a 10-minute meditation. There is nothing wrong with using meditation for even the smallest or most common of reasons if you feel it will add something to your life. If reducing stress, relieving emotional strain, or improv-

ing some other aspect of your everyday well-being is your only goal, you may skip chapter 8. If your intention for meditating includes increasing your spiritual connection to nature and mysticism, you are encouraged to read the entire book.

The information contained here also will include case studies from meditation teachers sharing their personal wisdom. Their insight will help the development of your practice. Last, consider using the resource and appendix information at the end of this book in addition to the subjects covered in each chapter. We hope you are excited about the possibilities of improving your life through meditation. The door to greater well-being awaits you.

The History and Science of Meditation

he word for meditation in Sanskrit is *shamatha*, which translates to "peacefully abiding." In his book, "Passage Meditation: Bringing the Deep Wisdom of the Heart into Daily Life," Eknath Easwaran defines meditation as the end of sorrow and mastery of the art of living. Meditation is the practice of reaching an intense state of awareness through the stillness of thoughts. It is a journey into the center of our own being. The word derives from two Latin words: "meditari" (to think or to dwell upon) and "mederi" (to heal). The Sanskrit derivation is "medha," which means "wisdom." The goal of meditation is to return the mind to its natural resting state. Without meditation, the mind is often a mass of confusion. Meditation allows us to develop internal peace and well-being while giving us the emotional resources to protect against disorderly states of mind. The simplest way to define meditation is to think of it as an experience that makes it possible for us to transform the mind. Beginning meditators should expect to practice:

1. Correct posture
2. Relaxed but deep breathing
3. Attention to thoughts, objects or sensations
4. Mindfulness of distractions

5. Present moment thinking
6. Open, nonjudgmental attitude

Harmful Effects of Stress, Anger, Anxiety and Depression

Meditation works because it restores the body's balance to where all its biological systems operate at functional levels. Stress, on the other hand, attacks and gradually destroys these systems, leading to a number of health-related issues. The regulatory systems affected by stress, bad habits and emotional distress include:

1. The nervous system
2. The immune system
3. The cardiovascular system
4. The gastrointestinal system
5. The musculature system
6. The lymphatic system

A body out of balance is very tough. In fact, most people are living proof that the body is capable of functioning under the difficulties of everyday living. Over time, however, these systems begin to fail if they stay stressed for too long. The nervous system is the body's regulatory system that maintains and manages your stress and relaxation responses to external events. When something stressful occurs in your life, your nervous system activates its stress response to adjust the body's functions to the situation. For example, when you are under stress, your nervous system will activate its *stress response*. The stress response is the body's transition from a resting state into a state of increased activity. During the stress response, adrenaline gives the body an enormous burst of energy, which allows it to function at a higher rate than normal. As adrenaline rises, muscle tension and blood pressure increase. Basically, your body is in a state of high alert and preparing to do battle with whatever has triggered the stress response. However, this

heightened state of activity burns energy in your body very quickly, so the nervous system stops digestion in order to use that energy itself.

When the stress in your life decreases, the nervous system activates the *relaxation response* by lowering your body's adrenaline levels, which softens your muscles and decreases blood pressure. The relaxation response is a physical state of deep rest that the body wants to achieve. Though the nervous system exists to help you deal with stress, its goal is to return the body to its natural resting state. When stress becomes chronic due to the constant pressures and demands of society, the body never lowers its stress response, and we carry tension into every aspect of our lives. The effects of the stress response will eventually show in our physical and emotional appearance and affect our relationships

Physical Ailments

When life keeps the body in a state of constant stress blood pressure remains high. This happens when the body's stress response pressures the cardiovascular system to increase delivery of blood, causing blood to thicken. The body's muscles, veins and arteries constrict, causing tiny rips in the lining of the arteries as greater amounts of blood are forced through narrower passageways. With time, blood clots can form, break loose and block arteries, which causes blood cells to die. Also when your muscles remain tense, you risk developing severe back pain. Relaxed muscles help move oxygen throughout the body, move out waste products and are vital in supplying every cell in your body with nutrients. When muscles tighten, reduced oxygen supplies and increased waste products begin to poison the body.

Don't forget that this heightened state of activity also takes energy from your digestive system. If digestion slows for too long, saliva and stomach juices dry up. Hydrochloric acid production jump-starts and you increase the chances of having problems such as ulcers, heartburn, gas pain, or constipation. When your body burns energy at unsustainable levels, you risk other types of cell damage. For example, when the immune system becomes

hyperactive, it begins to destroy healthy tissue, causing arthritic conditions and autoimmune disorders. According to registered holistic health practitioner of alternative medicine, Dr. Alka Khurana, "Meditation strengthens the immune system and cellular activity by enhancing the telomerase enzyme that protects genetic material during cell division."

When the musculature system tightens from stress, the lymphatic system (responsible for regulating the immune system and moving waste products) becomes impaired, causing your white blood cell count to drop. This can result in various types of cancer. Meditation counteracts all of this by reducing blood pressure, breathing rates, muscle constriction and adrenaline levels. In short, it helps the body return to its natural resting state where it can begin to heal itself from the effects of long-term hypertension and chronic stress.

Mental Ailments

If you have ever heard the yogic term "mind-body connection" you can probably figure out that it refers to the connection between the body and mind, and how they influence one another. Our thoughts and actions can have a powerful effect on the body's physical well-being due to the stress/relaxation response. How you think and act creates a reaction in your body that brings either harmony or disharmony to the entire system. The same holds true for mental diseases and disorders that afflict the brain. Research shows that symptoms typically begin to surface when the brain shows an abnormal balance of neurotransmitters, which help nerve cells in the brain communicate with each other. When the chemicals that regulate this process become unbalanced, the brain does not receive messages well. Likewise, certain infections can cause brain damage. As you now know, stress tightens the musculature system and causes the blockage of waste products. These toxins in these wastes become poisonous and create bacterial infections that eventually damage the brain.

Research also links bad diet to anxiety, depression and paranoia, which in turn play a role in the development of mental illness. Negative emotions such as these create blockages in the energetic openings of the body. These energetic openings, called *chakras*, alleviate emotions that cause chronic stress and keep the biological systems in a continual state of hypertension. Meditation unblocks the energetic openings, which then restores the mind/body connection and gets the biological systems of the body working again. In a study conducted at Massachusetts General Hospital, researchers found that individuals who meditated for about a half hour a day through eight weeks showed an increase in gray matter located in the higher brain called the neo-cortex. Research on these same individuals also showed a decrease in the size of the amygdala, the area of the brain that helps regulate anxiety and stress. Not only does meditation stimulate gray matter, it also accelerates white matter fibers, which increase connectivity between different biological systems and reduce brain degeneration.

Depression, Anxiety and Procrastination

If you consider how the body's biological systems deteriorate under prolonged periods of stress, it should come as no surprise why depressed people feel unmotivated. When people suffer from chronic stress, small tasks seem more difficult and larger challenges almost impossible to overcome. Likewise, depression can lead to problems with concentration and feelings of not being good enough. A mind focused on fear and anxiety prevents you from solving problems and properly responding to the obstacles of life. Therefore, once the mind becomes quiet at the beginning of your daily practice, the goal of meditation is focus. Focus serves to counteract the mind's desire to return to thoughts and emotions that cause depression. You might be surprised to learn that multitasking is actually *less* efficient than focusing on one thing at a time. The Journal of Experimental Psychology found that multitasking requires more time when it comes to concentrating on difficult or unfamiliar tasks because of the extra mental effort needed to break "flow state" (discussed further in Chapter 9) and shift back and forth

between different tasks. Humans have become so accustomed to multitasking that they almost never give their full concentration to *anything*, and the mind resorts to half measures as a means of solving its problems.

This is why chronic anxiety has become so common recently. The more the mind worries, the more overwhelmed it becomes. It is for this reason that fourth edition of the Diagnostic and Statistical Manual of Mental Disorders (DSM-IV) has classified generalized anxiety disorder as one of the most common forms of chronic stress. A person meets the criteria for generalized anxiety disorder when symptoms include:

1. At least six months of excessive anxiety
2. Difficulty controlling anxiety
3. Significant muscle tension and restlessness
4. Fatigue
5. Irritability
6. Lack of concentration
7. Lack of sleep
8. Dysfunction in daily life

Most teens across a variety of backgrounds have struggled against depression, anxiety and procrastination at one time or another. Few, however, are aware that they meet the criteria as someone with general anxiety disorder. If you suffer from the symptoms listed above, or if you have come to this reading with some other intention, this book will show you how a daily 10-minute meditation can lead to a variety of life sustaining benefits.

How Meditation Fosters Physical, Mental, Emotional and Social Well-Being

Daily meditation reduces production of epinephrine and norepinephrine, commonly referred to as "the stress hormones." When a person experiences stress on an ongoing basis, these stress hormones reduce immune system function, which can lead to high cholesterol levels and increase heart rate.

No matter what short-term or long-term intention you set for your meditative practice, you will begin to see improvements in your overall physical, mental, emotional and social well-being. Using concentration techniques, you will notice improvements in mental focus if you previously suffered from a wandering mind. You will experience reduced anxiety about the future if you are someone who tends to obsess about the unknown. Hurtful and regretful events of the past will no longer rule over your mindset. You will enjoy better relationships with friends and relatives as your sense of isolation from others disappears. Your mind will be free and clear to think problems and challenges through, and further improve your life choices. In short, gaining control over the mind involves a process in which the meditator learns exactly how the mind works.

When meditation quiets the mind, it becomes willing to receive both blissful and uncomfortable thoughts, emotions, and sensations without replaying the chatter that has formed its mindset. The chatter in the mind is the "life story" that the brain creates out of the experiences that occur over an individual's lifetime. When the mind buries the causes of inner disharmony deep within the unconscious, the individual begins to act out these root causes on the conscious level in an unexamined way. If you never examine or take time to understand the thoughts and actions that control you, you can never hope to free yourself of them. It is for this reason that meditation involves techniques that cultivate quieting the mind and present moment awareness, which forces the causes of inner disharmony to the surface.

Meditation does not support avoidance behavior. It is a means of confronting inner issues to reduce power over the mind, not a means of escaping pain. When the mind becomes quiet through meditative practice, the voice of judgment begins to settle down until eventually it stops talking. Now you are ready to move into a state of mindfulness where you can simply observe whatever thoughts or emotions come into the mind without judgment. In this heightened state of consciousness, the mind is able to examine

everything from a position of greater understanding and take the proper steps to repair its insecurities and learned behaviors of helplessness, blame, pessimism, judgment, and so forth. Meditative techniques are coping skills used for developing positive emotions and mind states that prevent negative and distracting thoughts from harming the mindset further. Mental clarity improves the mind's ability to make important distinctions between thoughts and emotions that previously went unexamined. Through concentration, awareness and mental clarity, you will begin to see more deeply into your true self and unravel what needs healing. The process of healing the mind/body connection is gradual; it takes time, and more important, patience. If you become frustrated when you set an intention that does not immediately appear in your everyday life, do not get discouraged or feel you are doing something wrong. The frustration you feel is merely the beginning of the mind's resistance to letting go of the mindset that no longer works for you. That you remain focused on the concept of success and failure in meditation is the first sign that your mind is still talking to you. Over the course of this reading, different techniques will address and provide solutions for the most common roadblocks and challenges found along the meditative journey.

The History of Meditative Practice

Archeological findings trace meditative practice as far back as 5,000 years when wandering holy men and women called *sadus* and *yogis* used meditative practice to connect with divinity and wrote scriptures called *Vedas*. Based on the Vedas, Vedic priests performed rites and chants that required concentration, prayerful meditation, and breathing control. Fueled by Vedic tradition, Yoga, Buddhism and Tantra were born. While meditation connects these practices to the same ancient root, Yoga aims to merge the physical body into the formless consciousness. Tantra, on the other hand, involves ritual and visualizations in connection to awakening *chakras*, as well as a powerful life energy called the *kundalini*.

Meditation in Eastern Religion

The foundation of Buddhism traces back to the Indian sage, Gautama Buddha, also known as Siddhārtha Gautama Shakyamuni whose name means "awakened one." As a Hindu prince who led a privileged life in the area now known as Nepal, Gautama felt a profound sense of compassion for human suffering after witnessing the poverty, sickness and death that existed among the less fortunate. He resolved to devote himself to uncovering a path to enlightenment that could end human suffering and rejected his privileged life. Eventually, he discovered a path to greater enlightenment through an examination of the spirit contained within his body and mind while sitting under a tree. By his late 20s, he became a spiritual teacher of the basic enlightenment principals that modern Buddhism is based on. Among Buddha's chief teachings is the belief that people suffer because they:

1. Falsely believe permanence is real and can be relied upon for happiness
2. Falsely believe the "self" forms our real identity and is independent of others

Buddhism, like its sister religions, agrees that everything in this world is deeply connecte, and that suffering is the result of the perceived disconnection to the union of all things. To liberate oneself from suffering, one must liberate the mind from the negative mindset formed by ego consciousness. It was by the third century B.C. that Buddha's teachings spread beyond the confines of India as other Eastern cultures began practicing the art of meditation. As Buddhism underwent significant changes in Sri Lanka and Southeast Asia, the newly formed approaches to Buddhism mainstreamed enlightenment beyond monks and nuns. From the roots of Buddhism came the practice of Zen, which blended traditional Buddhism with Chinese Taoism.

Meditation in Judeo-Christian Traditions

Meditation is not a religion, but rather a practice used by many religions, including those that originated in other parts of the world. While meditation is not traditionally associated with the Judeo-Christian and Islamic traditions that emerged from the Middle East, it is woven into its customs. While you may not recognize its presence, meditation in Christianity takes the form of prayer. The book of Matthew tells the story of Jesus as he meditated, fasted and prayed in the desert before starting his ministry. When Jesus retreated to the desert for 40 days and 40 nights, he meditated through prayer as a means of opening awareness to God. In fact, most modern English adaptations of the Bible contain more than 20 uses of the word "meditate." Joshua 1:8, for example, reads, "Do not let this Book of the Law depart from your mouth; meditate on it day and night."

By 300 A.D., Christian meditators in Egypt and Palestine began to follow Christ's meditative teachings. From these desert wanderers came the monks of the Eastern Orthodox Church and medieval Europe who used the scriptures as meditative prayer. In Judaism, interpreters of the Old Testament trace meditation back to Abraham, who entered into altered states of consciousness through fasting and strict practices. Even Islam shares a connection to meditative practice, as a group of mystical seekers known as Sufis engage in a meditative practice called *zikr*, which involves chanting a sacred phrase while rhythmically breathing.

Although there were some pockets of people who followed mediation in the West, it was not until an international conference in 1893 between religious world leaders that Asian priests and Zen masters were finally able to share their meditative concepts directly with Westerners. By the 1950s, Western societies began considering meditation as a means of helping citizens deal with stress, anxiety and depression. Meditation fully popularized into Western life when The Beatles began practicing Transcendental Meditation with the Maharishi Yogi, and Jack Kerouac's book, "The Dharma Bums," became an international bestseller. Within two decades, researchers

began testing the effects of meditation on the human psyche. As further scientific research solidifed the connection of meditation to wellness, more doctors began recommending it as a treatment in medical and therapeutic communities. Today's health industry officially recognizes meditation as a complementary alternative medicine (otherwise known as CAM).

Modern Schools of Meditation

Mainstream schools of meditation, such as Yoga, Tai Chi and Qigong, are now common in towns and sports clubs across the United States and the West. Qigong meditation allows you to practice in either a concentrative or mindful style. A concentrative practice provides a particular focus, such as a mantra, color or breath. As with any mindfulness practice, the goal is simply to notice or be aware of your breathing. At its core, Qigong is a series of standing or seated movements that release tension and build energy flow. The practice emphasizes the development of mind and spirit through body movement. Tai Chi allows you to find inner stillness using outer meditative movement that draws your "chi," or life force, through your body to create a feeling of relaxation, well-being and balance. Tai Chi can be challenging to learn on your own. If you cannot find a meditative school or class that suits your needs, consider purchasing a DVD to guide you visually through the movements. Yoga involves meditating through breathing, exercises and physical postures. Some of the more traditional forms — based on Hindu philosophy — include Raja, Karma, Bhakti and Jnana. In the United States, the most popular form of Yoga is Hatha, which places more emphasis on stretching, breath control and body poses to renew the body's energy source.

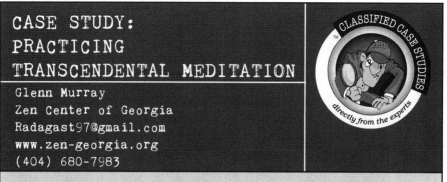

CASE STUDY: PRACTICING TRANSCENDENTAL MEDITATION

Glenn Murray
Zen Center of Georgia
Radagast97@gmail.com
www.zen-georgia.org
(404) 680-7983

When I was in my 20s, I began experimenting with transcendental meditation. When I was 40, I started taking Aikido and Zen meditation. I also currently practice Zen meditation in the Rinzai tradition and attend retreats three times a year. I train under my teacher Zen Master Miller Roshi, who is the Bishop of Daiyuzenji in Chicago. I now run our local school. I have no religious title or rank, other than as a student.

I do not really have a typical sitting session. If I had to describe the experience, I would use words such as "quiet," "meditative," and "centering." Sometimes the meditation comes very easy and deep; sometimes I struggle with it. The benefits of meditation depend on the individual. Sometimes, the outcome can be as simple as something that calms and reduces tension. Some meditators just want to reduce blood pressure and enhance their well-being. Some meditate to increase concentration. Some do it for religious reasons.

Meditation centers me and helps me to understand myself better. Perhaps one day it will lead to enlightenment, but that is not the reason I sit. I appreciate the way meditation enhances my ability to live in the moment and accept things as they are. I am Buddhist, so meditation is my primary religious practice. If feel it also makes me a better person. What people look for from meditation varies. Ultimately, meditation is personal in practice, both in its benefits and in its goals. The advice I would offer to someone beginning a meditation practice is simple: Do not be too hard on yourself. As simple as meditation is to learn, it is not easy to master. Learning to accept that you cannot be perfect from the beginning is part of learning to accept yourself as you are.

Environment is also an important consideration for beginners. Initially, a quiet environment free from distractions is important to learning how to meditate. As one gets more skilled, the environment becomes less important. Personally, I can mediate while hearing the noises from an Aikido class in the next room without it affecting my concentration. Ultimately, I would want to be able to enter any situation with complete equanimity. As beginners are developing a meditation practice, a guide or teacher can be helpful in offering feedback on breathing and posture. At the more advanced levels, it is important to develop a more mindful practice to deal with distractions created by the mind's ego.

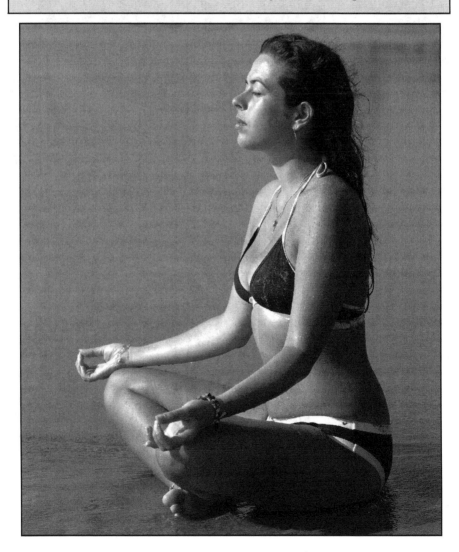

The second thing to understand about meditation is that it involves a process that requires two character traits: patience and non-judgment. If you expect results too quickly, if you expect results different from the ones you feel you get, or if you begin to judge and evaluate your progress, then you will begin to defeat your own intentions. Many beginning meditators who quit their practice do so because no one has informed them about what to expect or what not to expect as they progress. Those who do not leave behind their expectations about meditation are the ones most likely to ruin their commitment and quit their practice. This state of mind is what meditation gurus call *the beginning mind.* The beginning mind involves examining what attitudes you must shed and what attitudes you must adopt before you meditate. Therefore, this chapter will explore the necessity of understanding how the beginning mind creates the very anxieties, frustrations and judgments that work to undo the meditative process and eventually destroy the will to keep going. The purpose of understanding your state of mind is to develop the kind of mindfulness that identifies negative attitudes and judgments as they come up and to bring your focus back to meditation. The second consideration explored in this chapter is determining your motivation for beginning a meditative practice. As a third consideration, this chapter will provide an overview of the three core meditations and their corresponding techniques, as well as the aspects of well-being each one develops.

Pitfalls of Beginning Meditation

The meditation process requires the two character traits patience and non-judgment. The easiest way to understand the beginning mind and the pitfalls of starting meditation is to examine both of these character traits of the beginning mind. The beginning mind tends to bring disharmonious aspects of the outside world into a harmonious practice. Using these aspects, the beginning mind allows the inner dialogue that has been talking for most of the individual's life to form judgments destructive to the practice. Therefore, it is important to understand that inner conflict at

the beginning, and throughout various stages of meditative development, is unavoidable. The best way to deal with inner conflict is to understand when and why inner conflict occurs during meditation, that it is part of meditation's natural process, and be willing to let it go. A beginning meditator who encounters the first stage of inner conflict often misinterprets this conflict as failure to follow directions, failure of the instructor to give directions, or failure of practice to do what it claims.

Meditation involves a very simple instruction: *just sit and be.* Yet the process can be very difficult and the experience very complex. Beginning meditators who come to their first session expecting immediate physical or emotional results often find themselves frustrated when they fail to achieve them. What they fail to realize is that any evaluation of the experience in terms of success or failure is the first sign of an active, unquiet mind blocking progression. Some beginning meditators may find the initial results pleasing, only to later encounter negative thoughts and emotions they neither wanted nor expected. Such meditators cannot match these negative experiences with their expectation that meditation should never cause distress. These meditators fail to realize that negative thoughts and emotions are the result of meditation opening up energetic blockages. When beginning meditators evaluate their sessions and think in terms of results, they fail to understand the attitude necessary to achieve positive results. To successfully begin and continue a meditative practice, the beginning meditator must first:

1. Examine his or her present attitudes
2. Discard all expectations
3. Reserve all judgments
4. Learn to quiet the inner dialogue in his or her mind
5. Become open to whatever arises or does not arise during meditation

The easiest way to examine your present attitudes is to reflect on your life. To examine your present attitude, you have to examine your core beliefs

and examine the impact of those beliefs on your past actions, thoughts and decisions. Doing so will allow you to determine what attitudes you must shed versus what attitudes you must adopt before you meditate. You can make this your first meditative exercise by taking a few deep breaths, closing your eyes, and reflecting on past events important to you, or you can reflect by writing down your thoughts. There are no right or wrong answers in this exercise; simply imagine your life as if it were a movie. Start with your earliest memories, continue through the various stages of your life and note how the events in between have shaped your beliefs about yourself, about others, and about the world around you. As you play this movie in your head, think about accomplishments you feel good about - what makes these moments memorable, and what feelings do they bring up. Once you have finished replaying your life up to the present moment, consider how you might have lived life differently with the knowledge you gained so far from your life experience. (Do not read further until you have completed this exercise).

Now that you have completed this exercise, look at your answers to the question about what you might change about your life if you could go back to preschool and start over. The point of this exercise is to measure your sense of happiness about life without actually bringing up any negative thoughts. The larger the list of things you would change in your life, the more likely you are to have an unquiet, judging mind and an unhealthy attitude. In other words, this exercise is a way of predicting how your mind will react when finally asked to calm and quiet down. It will also determine the attitudes you must shed versus the attitudes you must adopt for your meditative practice. Gaining a sense of your mindset should not discourage you from practicing meditation or give you a false sense of confidence. It is merely a way to prepare you for the challenges beginning meditators sometimes face. The table below lists the character traits of a mind prepared for beginning meditation versus a mind unprepared for beginning meditation.

Prepared for Pitfalls	Unprepared for Pitfalls
Ability to understand that difficult thoughts and emotions are part of the process	Overreaction to difficult thoughts and emotions and inability to understand them as part of the process
Nonattachment to thoughts, memories and emotions	Tendency to dwell on thoughts, memories and emotions
Ability to quiet mind chatter	Inability to quiet mind chatter
Feeling a sense of connectedness	Feeling a sense of isolation
Ability to let go of external distractions	Inability to come back to focus
Present moment awareness	Preoccupation with past and future
Acceptance of reality	Resistance to reality
A mind that lets go of its tendency to judge and compare	A mind that judges and compares
Cultivated optimism	Cultivated pessimism

According to prominent Yogi scholar Tsultrim Gyamtso Rinpoche, "Being led by the thoughts is a waste of time in meditation… his continuous stream of thinking is *samsara* (perpetual wandering). Many people believe that since samsara is of such great suffering, we should try to leave it behind and try to obtain nirvana. They imagine that after practicing, one day will come when they see nirvana or emptiness and they will think, 'Now, I have attained realization and have been liberated.' In this way, they pursue and hope for some kind of appearance or phenomenon. Thus, in their meditation, they will always have a sense of waiting and expectation…these people are always pursuing some kind of meditative state and waiting for some state to appear…In general, people who are in [these] situations will be very tense in their meditation and have very strong attachments."

Exploring Your Motivation

Motivation is an important part of meditation. It not only establishes your reason for coming to your first practice, but also for continuing your practice over a period of weeks, months and years. More important, motivation

can make a difference between a halfhearted practice and a deep, meditative experience. Keep in mind, there is a difference between expectation and intention. Expectations are desires and beliefs that the ego drive tries to force into reality by its will. Intention is the focused attempt to accomplish something without the burden of attachment to success or failure. To explore your motivation, think about your goals. At this point, be honest and admit that your goals might concern your own well-being rather than others'. You might want to stop feeling depressed or worried. You might want to reduce the stress you feel about having to apply to college. You might want to stop procrastinating or kick another bad habit that causes problems for you. Spiritual leaders call these desires "lower intentions" because they are not the true intentions buried deep within your spiritual essence, but rather constructed by the ego drive. You should not be concerned with drawing a higher intention at the beginning. Meditation eventually will reveal the higher intention.

For now, focus on your lower intentions with the understanding that it is all right to have them. The natural energies you release during meditation will respond to your intention and improve your life. If you have a higher intention, such as developing genuine compassion for others or reaching higher levels of spiritual understanding, take that intention to your practice along with your lower intentions. To explore lower intentions, ask yourself what is lacking in your life and declare your desire to improve this aspect as your lower intention. Your lower intention might take the form of:

1. Stress relief
2. Improving performance in your school activities
3. Improving your health
4. Improving your creativity or concentration

Higher intentions are more difficult to name because the beginning mind is rarely aware of its true nature. Some people intuitively sense a hidden universal truth. They ask, "Who am I?" or "What is the meaning of life?" The answer given by the most enlightened meditators is quite simple: At-

tainment of the true self occurs when ego consciousness fades and you begin to identify with everything in being. Thus, higher intentions might take the form of:

1. Searching for meaning
2. Accepting and loving yourself/others
3. Expressing your inner perfection
4. Awakening others

Among all the higher intentions, Buddhists consider awakening others to be the most important intention of all. This higher intention, known as *bodhichitta*, is a selfless goal that advances the process of well-being because it offers a remedy to the ego-drive's need to acquire things for the self. Seeking the higher intention, the body and mind begin to radiate with love and affection for others and a genuine desire for their well-being. This is how the higher and lower intentions entwine. By connecting with your higher intention, you *amplify* the realization of your lower intentions.

Overview of different practices

This book identifies three core meditations and more than 20 meditation techniques that any meditator can apply to their practice. Both the techniques and the core meditations bring very specific benefits. As you read about the core meditations, you will discover that some overlap exists between the intentions they cultivate, so you might use one technique to serve two or even three core meditations. For example, if you want to enter a formless state of being, you first have to remove mind chatter. A mind quieting technique might serve to build your focus and concentration, which paves the way to a deeper meditative state. The purpose of this section is to define the three core meditations and provide an overview of the techniques that serve them.

Core Meditation is the meditative practice that allows you to shift your mental and emotional state as well as improve all areas of your life. Core

Meditation will help you relax, energize, release negative emotions, increase your positive outlook, clear and focus your mind, and strengthen your spiritual connection. What benefits you get depend on your motivation, intention and depth of practice. Higher intentions lead to deeper practices. Core Meditation comes from Qigong, Tao, and Kriya Yoga. The three core meditations are:

1. Concentration Meditation
2. Mindfulness Meditation
3. Lovingkindness Meditation

Core Meditation #1: Concentration Meditation

Concentration Meditation is the art of eliminating internal distractions so the mind can quiet the inner dialogue that clouds insight into the meaning of things. Internal distractions, for example, may take the form of past regrets and mistakes. People spend so much time focusing on the past that they never fully appreciate what they actually have, or they tell themselves they have nothing. They miss the gift of the beautiful moment happening right now. Hall of Fame football coach Mike Ditka once said, "You live in the past, you die in the past." Perhaps replaying the past has you already thinking about the things in life that you cannot go back and change. This is when the ego controlling the inner voice starts chattering. The ego's desire to protect the self it constructed may be well intentioned, but it only serves to cripple you in the present and beyond. Life experience shows that when the mind dwells in past regrets, it begins to live in fear of the future. A mind dwelling in the future might think, "I cannot let this happen again" or "What if I can't get back what I used to have?" Now fear controls the mind and the ego defense protecting it begins to imagine frightful scenarios where history repeats itself. The ego controlling the inner voice starts to chatter. For example, it might say, "Avoid this situation at all costs." In this sense, people who dwell in past regrets skip the present by moving directly

from past to future. The art of concentration allows the mind to quiet the inner voice by eliminating its concentration on past or future scenarios.

Deep concentration also serves to eliminate external distractions that can disrupt a deep state of meditation. Beginning meditators tend to have more mind chatter. Losing a meditative state to a noise from the outside world can be one of the most frustrating experiences for beginning meditators. They become so aware that they have lost a meditative state that the inner dialogue begins to work its way back into their minds. The mind begins replaying old stories about regret and fear. For example, it might say, "I lost my concentration because I'm easily distracted," and then it goes back to some past event where this mindset formed. If unchecked, the mind chatter jumps forward and pictures a future where it fears the same distraction will renew old hurts. When you develop strong concentration, you allow your awareness to expand into thoughts and emotions because the mind chatter quiets. Concentration occurs at the relaxation stage of meditation when you employ techniques such as body scanning, which helps the body relax and releases the mind from stored thoughts and emotions. Concentration also may occur at the internalization stage when you employ techniques such as the Breath Wave, which directs energy inward. The techniques used to cultivate the core practice of concentration include:

1. Mind quieting technique
2. The counting technique
3. Breath Wave technique
4. Breath motion synchronization technique
5. Naming technique
6. Releasing thoughts technique
7. Auditory technique
8. Thought release technique

Core Meditation #2: Mindfulness Meditation

The fact that concentration cultivates aspects of relaxation and internalization explains why some techniques for concentration also can cultivate mindfulness. Mindfulness is the second core meditation practice. It refers to the process of bringing nonjudgmental attention to the internal and external experiences that exist in the present moment. Since mindfulness deals with present moment awareness, you must achieve a meditative state in which your internal dialogue is not constantly returning your thoughts to past or future events. This is why concentration comes before mindfulness as a core meditation.

The best way to cultivate and improve mindfulness is through the regular practice of meditation. In recent years, health care practitioners have adopted Mindfulness-Based Stress Reduction (MSRB) as an official Complimentary Alternative Treatment (CAM). CAM Treatments describe practices recognized by doctors as effective treatments used along with conventional medicine. During mindfulness, a meditator should not ignore distracting thoughts and feelings that arise during Concentration Meditation. Rather, the meditator is encouraged to acknowledge and observe them in a nonjudgmental manner as they arise. In this manner, the individual detaches from internal and external thought in order to gain insight into what they represent. One key element of mindfulness includes the ability to stay in present moment awareness regardless of the emotional or mental content observed. In other words, Mindfulness Meditation does not block anything; it requires that you let anything in, even thoughts, feelings, or sensations you might consider very unpleasant. By exercising the quiet mind, concentration gives you the tools to observe the experience without the mind chatter triggered by an emotional reaction. The techniques used to cultivate the core practice of mindfulness include:

1. Body scan technique
2. Muscle tensing technique
3. Expanding to sensations technique

4. Walking technique

5. Drinking tea technique

6. Everyday activity technique

7. Thinking technique

8. Positive emotion technique

9. Self-inquiry technique

10. Habitual pattern technique

Core Meditation #3: Lovingkindness Meditation

Concentration and mindfulness share aspects of the internalization stage of meditation. The expansion stage of meditation occurs during the third core practice: lovingkindness. When self-concern dissolves into a feeling of genuine love and compassion for all living things, the meditator has entered a state of expanded consciousness. As the mediator radiates love outward, the body raises its state of communication with a universe that is now listening and ready to respond. The techniques used to cultivate the core practice of lovingkindness include:

1. Mantra (or chanting) technique

2. Altar technique

3. Compassion technique

4. Walking in nature technique

5. Third eye technique

Finding or Joining a Meditation Group

At this point you may be wondering if it is easier to learn and practice meditation in an individual or group setting. The answer depends on you. Some people feel more comfortable beginning a meditative practice alone; others prefer practicing with a group. Learning to meditate by yourself is not hard if you follow the principles outlined in this book. Where meditative sessions occur is not as important as the overall ambience of the meditative space. Creating a meditative space at home only works when

few distractions exist. If your home is located in a noisy neighborhood, or if you have younger siblings running around all the time, you could get distracted. If so, joining a meditation group could be a great opportunity to network with other like-minded people, especially if you are someone more motivated when working in a group setting and enjoy sharing experiences with others. Indian scriptures use the word, *satsang*, which means "in the company of other truth seekers," and believe the collective energy flow of a group enhances the experience.

In the opinion of integrated energy therapist Wil Langford, "The benefit of group meditation is that you are encouraged by the participation of the other people in the group. Some may help you by giving suggestions based on their own experiences. During meditation, the energy changes, and a group that is meditating together may help to increase each other's energy. It is also less expensive to join a group than it is to hire a private teacher or meditation guide. On the other hand, experiencing the energy radiated by a group may not be so good if the group has many negative members or people who are experiencing high stress due to their life styles and circumstances."

Group meditation classes have become common, so finding a local class has become easier than ever. The most popular places to find group sessions are in community recreation departments, sports clubs, local colleges, places of worship, meditation centers and private studios. If you already belong to a sports club such as L.A. Fitness®, your membership may include free Yoga sessions. Many meditation centers also offer free sitting instruction. For example, the Shambhala Meditation Center of Atlanta offers day and evening instruction twice a week. These instruction sessions are wonderful for beginners who have questions about posture, wandering minds or even shifting position in the middle of a sitting session. For a list of meditation centers across America, go to **www.freemeditationinfo.com** If you feel that a Buddhist monastery will have more experienced meditators, you can find a listing in 23 American states at **www.brandbharat.com/english/ religion/buddhism/buddhist_temple/usa_buddhist_temple_list.html**.

If you feel more comfortable with a more mainstream setting, private studios offer Yoga classes that often blend meditation with Yoga. However, before you contact any of these places, consider the following pros and cons of meditation classes to decide if group meditation is the right choice.

Pros of Meditation Classes

1. More likely to reduce stress in a shorter span of time
2. More likely to continue practice if motivated by others
3. More likely to receive encouragement
4. More likely to progress faster toward deep meditation with instruction
5. Less risk of sustaining physical injury from certain body poses with instructors present
6. Increased energy flow from collective meditation
7. Opportunity to network and socialize with like-minded people
8. Instructors can answer questions, provide added guidance, or correct issues that create roadblocks

Cons of Meditation Classes

1. More likely to face frustration if you begin looking around and comparing your efforts to others
2. More likely to lose focus due to external distractions
3. More likely to feel self-conscious if you are too concerned about your appearance
4. More likely to skip sessions and eventually stop your practice if you have to travel far
5. You may not like the instructors teaching style or technique
6. The schedule may conflict with some of your other commitments, disrupting your practice or causing you to quit

CASE STUDY: FROM TAKING CLASSES TO TEACHING CLASSES

Jim Malloy
Merida, Yucatan, MX, 97130
jmalloy@meditationcenter.com
www.meditationcenter.com
052-999-272-8968

I came to the practice of meditation relatively early in life. I had just graduated from high school and a good friend suggested we go to a lecture on meditation. The speaker appeared very peaceful and said that meditation would change our lives in many wonderful ways. So we signed up, learned how to meditate, and sure enough, it did. I started practicing mantra meditation, but after about ten years, I started following more of an intuitive path where I found myself drawn to meditations that aligned with whatever phase of spiritual growth I happened to be in at the time. After practicing Transcendental Meditation for seven years, I spent ten months on the southern coast of Spain, where Maharishi Mahesh Yogi trained me. After teaching within the TM organization for a few years, I began teaching independently.

Sitting sessions for students often vary. For most, it is relaxing and peaceful. I teach students how to find deep states of inner quietness known as Yoga nidra, which generally feels like sleeping or dreaming. Some struggle with mental distractions until they come to accept that it is not necessary to fight thoughts or try too hard to stay focused. I think the need for relaxation and stress reduction is very important. However, what I believe is even more important is learning to elevate one's consciousness, which reconnects one with the innermost self or spirit. Nowadays, most people come to meditation looking for relaxation, stress reduction, improved health and better sleep. Only a small percentage of students in my classes seek spiritual development. My advice for someone just beginning a meditation practice is simple. Put aside all your expectations about what you want to happen and what you think is supposed to happen when you meditate and simply accept whatever does happen.

Also, commit to staying with it. If you are just beginning a meditation practice, it is helpful to give careful thought to the environment. It helps to have a quiet place with no potential interruptions. Having a place specially designated for meditation helps with one's practice and tends to build up the peaceful energy generated through meditation. However, after someone has been meditating for quite a while, the environment becomes less important. I believe it is very helpful for most people to have a teacher to help them get started, but I do not think it is essential for everyone. Some individuals can develop new abilities well on their own.

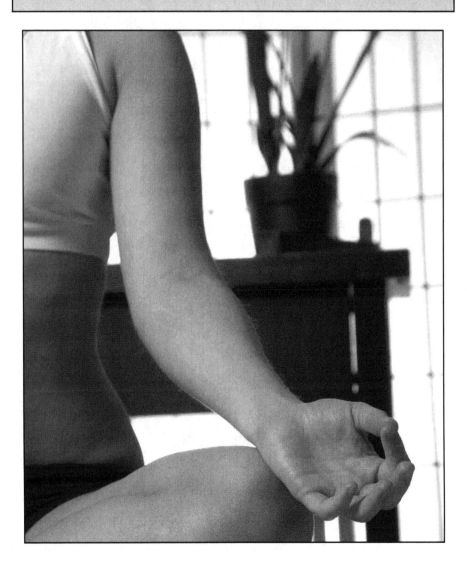

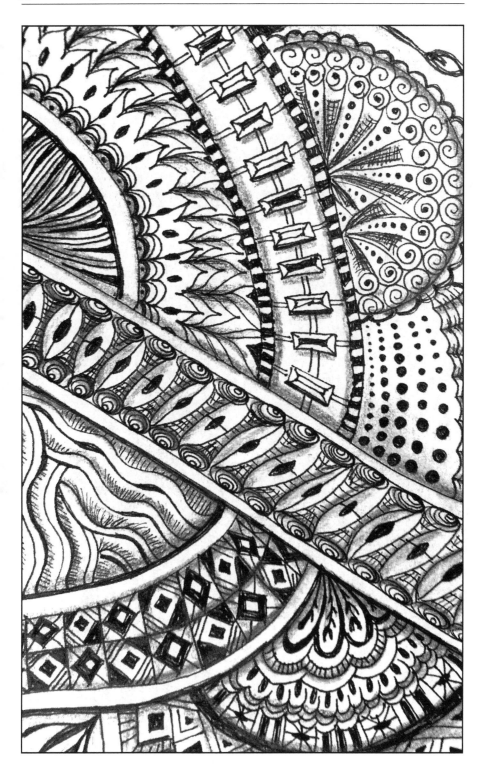

How to Create a Regular Meditative Practice

editating in the private space of your home is a great way to begin a practice if you decide not to join a group practice. To create a regular meditative practice, it is important to select one or more core practices and then customize that practice with the techniques that fit your needs. When thinking about what you hope to get out of meditation, contemplate or re-read the core meditation overview provided in Chapter 2 after finishing this book. After deciding which core meditation to use, consider or re-read the corresponding techniques described in greater depth in chapters 5, 6 and 7. In addition, look at the 10-minute exercises in those chapters, which may help to customize your own practice. Generally, experts recommend practicing all three core meditations. However, if your intention is to relax and reduce stress, Concentration Meditation will suffice. To improve memory and unravel bad habits, use concentration and mindfulness. To expand your consciousness, start with concentration, continue to mindfulness and finish with lovingkindness. Once you know

which core meditations you plan to practice, it is time to consider several important factors that may affect a daily routine. Those factors include:

1. Choosing the best time to mediate
2. Deciding how many times a day to meditate
3. Choosing what to wear
4. Choosing what kind of atmosphere to create
5. Choosing what type of accessories may enhance the experience

Choosing the Best Time to Meditate

There is no perfect time of day that works best for meditation because it varies from one person to the next. What matters is creating a routine that fits with your daily schedule and provides enough flexibility to move your session to a later or earlier time if your daily schedule at school or home suddenly changes. Some people prefer to meditate at dawn, others prefer the afternoon and others still prefer to meditate at night. People with little time to spare may not have the option of choosing a time of day or night, so they have to meditate when they have time. The good news for these people is that meditation is a mobile practice, performed any time — and, as advanced practitioners will testify — in any place. For example, you can start a session in a car, on a train, on a plane, or while walking somewhere. For busy people always on the go, it might be possible to squeeze a session in during lunch hour at school or even during a study break. It also might be a good idea to build a routine in right after school before starting home-work or other extracurricular activities.

On the other hand, meditative exercises do not require a lot of activity. In fact, most of the principles involve being still in mind, body and spirit. However, developing different thought patterns does require a considerable amount of concentration, especially early on in the process; therefore, you should not begin certain meditative techniques while driving or perform-ing another task that requires your attention. Meditating to achieve a high-energy state should go with techniques that produce more energy, while

meditating to achieve a relaxed trance state should go with techniques that produce relaxation. The best meditative practice combines both states to achieve a balance of relaxation and energy. To explore which energy state fits your schedule, goals and intentions, begin the evaluation process by considering the benefits of meditating at different times.

Morning Meditation vs. Night Meditation

Advanced meditators in Eastern cultures who practice body and mind exercises usually fit their sessions into the early hours of the morning between 5 and 5:30 a.m. Morning meditation works for early risers who like to get a head start on their day. It also works for people who feel groggy in the morning and need an influx of energy to wake up and face the day that lies ahead. Most young adults need roughly nine hours of sleep to function well throughout the day. As a rule, the best time to meditate in the morning is one hour after you wake up. Meditating within this time frame can heighten the meditative experience by drawing from the energy collected after a full night of sleep. The mind also tends to be quieter since it has just come out of an nine-hour resting state, in which case it will take less time to reach the internalization stage of meditation. Meditators who prefer to practice at sunrise typically feel a heightened sense of peacefulness and self-awareness. That alone makes the idea of altering your sleeping patterns something to consider. The best way to alter any routine sleep pattern is to shift the hours of sleep back enough for a proper waking at sunrise. Decide how much sleep is necessary to function the next day and count backward. If time does not allow you to make this type of shift, set the alarm clock an hour back from your normal walking hour and count backward to determine what time you will need to fall asleep in order to meditate in the morning.

On the other hand, some people prefer night meditation. The same principle for night meditation applies: it is best to do so one hour before bedtime. Using the right techniques can usher the body into a deep, relaxing sleep. The reason that meditators use certain techniques to induce greater

drowsiness or greater wakefulness has to do with the effect that meditation has on brain waves. Explored further in Chapter 5, the four types of brain waves measured by EEG are *beta, theta, alpha* and *delta.* Sleep occurs in four stages: transition to sleep, light sleep, deep sleep, and dream sleep. Meditation can cure insomnia by helping your body transition to a sleeping state. At night, your mind is most likely to be in beta. In beta, your mind is agitated and constantly thinking about what happened over the course of the day. A nighttime meditative practice helps the mind go from beta to alpha. An alpha state is a deepening state of relaxation in which the brain's activity becomes more settled and the brain wave amplitudes grow bigger, slower and more rhythmic. As brain waves slow down further, the body enters a theta state of light sleep. Theta lasts from 10 to 25 minutes, during which all eye movement, heart rate and body temperature decreases. After 25 minutes, the body enters a delta state of deep sleep. About 70 to 90 minutes after falling asleep, the body enters Rapid Eye Movement (REM) sleep, where dreaming occurs. Keep in mind that the quality of hours spent sleeping is more important than the number hours of sleeping.

The stages of REM and non-REM sleep form a complete sleep cycle. Each cycle lasts about 90 minutes and repeats four to six times during the night. Most young adults spend about half their sleep hours in a non-REM state, about 20 percent in REM state, and 30 percent in the remaining stages, including deep sleep. Deep sleep repairs the body and builds up energy. It plays a major role in growth, repairing muscles and tissues, and boosting the body's immune system. Getting enough deep sleep is an important part of reenergizing the body Walking up in the middle of the night decreases the body's ability to go through the cycles of sleep necessary to repair and energize itself. If you have trouble falling asleep or frequently wake up in the middle of the night, you increase the chances that your body is not spending enough time in the different stages of sleep. In this case, night meditation would be more helpful than morning meditation.

Creating a Flexible Schedule

The majority of students have a strict class schedule that takes up the better part of their day. To create a more flexible schedule, some beginning meditators will keep a journal and record the times of day they feel most relaxed and open to meditation. Try this for three to five days and find as many periods during each day where you feel relaxed and have free time, then write them as options in descending order. That way, if something interrupts your daily routine, you can look down your list and choose the next best option. A journal is also a good way to reflect on meditation and track improvements in your thoughts, outlook or energy level. Experts recommend that beginning meditators practice at the same time each day once they decide upon an optimal time, since it helps establish a practice that becomes ritual. Home meditators should practice their sessions when family members are either not home or busy with other things, to keep distractions to a minimum. Ideally, this free stretch of time should happen while the body feels at peak energy.

Meditation takes time to become ritual. A routine often feels forced and takes effort to return to every day. A ritual, however, feels more like a necessity. Meditators who commit to a schedule and leave enough flexibility in their day to make meditation a regular practice eventually see their practice as a ritual they cannot live without. Many beginners succumb to the pitfall of negatively judging their initial practice. It is important to remember some practices are going to flow better than other times and spending some time practicing meditation is better than not doing it at all. It is important to remain committed to that time and try not to plan other activities within that block of time. This is especially important during the early stages of creating a routine, as consistency is key in forming a strong, regular habit that feels like a natural part of your day.

Eating habits are another consideration for creating a flexible schedule. When the body processes food, digestion draws energy away from other areas. Bigger meals, especially meals high in carbohydrates, require greater

digestion which requires larger withdrawals of energy, causing sleepiness. Meditating is a difficult task to perform on a full stomach. Digestion will often get in the way of the process of meditation because it requires so much mental focus and energy. This is also another reason that meditation experts recommend practicing in the morning before breakfast. You can either wait at least one hour before starting a session, create an alkaline diet (discussed later in this chapter), or eat smaller portions. You should also avoid substances that raise the body's acidity levels. This includes coffee, cappuccino, and any other caffeine-based beverages.

Creating a Meditative Environment

Ambiance is a specific environment defined by mood, character, quality, tone and atmosphere. Meditation does not require ambiance. However, some people feel that ambiance allows faster entry into meditative states; others believe it adds something to their practice. Because more distractions and gadgets now compete for people's attention, serious meditators have turned to creating a specific environment for their practice. Meditation should occur in a calm environment that promotes a sense of peace. Eliminating the possibility for any loud sounds to occur is the first step toward creating an good environment. This means shutting off cellphones or removing them entirely from your space. If you want to keep track of the time without having it hang over you as a distraction, buy a meditation timer.

Removing Distractions

Practicing during the daylight hours might mean blocking out bright sunlight with heavy curtains or some other fabric. Softer lighting promotes relaxation, while bright light creates intensity. Light as it relates to creating mental states of relaxation and intensity explains why romantic dinners are candlelit and operating tables have lamps with bright lights. A space devoted to daily meditative sessions should be free of distractions, but as you progress further into practice and gain concentration, disturbances will

lose their effect. For now, it is best to aim for a dark space with only a small amount of light unless you plan to practice Open Eye Meditation. Open Eye Meditation allows for greater amounts of light within a meditative space, but too much light can prevent the eyes from relaxing. Most beginning meditators find it more productive to close their eyes to block out light. Keep in mind that some light will enter through the eyelids during closed eye meditation. You want to keep your eyes closed but also relaxed, which means that some light will penetrate into your experience. Therefore, a small amount of incoming light is acceptable for meditative purposes. If too much light distracts your focus, choose a very small space with no windows or openings, such as a garage or closet. Complete darkness works well depending on the type of meditation. For example, third eye meditation activates the pineal gland located in your midbrain. The pineal gland is an organ that projects light into your mind's eye and works better in complete darkness. Even a small space such as a walk-in closet, pantry, or nook is enough room for a daily practice.

Ambient Music and Sound

When it comes to selecting a room with a dual purpose, such as a den or bedroom, make sure the room has nothing noisy or visually loud that can create a distraction. However, some advanced meditators purposely choose rooms where these distractions exist as a way of cultivating a core meditation. For example, if you live in an urban area where traffic is always part of the background noise, you might use the background noise as an object of focus in your concentration technique. If you do live in an urban area and want to block out these background noises, it might be better to substitute one noise for another. In other words, use headphones and ambient music to override the sounds of traffic. Ambient music might include anything from binaural beats, to white noise, nature recordings, instrumentals, or some other digitized sound that draws your focus.

Even if you prefer meditating in complete silence, using certain techniques may require connecting to something that develops concentration or mindfulness. In his book, "Teach Yourself to Meditate in Ten Simple Lessons," Eric Harrison writes, "One advantage of ambient music is that when your mind wanders, it tends to fall into the music rather than back into thoughts. The music acts as a safety net. Another advantage is that the sensual and rhythmic qualities of music augment the sensory component of your meditation." However, any music played in along with breathing techniques should be monotone or bland since interesting music can create a distraction. Do not choose music with lyrics, because the words may provoke thinking, and do not choose anything jarring, like rock or rap music. A monotone sound will not dominate your consciousness or jolt you with auditory peaks and valleys. The volume, likewise, should not be so loud that it takes up your entire focus. As a rule, keep an ambient noise to a background level by turning the volume no more than halfway up. Some of the most popular ambient recording artists include Biosphere, The Orb, Tim Hecker, Darshan Ambient and Gandalf. For a list of the top 25 ambient music albums of the last 20 years, go to the resource section at the end of this book.

Although it is important to give some thought to creating the right environment for each meditation session, it is more important to maintain an open mind. Sometimes distractions and interruptions will occur despite your careful planning. That is all right; let the distractions come and go without becoming angry or judgmental. Just do not allow distractions to distract you. Simply notice what is happening and then gently return your attention to the meditation object (e.g. your breath, a mantra, or a sacred passage).

Using Candles, Crystals and Incense

Candles emit just the right amount of light for meditation. They not only create a peaceful ambiance, but can also serve as a focal point during Concentration Meditations. Scents work as powerful mind-centering tools.

Aromatherapy, for example, uses oils to relieve stress, anxiety and depression. If you decide to light candles and burn incense as part of a ritual, use candleholders and position the incense in a place where nothing can spill. Avoid using heavy perfumes or other overpowering scents that might sting your nose or create distractions. If you want to decorate your meditative space with objects that inspire focus, look for earthy objects that naturally strengthen your energy chi such as pyramid crystals and orgonites. You might also consider creating an indoor Zen garden. To brainstorm decorative ideas for a meditation space, consult the online stores listed at the end of this book. If you follow a religious faith, consider creating an altar dedicated to a famous spirit guide, such as Jesus, Buddha, or Mohammed.

Regardless of how you decorate, make sure the space is clutter free with a minimal amount of wall paintings, framed photos and posters. Focusing on these items can cause the mind to wander away from centered, present moment awareness. If you have any pets, find something to keep them safely occupied for at least 10 minutes.

Keeping a Tidy Meditation Space

Every meditation space should be free of clutter. Meditating in a messy room filled with dirty clothes scattered about offers the mind an opportunity to start mentally organizing the room. Cleanliness symbolizes order and discipline. However, picking the clutter up off the floors might not be enough. In some cases, it might be a good idea to vacuum rugs, wipe down dusty areas, organize schoolwork, and open the window. A fresh, clean room will be one where you look forward to spending quiet time. The more you come back to your practice, the more your meditation space will generate and store positive energies.

Choosing Comfortable Clothes

Wearing the proper clothing is just as important as choosing the proper ambience and a regular time to practice each day. Anything tight or constricting will prevent the body from reaching its relaxation state. If you

incorporate yogic poses into meditative practice, you may wind up ripping your clothes or limiting your own movement. The right clothing should be breathable clothes designed for absorbing sweat, and they should either fit loosely or feel expandable. Heavy or uncomfortable clothes will get in the way of meditating since they will make breathing challenging. Loose, comfortable clothes will make it far easier to concentrate.

Clothes made with natural fabrics such as cotton are best during meditative sessions. If you ever wondered why pajamas are made of these materials, it is because these threads feel smooth against skin. Not all fabrics and clothing accessories are the same, so choose what is more comfortable over what looks better. Beginning meditators often make the mistake of being more concerned with the latest fashion trends and less on wearing clothes that feel comfortable. Most meditators wear sweatpants and other related types of drawstring pants during a session because they allow for movement and flexibility in a seated position. A variety of different drawstring pants and other types of flexible, athletic clothing articles are available in an assortment of styles from retailers. Going shopping with friends or family and adding this type of clothing into your regular wardrobe might be well worth it.

Room temperature is another consideration to make as it relates to personal comfort. Some people react differently to temperature than others, so be sure to adjust the temperature to a level that feels unnoticeable. If you cannot control the temperature of the room, always keep handy an article of clothing that meets the conditions described above. Some meditative states can cause a drop in body temperature and blood pressure, so even if you begin a practice feeling comfortable, you might begin to feel chillier than usual. You can find clothes that work well for meditative practices at many sporting goods stores. Additional store supplies include meditation mats, instructional videos, scented candles, meditation music, meditation timers, Yoga bolsters, incense and altar paraphernalia. For a list of stores

that carry additional supplies and accessories, consult the resource section at the end of this book.

Body Support Accessories

Choosing the proper meditation cushion depends on several factors, including how your body responds to certain postures, what postures and alignments you plan to use, what area of the body the cushion provides support, and how comfortable the cushion feels. Each person's spine is different. Without proper support, you risk injuring your body on an unsupportive surface. Improper body support can misalign the body, create discomfort, or promote injury. If you require constant body support, you may need more than one type of cushion. Meditation in any sitting or kneeling postures requires strength and flexibility of the ankles, knees and hips. If you have aches and pains, or have previously injured any of these parts of your body, contemplate getting a cushion that offers direct support there.

Cushions come in a variety of shapes, heights, sizes, colors and materials. Depending on personal belief, the color of the cushion may not be too important, though most people look for a color that matches the colors of their meditation space. Some cultures believe that colors promote harmonization with the surrounding environment. The Chinese call it *feng shui*. For example, red relates to fire energy, which they believe elevates energy. Violet restores balance, yellow elevates mood, blue calms the body, black induces deep inward focus, orange promotes healing, and green encourages slow, deep breathing. If you buy a cushion online or in a store, try to find out of the material is made of either kapok or buckwheat hull. Kapok is a cotton-like material that does not compress like other cushion products. It is also lightweight and conforms to the shape of the body in a supportive manner. Buckwheat hulls weigh more than kapok cushions, but they also conform well to the shape of the body and create a grounded feeling. Generally, more people prefer buckwheat hull cushions because they feel more stable than

kapok cushions. So what is the best body support accessory to choose? The most common body support accessories include:

1. Cotton Yoga mats
2. Zabutons
3. Zafus
4. Gomdens
5. Meditation benches

Cotton Yoga mats work well for lying postures. However, if you plan to sit for long periods, *zafus* are the most commonly used apparatus among Zen and Buddhist meditators. Zafus look like plump round cushions, sometimes accompanied with a soft square base called a *zabuton*. Depending on what posture you need or want to achieve, try interchanging the *zafu* and the *zabuton* to see which feels best. *Zafus* may also come with a padded bench for beginning meditators who expect to do a lot of kneeling. The figure on the left illustrates the look of a typical *zafu* with its *zabuton* underneath.

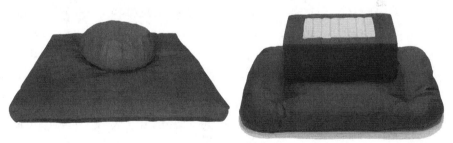

The *Gomdens* are also meditation cushions that come with *zabutons*, except they are square. Most meditators use *gomdens* for cross-legged postures that require the knees to be up off the *zabuton*. The figure above, on the right illustrates the look of a typical *gomden* with its *zabuton* underneath.

Lifestyle Tips for Mental Well-Being and Physical Health

Finding balance between work and play is critical to achieving a successful lifestyle. School and work are important, but not the sole points of living. People who bring their stress home and allow it to affect their home life have no balance in their lifestyle. People who master meditation and present moment awareness know how to reduce stress so that the responsibilities and stresses of school and work never come home with them. In short, they have balance. Their siblings never feel neglected and their parents don't complain about a lack of interest in home life. Being truly in the moment with someone you care about is one of the great joys of life. Meditation teaches people how to push distractions away so they can deepen relationships and enjoy the social interactions that make life worth living. As you progress through your practice, you will begin to feel more open to new experiences. If you want to bring positive energy to your lifestyle, think about volunteering with a charity organization, such as a nursing home or animal shelter. Make a "bucket list" of things you would like to do in the future. Keep in mind that whichever new experience you choose to pursue, none may be more important than changing unhealthy eating habits, especially if stress is causing you to choose comfort foods over foods that supply the energy needed to balance your body and mind.

Healthy Eating

Returning to an earlier discussion about foods that cost the body large amounts of energy, it makes sense to consider changing your diet if you want to promote wellness and bring more energy to the practice of meditation. To recap, bigger meals, especially meals high in carbohydrates, require greater digestion, which requires larger withdrawals of energy, causing sleepiness. For this reason, starting an organic-based alkaline diet has become one of the more popular trends promoted by nutritionists, meditators and people who need more energy to function in their daily lives.

Acid Foods vs. Alkaline Foods

One of the most important balances the human body strives to maintain is the need to maintain a proper acid-alkaline state called pH level. The term "pH" is an abbreviation for "power of hydrogen." What pH measures is the level of hydrogen ion concentration in a water-based solution. Since the human body counts as a water-based solution, the kidneys serve to monitor the pH levels by filtration. This filtration process helps the body balance blood pressure, salt and water levels. Thanks to the kidneys, the pH level of the blood does not change. However, in a highly acid state, the pH level of the cells *can* change. Your cells have energy cycles, so when the pH level of cells become more acid, chemical reactions happen too fast and the body cannot receive the proper nutrients. When the pH level of cells become too alkaline their chemical reactions become too slow and the body does not absorb minerals. To measure the body's level of pH, scientists constructed a pH scale ranging from 0 to 14. Illustrated in the chart below, the number "0" indicates a purely acidic state, the number "7" indicates a neutral state (equal parts acid and alkaline), and the number "14" indicates a purely alkaline state. Different areas of the body require different pH levels. For example, the stomach should be very acidic (between 1 and 3), as should urine. Sweat should be slightly acid while fluid outside the cell should be slightly alkaline. Brain fluid should be slightly alkaline (roughly 7.5), and bile and pancreas should be very alkaline to neutralize stomach acid. At the cellular level, Australian author and nutritionist Barbara O'Neil recommends a slightly acid state of 6.5 because it facilitates the speedy uptake of chemical reactions. Other nutritionists believe the ideal pH level for a person is 7.3—or very mildly alkaline.

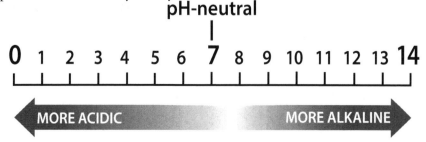

To maintain a balanced acid-alkaline balance, the total pH of food consumption should be roughly 80 percent alkaline foods and 20 percent acidic foods. However, since most Western meals consist of meats, sugars and carbohydrates, the average person's diet is more like 80 percent acidic foods and 20 percent alkaline foods. As an example of how acidic Western diets have become, Barbara O'Neil notes that sugary beverages like soda and root beer have a pH level of 2.7 (highly acidic). So how does a highly acidic state affect the body? When the lungs and kidneys come under intense pressure to filter high levels of acid, they begin to pull calcium phosphate (an alkaline compound stored in your bones) out of the bones and into the blood to combat the "acid crisis." The calcium phosphate restores the pH balance, but at a high cost. If the body draws too much calcium out of the bones, the blood becomes too alkaline, which creates calcium deposits and bone spurs. If you factor in emotional states like stress, worry and anxiety, the body is fighting a two-front war to combat a rising acid-alkaline imbalance. Other behaviors, such as lack of sleep, lack of sunshine, and lack of exercise create acid conditions. This is why adopting a healthy lifestyle will promote the very things you are trying to accomplish through meditation. To this end, Barbara O'Neil notes, "There is nothing wrong with stress; it is *distress* that creates an acid condition." The result of an extended acid-alkaline imbalance includes:

1. Loss of energy
2. Inflammation
3. Mucus congestion
4. Hardening of arteries and soft tissue
5. Ulceration
6. Degenerative diseases such as cancer, heart disease, stroke, ALS and diabetes

Depending on your level of stress, you may not notice these symptoms until they have had time to evolve and cause serious damage. The chart below lists the physical symptoms that appear when a body is too acid or too alkaline.

Too Acid	Too Alkaline
Excessive coughing	Eyelid Twitching
Irregular heartbeat	Hyperventilating
Feeling weak	Arthritis
Feeling nauseous	Allergies
Feeling sleepy but wired	Bone spurs
Frequent sighing	Low thyroid
Feeling anxious	Calcium deposits

The best way to support your meditative practice is to eat right, exercise daily, sleep 8-10 hours a night, consult a nutritionist and get your pH level tested the next time you visit the doctor. Since time constraints prevent many people from exercising or sleeping enough, changing your eating habits can be the easiest way to adopt a lifestyle that supports meditative practice. To restore or maintain your body's energy level, consider adopting an acid-alkaline diet that consists of foods that balance the acid-alkaline levels and energize the cells. For a list of acid and alkaline producing foods, consult Appendix E.

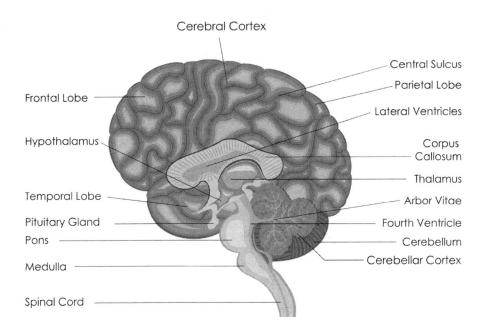

Cerebral Cortex

Central Sulcus
Parietal Lobe
Lateral Ventricles

Frontal Lobe

Hypothalamus
Corpus Callosum

Thalamus

Temporal Lobe
Arbor Vitae

Pituitary Gland
Fourth Ventricle

Pons
Cerebellum

Cerebellar Cortex

Medulla

Spinal Cord

Additional lifestyle tips to consider:

1. Buy local, organic produce

2. Stop eating fast food (it is processed with unnatural chemicals)

3. Replace artificial sweeteners with stevia

4. Avoid soda, diet soda, foods with hydrogenated oil and fructose corn syrup, and fat free and low carb labels

5. Eat dark chocolate if you crave chocolate

6. Reduce the amount of time watching television (especially programs that make you feel negative)

7. Listen to uplifting music early in the morning

8. Make time for friends and loved ones

9. Practice random acts of kindness

10. Get a gym membership

11. Try acupuncture

12. Buy an alarm clock with natural earth tones

13. Create an important goal for yourself in the future

Detoxing Herbs

Detoxification happens naturally when meditation becomes a regular practice. The body's chi energy starts pushing poisons out of the body so it can flow without obstructions. However, the chi only purifies when the body purifies. You can accelerate the body's purification process by detoxing with natural herbs. The areas of the body that need purification are the arteries, kidneys, liver, connective tissue and blood. For non-herbal dietary supplements, go to the resource section at the end of this book. For herbal supplements, **http://detoxsafely.org** lists the following remedies and their cleansing effects, which include:

1. **Alfalfa:** Breaks down poisonous carbon dioxide

2. **Black cohosh:** Loosens and expels bronchial tube mucous

3. **Black walnut:** Oxygenates the blood, balances sugar levels, burns excessive toxins

4. **Burdock root:** Reduces joint swelling, calcification deposits, clears blood of acids

5. **Cayenne pepper:** Used as antioxidant, antiseptic and circulatory stimulant

6. **Chlorella:** Reduces body odors; can be used as a mouthwash

7. **Cascara sagrada:** Increases stomach, liver and pancreas excretions; helps gallstones and hemorrhoids

8. **Chickweed:** Helps heal stomach ulcers

9. **Cranberry:** Treats bacterial bladder infections

10. **Dandelion:** Detoxifies the liver and promotes healthy circulation

11. **Echinacea:** Stimulates production of white blood cells; removes blood toxins

12. **Fennel seed:** Improves digestion as a diuretic

13. **Fenugreek:** Softens and dissolves accumulated mucous, phlegm and infections from the lungs

14. **Gentian root:** Helps in the breakdown of protein and fats

15. **Ginger root:** Cleanses the bowels, kidneys and skin

16. **Guar gum:** Used therapeutically to lower cholesterol and curb appetite

17. **Hawthorn berries:** Strengthens the heart muscles

18. **Hibiscus flower:** Used as antibacterial, mild diuretic and anti-parasitic

19. **Horsetail:** Used in urinary tract disorders

20. **Irish Moss:** Soothes an irritated gastrointestinal tract

21. **Licorice root:** Soothes irritated mucus membranes and nourishes the adrenal glands

22. **Marshmallow:** Removes hardened phlegm in the intestinal tract

23. **Milk thistle:** Prevents liver destruction and enhances liver function by inhibiting free radicals

24. **Mullein leaf:** Soothes irritated tissues

25. **Oat straw:** Helps provide minerals to nourish bones, skin, hair and nails

26. **Papaya:** Aids digestion

27. **Passionflower leaf:** Helps to calm stress and slows the breakdown of neurotransmitters

28. **Peppermint:** Brings oxygen into the bloodstream

29. **Psyllium husk:** Used for all intestinal troubles

30. **Psyllium seed:** Used as a laxative agent and sweeping the gastrointestinal tract of toxins (Drink lots of water with psyllium.)

31. **Pumpkin seed:** Helps the body expel parasites

32. **Red clover:** Used as a tonic for the nerves and as a sedative for nervous exhaustion

33. **Slippery elm:** Neutralizes stomach acidity and absorbs foul gases and toxins

34. **Yarrow:** Acts as a blood cleanser, helps to regulate liver function and heals the glandular system

35. **Violet leaf:** Used as an antifungal, demulcent, diuretic and laxative

36. **Witch hazel bark, twigs, and leaves:** Helps heal damaged blood vessels

37. **Yellow dock:** Used as a blood builders and stimulates waste elimination

38. **Yucca root:** Helps break down organic waste in the body and relieves inflammation associated with arthritis

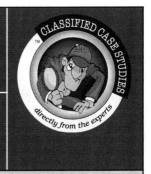

CASE STUDY: CREATING YOUR MEDITATION ROUTINE

Travis May
The St. Petersburg Shambhala Center
travismay108@gmail.com
www.travismay108.wordpress.com

I think the best time to meditate varies from person to person. I have no strong preference for any particular time of day, so I often practice at very different times. I do, however, like practicing in the morning because it is a good way to set the tone for the day. If I have to be somewhere early in the morning, I will shift my practice schedule to the middle of the day because that is when I need the most energy. At the Shambhala Center, we have classes in the early evenings. If my schedule prevents me from meditating in the morning and at noon, I will go there for a session. Early evening is a good time because I feel relaxed and ready to practice without it being late enough where I might feel too tired .

I will sit late at night as a fourth option if I have not meditated in the morning, noon, or early evening at the center. I may feel more tired, but knowing that meditation creates the right conditions for a deep sleep is what motivates me to practice right before bed.

If you want to create a flexible schedule to fit your lifestyle, I recommended setting a time every day. If it becomes a normal part of your routine — like taking a shower, exercising and brushing your teeth — you will be more likely to do it. If your goal is to sit for 15 minutes a day, start getting up 15 minutes earlier than you normally do and add the sitting session to your morning routine. Perhaps it is better for you to sit when you get home from school, or during your lunch period. We each have to find what works best for us. The key is that we actually do it.

Some people prefer an elaborate ambiance. I recommend that you find a nice, comfortable, safe, quiet spot. It is good to have a space in your house dedicated for meditation practice. How you set that up will likely depend on your available space, connection to the practice, and budget.

I have a setup at home similar to what we have at the meditation center. I use candles and incense to emulate the practice environment at the center. Everything in our shrine is symbolic, and I think it is good to understand the meaning of your shrines rather just doing it as a gimmick or because you think it might magically make you meditate better.

I would recommend just wearing light, loose fitting, comfortable clothing. In other words, what you would normally wear for any physical exercise. Wearing tight jeans can cut off your circulation and cause your leg to go to sleep, or it can restrict you to an uncomfortable sitting position. Many meditation centers recommend wearing layers so you can adjust to different temperatures, too. Ultimately, it is not necessary to go out and purchase a new wardrobe to meditate, but if it gets you focused on maintaining a schedule, then go ahead and do so.

I would not say that any support accessory works best because they are highly individualized. Our size, flexibility and health can affect which cushions or chairs we might use to practice meditation. When working with posture, people often try different heights by stacking cushions on top of each other, or using a cushion plus a smaller support cushion. To figure out which accessory works best for your body type, visit a meditation center. They will probably have several kinds of body support cushions that you can try out with the help of a qualified instructor who can give you advice.

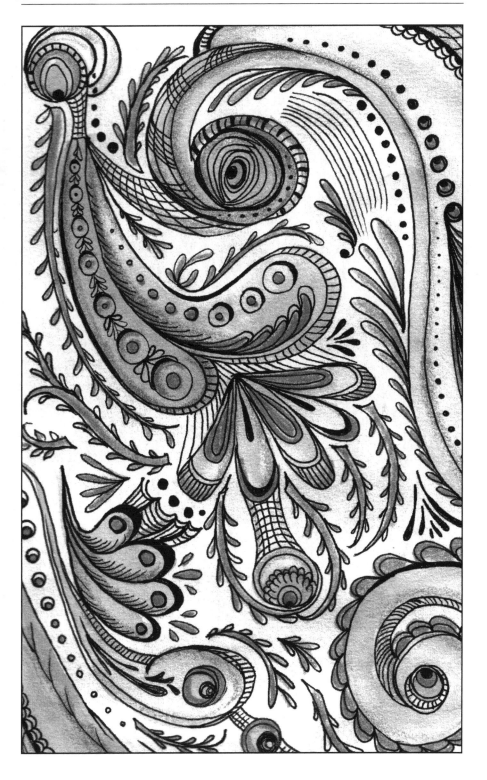

Preparing the Body for Core Meditation

In addition to ambiance and environment, preparing the body for core meditation involves looking at the current state of your physical health. While much of meditation involves sitting, how you sit can often determine the effectiveness of your practice. Using a zafu or zabuton as a body support will encourage proper body alignment, but if you become lazy in your posture, you will begin to strain your back, hips and joints. Beginning meditators who strain these areas long enough will begin to risk injury if the physical core of the body's midsection (not to be confused with core meditation) is not strong enough to support a long-held posture. Therefore, having strong core muscles in your body's midsection will reduce the possibility of straining areas not designed for sustained pressure.

Having a strong core midsection gives beginning meditators confidence that they can sit in basic or more advanced positions. Having confidence in posture means not having to think about posture during mind quieting or concentration exercises. Having a weak core midsection means worrying about injures while trying to meditate. Out of

this fear of being injured, your inner dialogue will try to begin talking you out of your practice. It might replay an old injury that had nothing to do with sitting. It might recall the pain your body experienced when this injury occurred. The more you think about past hurts, the more you may begin to associate pain with your meditative practice until you become discouraged from returning to your practice. It is for these reasons that the different forms of yoga practice all incorporate poses called asanas with their meditative disciplines. Your body's core midsection consists of:

1. The transversus abdominis (the muscle layer of the abdominal wall)
2. The pelvic floor (the muscle fibers underneath the pelvis)
3. The diaphragm (the sheet of muscle extending along the bottom of the rib cage)
4. The multifidus (the muscle protecting the spinal column)

To strengthen the core midsection, consider buying a medicine ball and follow the exercise instructions that typically come with them, such as calf stretches, inversion stretches, ab crunches and reverse back crunches. During these exercises, remember to exhale coming up (keeping your midsection tight) and inhale on the way down. The range of motion in the exercises performed on a medicine ball can really build the necessary midsection strength for supporting meditative poses and maintaining balance.

The Importance of Proper Body Alignment

Proper body alignment is important because meditation is about achieving balance and staying centered in the body and mind. Meditation starts with achieving balance in the core midsection through proper posture and alignment. When the midsection loses balance, other areas of the body not meant to support posture begin to compensate for it. When other areas of the body become strained, joints

and muscles eventually tire and begin to break down from improper use. Good body alignment harmonizes the relationship between mind, body and spirit. Since the goal of meditation is to create a connection between all three, your body's alignment is the first step in building this bridge. Correct body alignment also increases circulation to vital organs, which helps bring balance to your emotional and physical state. Proper body alignment also increases the efficiency of your meditative exercises. If you become physically frustrated with meditation, examine your preparation. It may be that improper alignment of your body is causing you to work harder with less benefit. Proper alignment means working the body less and maximizing results.

The best way to determine the strength of your body's core midsection is to attend a yoga class for beginners. Taking a yoga class can give you a feel for your body's flexibility, which poses come easy and which postures your midsection struggles to maintain. Whether you settle easily into each posture or not, pay attention to the instructor's directions about maintaining posture so you can apply these tips to your regular sitting practice. Another way to strengthen your core muscles is through breath work. Train your abdominal muscles, lie on your back with both knees bent and place your palms at the bottom of your rib cage. Take a breath in through your nose and breathe deeply, allowing your diaphragm to expand your stomach while keeping your chest still. After your stomach rises to its highest point, exhale through your mouth and repeat the process.

Sitting Postures for Meditation

Sitting in a meditative posture is the most common type of stationary practice because it creates a stable position that roots deeply into the heaven and earth. Standing meditative stances may serve different but equally effective purposes. Some meditators use the horse stance, for example, to prevent or ease panic attacks. Lying down positions, such

as the corpse pose, work best at the end of a yoga practice for allowing the body to release its tension and settle into an even deeper state of relaxation. For the purpose of most beginner meditations, however, sitting postures may create the best experience. When you sit upright, keep each part of your spine stacked evenly. If it helps to visualize your spine (from the base to the top) as a skyscraper in order to keep it upright, then do so. The point of rooting yourself firmly between heaven and earth is to create a link between the physical and spiritual dimension of existence.

The seven basic points of correct meditative posture include: crossing the legs, placing both hands in the lap, keeping the back and neck straight, maintaining shoulder balance, relaxing the tongue and mouth, and keeping the eyes relaxed and either closed or semi-closed. If you wish to stand during meditation, consider using the sun salutation exercise, putting both feet together with both hands at the side. Variations of standing meditation also include the horse stance (a common standing meditation used in Tai Chi), or the empty stance (a common standing meditation in Qigong to relieve back pain). Using the horse stance, stand with both feet shoulder width apart, keeping the back straight and feet pointed straight ahead. Bend the knees and hips as if you are about to sit down, raise both hands, and maintain that position for the duration of your practice. The horse stance is commonly used when you want to combine meditation with a physical workout that gets the blood flowing. To use the empty stance, stand with the knees slightly bent, keeping the legs six inches apart, and move one foot ahead of the other. Next, shift most of your weight to the foot closer to you, then lift the other foot and let it barely touch the ground. Raise your arms in front and begin meditation.

As an advanced alternative to standing or sitting, the bow position is an inverted pose that offers a great way to reverse stress and relax the mind before practicing meditation. To complete the bow position, lie

face down on the floor with your hands at your side and bend your knees. Using your arms, reach behind you and cuff your ankles with both hands. Once you have the right hand cuffing the right ankle and the left hand cuffing the left ankle, lift the upper half of your body by pulling on the ankles to form a "U" with your body. If you prefer to sit, the most common types of stationary sitting postures are:

1. The seated position (in a chair) — helps prevent slouching
2. The kneeling position (on a stool or seiza bench) — difficult without support
3. The lotus positions (half, full, Burmese) — most stable posture for beginners

Using Yoga to Improve Body Alignment and Posture

Stretching the body before each meditative practice can also help the muscles in the body to become more limber. When you start a car engine in the middle of winter, you want to warm up the engine to prevent the engine from breaking down. The same concept applies to muscles before meditation. If you attend a yoga class, look around at other meditators to see how they stretch the muscles in their body before class begins, or simply ask the instructor for stretching tips after class. Stretching before a yoga class is not always necessary since a good instructor always starts the practice slow to prepare the muscles for deeper stretches and postures. Good instructors also take notice of their students' posture problems and work to correct misalignments as they occur. In addition to stretching, yoga helps build core muscles through breathing and resistance. Yoga poses useful to strengthening the body's core muscles include:

1. The child pose
2. The cobra
3. The plank pose

4. The downward dog
5. The spine rotation
6. The bridge pose
7. The boat pose with variation

The Child Pose

The child pose is a yogic position that stretches the core muscles by extending the hips and spine. To get into this position, sit on your knees and let your toes point backward, then spread both knees a little wider than your shoulders, and lean forward with your forehead on the floor. Two variations of the child's pose exist. In the first variation, place the back of your hands on the floor just outside your feet and hold this position for ten deep breaths. In the second variation (illustrated below), you would extend your arms in front of your head to get a diaphragm stretch. With your arms extended, both palms should lay flat on the floor. Hold this position for 10 deep breaths. Repeating this stretching and breathing exercise over time will improve the overall strength of the core muscles and make your body more capable of handling meditative poses in proper alignment.

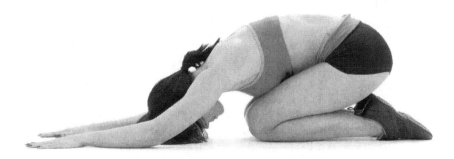

The Cobra

The cobra (illustrated on the following page) is a yogic position that stretches the muscles that flex your spine. To assume this position, lie

on your stomach, palms on the floor, elbows bent and fingers pointing straight ahead. Using your arms, push up the top half of your torso and hold this pose for 15 to 20 seconds, making sure your arms stay close to your sides. Keep your toes pointed backward, and lift your head up, keeping the spine arched until you feel the abdomen begin to stretch. After 15 to 20 seconds, lower the top half of your torso back down until it is on the floor again.

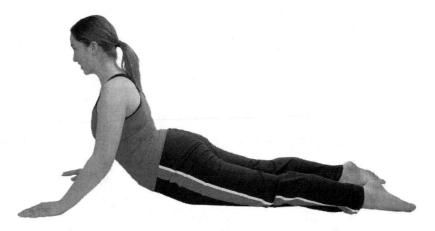

The Plank

The plank (illustrated below) is a yogic position and form of resistance training that builds strength in the lower lumbar of the back and in the abdominals. A weak lower lumbar will strain and eventually collapse during long sitting periods, causing the body to misalign and shift weight into areas that cannot support the position. Building

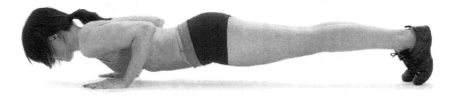

strength in the lower lumbar means the body is more likely to stay properly aligned. You can use the cobra position to come into the plank pose by slowly lowering the top half of the body's torso to face the floor again and then pushing the body up off the ground, keeping the elbows bent and the back completely straight. Hold the plank pose for 30 seconds. To maintain proper positioning, make sure the lumbar stays straight and does not begin to drop toward the ground. To keep the lumbar from dropping, tighten the stomach's abdominal muscles. The longer the body remains fixed in this position, the stronger the abdominal muscles become.

The Downward Dog

The downward dog (illustrated below) is a yogic position that helps the body maintain a neutral spine alignment, which is important for creating balance in your meditative position. You can come into downward dog from the plank pose by walking the hands back to the feet and raising your hips upward until your body forms a triangle. To come into this position first, get on your knees and lean forward on your hands, then shift the bottom half of your weight back onto your feet and walk your hands backward until your body forms a triangle shape.

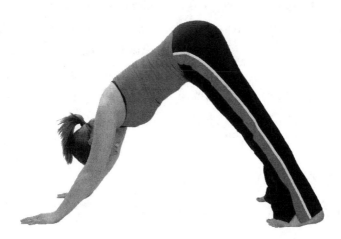

The Spine Rotation

The spine rotation (illustrated below) is a yogic position that stretches the abdomen and lower back muscles that twist the torso left and right. If you have stiffness in the lower back before or after assuming a sitting position in meditative practice, using the spine rotation can help realign the spine and reduce stiffness and discomfort. To assume this position, sit on the floor and place your right hand flat and behind you, fingers pointing away from the body. With the right hand stabilized and the arm remaining straight, fold the left leg into the groin area with the left arm and cross the right leg over the folded left leg. Next, bend the elbow of the left arm, rotate your torso and place the bent elbow against the right knee. Tense your core muscles for about 10 seconds, then release the tension by rotating back to the original position. Repeat this position several times, then position yourself for a spinal rotation in opposite direction, and rotate and tense the torso muscles to the left.

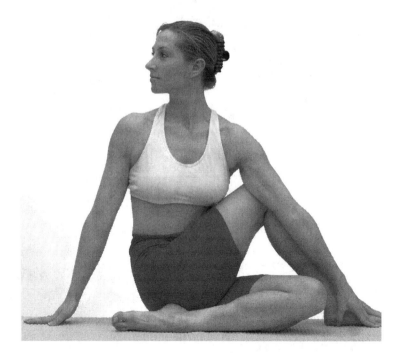

The Bridge Pose

The Bridge Pose (illustrated below) is a yogic position and breathing exercise that can relax tension felt in the spine, breathing structures, and pelvic floor as well as activate the energy openings in these areas. The bridge pose is especially useful if energy blockages in the pelvic area create strain through long sitting periods. It also lowers pressure in the thoracic cavity (area around the lungs). To assume this position and practice the breathing movements, lie on your back, and slide your feet closer to the buttocks until your knees are bent and in the air. On the next inhale, keeping your arms on the floor, raise your buttocks and pelvic region to the air. On the exhale, bring the buttocks and pelvic region back to the ground. Repeat this breathing exercise for 20 or 30 seconds.

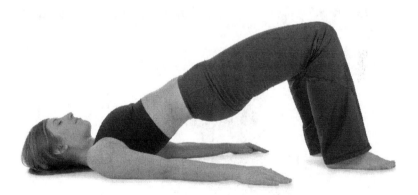

The Boat Pose

The Boat Pose (illustrated on the following page) is a yogic position and form of resistance training that strengthens the spinal muscles against the pull of gravity. It also protects the lumbar from straining and losing support during long sitting periods. To assume this position, lie down on your back with your legs slightly apart and slowly raise your upper and lower torso at the same time until you are balancing

on your buttocks. As you balance, keep the abdominals tight and both arms pointed straight ahead and locked at the elbows. The boat pose creates a resistance similar to sit-ups. If you decide to do sit-ups as a form of resistance training, consider placing a light weight on your upper abdomen as you gain more strength. For reverse sit-ups, use a slant board to build core strength in the muscles around the spine. The boat pose is ideal for meditators looking to build core strength because it builds core strength in both the abdominals and around the spine at the same time.

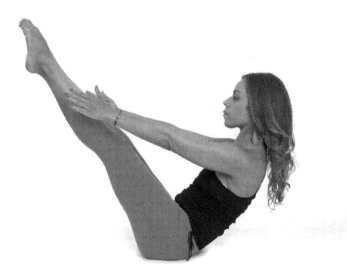

Gravity is a challenge in this position, but your balance will improve as core muscles become stronger. Physical balance is an important aspect of any meditation because it will keep the body in proper alignment and reduce stress that can often break concentration. Keeping the back straight is the most important part of this pose, so if you begin to slouch, straighten the back. The boat pose is a more advanced pose, so to avoid risking injury, consider building core strength through the other exercises before attempting to balance in boat pose.

Building core strength is important for reasons that go beyond meditation. Millions of teens in America and throughout the world spend a bulk of their time at school sitting at a desk or in front of a computer screen. Without strengthening these areas of the body, a significant number of these people will probably experience a gradual weakening of the spine. The answer to avoiding these physical problems is building strength through breathing exercises, resistance training or stretching. By implementing all three techniques, you will not only prepare your body for meditation, but activities in everyday life that require support from these areas. "Yoga Anatomy" by Leslie Kaminoff and Amy Matthews offers a greater examination of yoga's strengthening effect on the physical anatomy as well as a number of useful illustrations.

The Most Common Forms of Yoga

The word yoga means union, which refers to a union between the body, breath, mind and spirit. Many people in the world today practice different kinds of yoga for different reasons. The most common forms of yoga differ to some degree in their practice, their intention and their results. Before committing to yoga as a meditative practice, you should learn their differences and think about which might best fit your meditative intentions. Although each form of yoga differs in many respects, they all use asanas (poses) in their disciplines. The original intent of yoga, as written in "Yoga Sutras" was to reach a higher state of consciousness known as Samadhi, or oneness with God. The use of asanas is one of seven paths taken before reaching the eighth path of Samadhi (charted in Appendix D).

The best form of yoga is whichever form suits each individual person. Once a person finds his or her style of yoga, the benefits are virtually limitless. Some benefits include becoming more peaceful with oneself and with others, as well as achieving contentment and attainment of Samadhi.

Improvements involve posture, mental attitude, concentration, strength, flexibility, balance, lung volume, spirituality, well-being and a healthier immune system. Following the path of yoga as originally intended through all eight paths (otherwise known as sutras), purification of the mind and body will occur over time. Practicing asanas may help detoxify the body, but many yoga masters believe that practicing only one path of yoga is not really practicing yoga. The eight paths of yoga are:

1. Yamas — non-violence, truthfulness, moderation in all things and non-covetousness
2. Niyamas — keeping the body and mind free of impurities, being austere and studying the sacred texts
3. Asanas — postures for internal discipline
4. Pranayama — regulation and control of the breath
5. Pratyahara — withdrawal of the senses in order to still the mind
6. Dharana — concentration
7. Dhyana — meditation
8. Samadhi — achieving unity of self with all things

The first two paths of yoga involve making a determination to set oneself on the yogic path, which begins with a commitment to positive living and being. Although practicing asana only constitutes the third path, they are very useful to everyday meditators when combined with the breath (referred to as prana) and a focused mind. Moving through a series of poses is called a vinyasa. Where breath goes, energy will follow. In yoga, energy is referred to as shakti, and the meditator's body is called sushuma. Being able to direct or control energy through the body by using the breath is what constitutes the fourth path, pranayama. The healing power of shakti can be very powerful once a yogi has perfected pranayama because the yogi can direct healing to any part of the body. This is why yoga masters do not believe that a yogic pose by itself is yoga, but rather, a combination of various paths that heals the body. Yoga is more effective if you have more than 10 minutes a day to meditate, so if you do not have more than ten min-

utes a day, consider learning some yogic poses to aid your meditation and combine the third path (asanas) with the fourth path (pranayama), as this will help you eventually learn to direct energy throughout the body. This will prepare your body and mind for the fourth and fifth stages of the yogic path — quieting the mind (pratyahara) and concentration (dharana). Some of the more common forms of yoga in the U.S. today are:

1.   Hatha yoga combines poses with pranayama (lengthening of the breath) and relaxation techniques. The most common reason people use Hatha yoga is to reduce stress and achieve mental peace. Certain types of yoga, such Kripalu yoga and Lyengar yoga are derivations of Hatha yoga.

2.   Kundalini yoga helps open the energetic blockages that cause tension and other physical and emotional maladies. Kundalini yoga involves meditation for the chakras, which combines poses, chanting and pranyama.

3.   Ashtanga Vinyasa yoga helps build strength and power. Its exercises are useful for strengthening core muscles to prepare the body for longer meditative periods. Certain types of hot yoga practices are derivations of Vinyasa yoga.

4.   Bikram yoga is considered the original form of hot yoga, which involves a series of postures and breathing exercises in a room with a temperature set to 105 degrees Fahrenheit. Setting the room to 105 F opens the pores and helps flush out toxins, increases oxygen flow to the cells and improves blood flow in the body. To avoid confusion about hot yoga, the general rule is that all Bikram is hot yoga, but not all forms of hot yoga qualify as Bikram yoga. Be advised that dehydration is a potential danger that exists with Bikram or any other form of hot yoga.

Setting Up the Energetic Openings

Negative thoughts, feelings, emotions and behaviors diminish the body's natural energy and cause disease. Positive thoughts, feelings, emotions and behaviors expand and generate the body's natural energy for healing. Where breath goes, energy will follow. The more you breathe, stretch, exercise and meditate, the more energy will begin to accumulate in your body. As energy begins to build-up, the closer you come to tapping into a seemingly limitless energy source. The concept of healing the body through the accumulation and redirection of energy is what some meditation experts call energy medicine.

Balancing the energy centers in the body requires treating energetic blockages wherever they exist. Old hurts and negative emotions create energetic blockages that imbalance the body intellectually, physically, emotionally and spiritually. One goal in your meditative practice should involve unblocking these energetic openings so that energy can flow free to do its healing work. For instance, kundalini yoga involves the practice of awakening the divine feminine energy called the kundalini, which resides at the bottom of the spine. Once activated, the kundalini rises up through the spine and unblocks the energetic openings. The seven energetic openings along the spinal channel are called chakras. Each chakra is located at a different nodal point along the spinal column. Meditators who awaken the kundalini typically describe it as a wellspring of energy that rises up the spine and bursts through the top of the head, causing a feeling of ecstasy.

The Seven Chakras

Each of the seven chakras that exist along the spinal column influences the glands and organs surrounding it. The chakras are called energetic openings because they draw their energy from the universe. The word chakra means "wheel" in Sanskrit because the mystics believed the energy in them revolved as spinning energies. An energetic blockage in one chakra can lead to blockages in the other chakras and interrupt their functioning. The following diagram illustrates the seven chakras, along with their name, location and purpose.

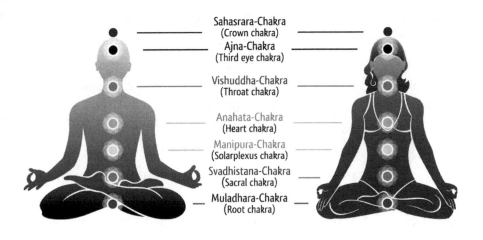

Sahasrara-Chakra
(Crown chakra)
Ajna-Chakra
(Third eye chakra)
Vishuddha-Chakra
(Throat chakra)
Anahata-Chakra
(Heart chakra)
Manipura-Chakra
(Solarplexus chakra)
Svadhistana-Chakra
(Sacral chakra)
Muladhara-Chakra
(Root chakra)

MAN MEDITATION
Padmasana/Lotus

WOMAN MEDITATION
Siddha Yoni Asana

Some meditators report being able to open the higher chakras, while the lower chakras remain closed. The lower chakras represent issues related to lower intentions, such as personal safety and well-being, while the higher chakras relate to higher intentions such as spiritual oneness and unconditional love. Lower chakras actually may be more difficult to open because of the personal issues associated with them. The first (or root) chakra is located between the anus and genitals, and

it concerns personal safety. If the body is in a state of fear, this chakra will not open until the mind-state of fear subsides. The second (sacral or splenic) chakra is located at the base of the spine (called the sacrum) and concerns creativity and emotional attachment. If the body is clinging to either someone, something, or past regrets, then this chakra will not open until the person becomes present and releases from negative emotional attachments. The third (or solar plexus) chakra is located at the solar plexus and concerns feelings of empowerment. A body in a state of disempowerment cannot find a way to release emotions that make the person feel small and insignificant. The fourth (or heart) chakra is located at the center of the chest near the heart. It is associated with love and self-esteem. If the body is in a state of self-hatred, this chakra will not open until the person learns to stop punishing him/herself. The fifth (or throat) chakra is located at the center of the throat. It is associated with communication, self-expression and confidence. A body in this state cannot find a way to understand or deal with feelings such as mistrust or anger. The sixth (or third eye) chakra is located between the two eyes and relates to mental clarity and intuition. A body in a state of mental cloudiness cannot make plans or solve problems. The seventh (or crown) chakra is located at the top of the head and relates to spiritual transcendence. A body in a state of disconnection to spirit sees no spirit, no meaning in anything and no connection to anything but him/herself. Opening the seven corresponding chakras raises the levels of each energy body. Over time, or perhaps immediately, blockages fade and the meditator begins to experience an increased sense of security, creativity, detachment to emotional hurts, self-empowerment, self-esteem, confidence, mental and psychic clarity, and connection to spirit.

Because chakras govern certain parts of the anatomy, certain illnesses correspond with energetic blockages of certain chakras. If you have a particular illness and your doctor has identified where the problem is, consult the chart above to see which chakra might need unblocking. To set up the

energetic openings for optimal functioning, the meditator needs to rebalance the chakras. For advice on awakening the kundalini to unblock the energetic openings, see the case study at the end of this chapter. Otherwise, try opening the chakras by using the following steps:

Step 1 — Opening the root chakra: Sit down in a chair or in a lotus position. Keep your back straight, your spinal column stacked upright, and avoid slouching. Bring your thumb and index finger on your right hand together and do the same for the left hand. To stimulate the root chakra, begin flexing the muscles located between the genitals and anus. With your mind, visualize the first chakra opening within this part of your body and repeatedly chant the sound "LAM."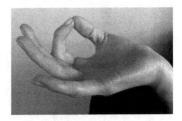

Step 2 — Opening the abdomen: While sitting in a chair or in a lotus position, place both hands on your lap. Face both palms upward, with one hand underneath the other and the tips of both thumbs touching each other. With your palms up and your hands near the abdominal or sacral area of your body, begin chanting the sound "VAM" and visualize the sacral chakra opening within your abdomen. Also, with the 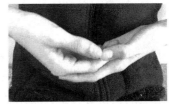 help of a yoga instructor, try several hip opening postures, as these stretching techniques directly connect to the second chakra. The full lotus position is one such hip opening posture. Other hip opening exercises include the reclining butterfly, wide-legged forward bend, and warrior II (for a description of these hip exercises, see Appendix F).

Step 3 — Opening the solar plexus chakra: Raise both hands in front of your stomach. With fingers remaining straight, touch both hands together at the fingertips to form a triangle, and cross one thumb over the other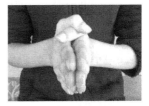

thumb. Now close your eyes and visualize the third chakra opening within your solar plexus while repeatedly chanting the sound "RAM."

Step 4 — Opening the heart chakra: Sit with your legs crossed in a lotus position. Let the tips of the index finger and thumb on your right hand touch; then do the same for the left hand. With the index finger and thumb on both hands forming circles, place the right hand to the center of your breastbone. Next, place your left hand on your 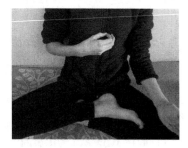 left knee, fingers still touching and the palm facing up or facing down. Close your eyes, smile, visualize the fourth chakra opening within your heart, and chant the sound "YAM." If you want to add a variation to this technique, obtain a piece of rose quartz (considered to hold a love energy) and hold it to your heart chakra as you say the words, "I accept and deserve love." Chant the mantra "Hu" repeatedly, bring the quartz to your lips, inhale, exhale and say, "Thank you."

Step 5 — Opening the throat chakra: Sitting in kneeling position, let the tip of your left thumb touch the tip of your right thumb; then let the fingers of your right interlock with the fingers of your left hand. Close your eyes and visualize the chakra opening within your throat while chanting the sound "HAM."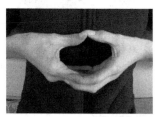

Step 6 — Opening the third eye chakra: This chakra tends to close more than the other chakras due to issues with pineal gland. First, sit in a lotus position and let the tips of both middle fingers touch each other to form a triangle; let the thumbs touch each other as well. Then fold both index fingers down, allowing them to touch. Bring this hand forma-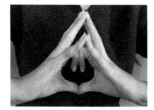

tion to the lower part of your chest (roughly the same spot you brought your hand in the heart chakra opening). Close your eyes and visualize the third eye chakra opening between your eyes while chanting the sound "OM." As an additional technique, consider using binaural beats instead of chanting. Binaural beats are useful for chakra tuning, especially for third eye meditation.

Step 7 — Opening the crown chakra: The seventh chakra is the most spiritual. You need a strong foundation to open this chakra, so do not attempt to open it unless you have already opened the root. In fact, you should not attempt to release the kundalini through kundalini meditation unless you have opened the root chakra. Many yoga masters warn of dangers associated with following short cuts to third eye opening and improper kundalini release, so follow these instructions and consult with your teachers. Once you are ready to open the crown chakra, remain seated in a 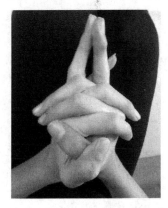 lotus position, place your hands at stomach level, clasp the fingers of your right and left hand together, and let the tips of your ring fingers touch to form a triangle. Close your eyes, chant the sound "NG," and visualize the seventh chakra opening at the top of your head.

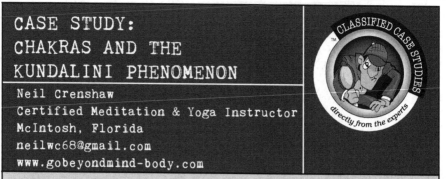

CASE STUDY:
CHAKRAS AND THE
KUNDALINI PHENOMENON

Neil Crenshaw
Certified Meditation & Yoga Instructor
McIntosh, Florida
neilwc68@gmail.com
www.gobeyondmind-body.com

My favorite meditative posture is sitting with my legs crossed and wearing gloves, a blindfold, and earplugs to isolate myself from outside stimuli. I believe it is best to sit in an upright position and be as comfortable as possible. If this requires cushions, pillows, bolsters, etc., that is fine. It is best not to sit in a bothersome position that distracts from the meditative process. Sitting in a comfortable position reduces any possibility of injury to the spine. When the spine is stacked in vertical position, energy flows more freely. I begin every meditation with chakra breathing. This practice begins with the first chakra at the base of the spine. I visualize the chakra as a wheel with the axle of the wheel lying horizontal, from left to right, and the chakra looking much like a water wheel. The breath flows in at the bottom of the chakra and out at the top. Each breath turns the chakra and opens it further as I continue breathing.

The first chakra is very important because it lays the groundwork for the remaining chakras. It may take ten or 20 minutes of slow, rhythmic breathing at the first chakra before the breath moves up to the second chakra. For me, moving up the chakra system becomes automatic once the first chakra opens. Once I reach the seventh chakra, energy expands out the head into universal consciousness. I do not use a timer because I feel it would disturb the natural flow of energy. It may take 30 or 40 minutes to open all the chakras and about an hour or so remaining in universal consciousness. Afterward, I usually come back into my body and go about my daily activities while attempting to stay in pure awareness as much as possible.

The first time I experienced the kundalini phenomenon was about ten years ago. I was meditating in a chair when a sudden a surge of energy rushed up my spine and out the top of my head. I have not had such a dramatic experience since that time, but I do experience smaller and varying degrees of kudalini almost every night. Typically, I will stand, press an acupuncture spot with my fingernail, and take short inhalations through the nose. After about 25 to 30 breaths, the kundalini moves up my body and finally out the top of the head. It is a very relaxing and energizing experience.

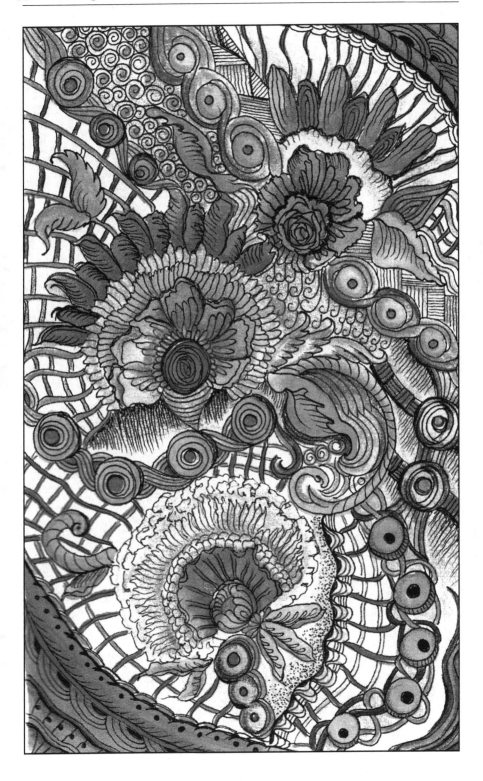

Beginning Core Meditation with Concentration

O nce you have created an ambient environment, hammered out a flexible schedule, and prepared your body for meditation, it is time to begin your core meditation with concentration. In Chapter 2, we identified Concentration Meditation as the art of ridding yourself of internal distractions so the mind can quiet the inner dialogue. The 10-minute meditation format available at the end of this chapter is a good starting point for your meditative journey. However, the purpose of this book is not to confine you to a specific practice, but to provide enough techniques to mix and match according to their individual benefits and your personal needs.

Chapters 5, 6 and 7 will cover the three core meditations (concentration, mindfulness and lovingkindness) respectively. For now, practice the 10-minute format provided in these chapters before you begin to mix and match with your own 10-minute meditative recipe. For example, when you finish this chapter (or book depending on your preference), try practicing one core meditation per week over a period of three weeks. In week one, practice Concentration Meditation using the techniques you learned

in this chapter. In week two, practice Mindfulness Meditation using the techniques you will learn in Chapter 6. In week three practice Lovingkindness Meditation, techniques you will learn in Chapter 7. However, before beginning this exploration into the core meditations, it is important to understand the states of consciousness you will find yourself entering as you meditatively awaken.

The Four States of Consciousness

While Chapter 3 briefly covered the four types of brain waves measured by EEG (*beta, theta, alpha* and *delta*), this chapter will define these states of consciousness further. To recap, beta is the state of consciousness where the mind is constantly thinking about what happened over the course of the day. An alpha state is a deepening state of relaxation in which the brain's activity becomes more settled and brain wave amplitudes grow bigger, slower and more rhythmic. Theta is the point at which brain waves slow to where the body enters a state of light sleep. Delta is the point at which the body enters a state of deep sleep and the mind eventually begins dreaming. The table below illustrates the frequency and mental state of each EEG type.

EEG type	Occupied frequency bandwidth	Mental states & conditions
Delta	0.1Hz ~ 3Hz	deep, dreamless sleep, non-REM sleep, unconscious
Theta	4Hz ~ 7Hz	intuitive, creative, recall, fantasy, imagery, creative, dreamlike, switching thoughts, drowsy
Alpha	8Hz ~ 12Hz	eyes closed, relaxed, not agitated, but not drowsy, tranquil conscious
Low Beta	12Hz ~ 15Hz	formerly SMR, relaxed yet focused, integrated
Midrange Beta	16Hz ~ 20Hz	thinking, aware of self & surrounding
High Beta	21Hz ~ 30Hz	alertness, agitation

A person who has mastered meditation will typically fall within the theta category. With enough practice, these meditators can easily fall into theta states within 10 minutes. Beginning meditators might need more time to

focus and clear the mind. This is why focusing on one practice at a time — concentration in the first week, mindfulness in the second week and lovingkindness in the third week — makes more sense than trying to do different things in one session. Without practicing concentration, beginners also tend to fall asleep in the middle of meditating. However, this can happen for a number of reasons that may have nothing to do with depth of practice. For example, a meditator might be dealing with sleep apnea, jumpy legs syndrome or physical exhaustion.

Beta Consciousness

The purpose of understanding brainwave consciousness is to be able to identify the moments when your consciousness has shifted into a new pattern during meditation. This will become especially useful during Mindfulness Meditation . Brainwaves are also important to Concentration Meditation because noticing a shift in consciousness can often be your signal to begin a new technique. It can also serve as a signal to shift from Concentration Meditation to either mindfulness or lovingkindness. When you begin a meditation, you will most likely always begin in beta consciousness. The purpose of Concentration Meditation is to quiet the mind and move your brainwaves out of beta. While thinking is an important part of life and problem solving, its consequences come in the forms of distractions and emotional disturbances. Beta consciousness is the mind-state that the average person experiences shortly after waking until just after bedtime. It is also characterized by high energy use. At the same time, it often inspires fear, anger, and ego drive. This, of course, is not an ideal state for meditation. Most people spend most of their lives in beta consciousness.

Not everyone, however, spends most of their time in beta consciousness. Depending on how stressful your life is, you may actually alternate between beta and alpha. For example, people who experience periods of stress throughout the day marked by short periods of relaxation typically shift from beta (alert and active) to alpha (relaxed and tranquil), back to beta,

and so forth. During the day, it is important to try to set aside moments of relaxation, even if you experience high levels of stress at school. The reason for this is simple. The body naturally experiences 90-minute cycles of high and low energy during the day. If the body does not rest during the low ebbs, mental and physical fatigue will set in more quickly. If you are someone who values productivity, you could wind up being more productive and less exhausted by simply recognizing when you have hit low energy and taking five minutes to complete a breathing exercise.

Alpha Consciousness

You may remember an earlier discussion about when the body is engaged in the stress response, it is always striving to return to the relaxation response. The same concept holds true for the body's brain waves. When the mind is in beta, it is always striving to return to alpha. Alpha consciousness is the point at which the mind begins to relax and burn less energy. The mind wants to descend back into alpha consciousness because that is the mind-state where it can become so inactive that it rejuvenates itself. Even if your only goal in meditation is to serve a lower intention (such as recharging for mental clarity), meditating for 10 minutes will accomplish just that.

The shift into alpha consciousness can happen very rapidly by slowly inhaling and exhaling a few deep breaths. Difficulties that come with trying to fall into alpha usually happen when the mind is trying to focus on two different things. For example, if you attempt to have a conversation with another meditator while listening to ambient music, your mind will remain in beta because you are keeping the mind's beta components active. Alpha is a state of "being" rather than a state of "doing." In a state of "being," the mind has no concern of the past or the future, where the ego creates worry and inner dialogue as a form of defense. This is why Concentration Meditation comes first in meditative practice. Alpha consciousness is the gateway into the meditative state. If you cannot concentrate and keep the mind focused on a mentally simplified state, you cannot enter alpha

consciousness. If you cannot enter alpha consciousness, every technique you attempt will fail in its purpose.

This is not to say that awareness in alpha consciousness is nonexistent. In actuality, awareness develops in several stages as you move through different states of consciousness. One familiar characteristic of alpha is the way thoughts begin to enter the mind in more random fashion. It is important to be aware of these random thoughts in an equally detached manner. Even in deeper states of beta consciousness that begin to border alpha, the mind is still aware of its own thoughts as being distractions. For example, you might say to yourself, "I can't forget to finish that homework assignment tomorrow." In beta, you can choose to continue thinking about that bill you have to pay, or you can choose to let the thought go. As we will see in our exploration of Concentration Meditation, naming a distraction during beta consciousness is an effective technique for letting go and returning to focus. Another way to get away from thoughts during beta is to return your focus to your breath. Focusing back to the breath means turning away from beta thoughts and returning to the beginnings of alpha consciousness sensations.

Theta Consciousness

In beta consciousness, the mind is unable to focus on two different things without triggering ego and inner dialogue. In alpha consciousness, the mind can focus on multiple thoughts and sensations without feeling taken away from true focus. In theta, the mind becomes more expansive. As the mind becomes disengaged from the body, internal and external stimuli cease to become distractions. Meditators in theta consciousness often report lucid dream imagery, the rise of deeply buried emotions and memories, timelessness, and self-revelations. You will know you have entered into the initial stages of theta when focus becomes effortless and nothing takes you away from it. However, it is during mid-range theta frequency that the body and mind is at most risk of falling asleep. For this reason, the focus of meditation should shift from concentration to awareness. As we explore

Mindfulness Meditation in the next chapter, you will begin to see how to avoid the pitfall of falling asleep during this dream-like stage.

Delta Consciousness

Delta consciousness exhibits the lowest frequency of the four brainwaves. This is the point at which astral project and third eye meditation are all possible. Buddhists describe third eye meditation as the spiritual channel of the inner mind's eye and astral projection as an out-of-body experience where your spirit encounters other spirit entities. During astral projection you might float through walls, penetrate other dimensions, or instantly teleport to other parts of the universe. During dream sleep, Buddhists believe that this is what our spirits are doing anyway. As the mind leaves theta and enters the early-range delta frequency, not falling asleep becomes even more challenging, and requires maintaining awareness and mindfulness. This is where meditators often begin their Lovingkindness Meditation. Not only can the practice of lovingkindness help maintain awareness as the mind enters early-range delta frequency, it also can deepen the practice of sending and receiving love. You can practice lovingkindness in alpha too, but the effect of Lovingkindness Meditation is generally larger in delta consciousness.

Using Binaural Beats to Alter Consciousness

Another way to move your consciousness into different states is by using headphones and listening to binaural beats. Binaural beats are auditory tones that create two slightly different audio waves in each ear. Listening to both tones together generates a specific brain wave pattern, which correlates to each of the four states of consciousness (beta, alpha, delta and theta). Discovered by Heinrich Wilhelm Dove in 1839, binaural beats became the subject of scientific experimentation in the early 1970s when physicist Thomas Warren Campbell used them to alter subjects' mental states. During this time, Dr. Gerald Oster presented a paper in Scientific American with findings that showed binaural beats improved medical conditions such

as Parkinson's disease. The use of binaural beats became a mainstream phenomenon when research in the '90s linked the use of binaural beats to:

1. Weight loss
2. Quitting smoking
3. Sleepiness
4. Detached awareness
5. Reduction in depression and stress
6. Changes in consciousness
7. Increased energy flow
8. Heightened focus and memory
9. Heightened creativity
10. Heightened intuition

Binaural beats can help you achieve a deeper state of consciousness or a more alert consciousness if you so choose. How can you tell which binaural beats create beta, alpha, theta and delta mind-states? While most online stores that sell binaural beats will provide the information, the best way to tell is to find out, if possible, the frequency of both tones and divide the difference. For example, if one audio wave registers at 240 hertz and one at 244 hertz, the difference between the waves is 4 hertz. To determine which state of consciousness this beats produces, you would refer back to the frequency table provided earlier in this chapter. In this case, 4 hertz is a late-range theta wave bordering on delta consciousness. Therefore, a mental state of intuition and creativity bordering on a feeling of universal love is the effect produced by the beats. If your intention is to become extremely alert and awake, you might look for binaural beats producing beta consciousness. If your intention is to practice Concentration Meditation in an alpha state, you might look for binaural beats that produce alpha consciousness. For Mindfulness Meditation, binaural beats that produce theta might be most effective. For Lovingkindness Meditation, you might look for beats that produce delta waves. Keep in mind that binaural beats only form when two tones are less than 26 hertz apart. Some binaural beats specifically work

for the purpose of opening and balancing the seven chakras. Using binaural beats for this is a great way to prepare the body for core meditation. Binaural beats designed for opening and balancing the seven chakras will contain a different frequency for each chakra, starting with the root and working up toward the crown. If you listen to beats for chakra cleansing, direct your concentration to both the sound of the beat and the corresponding chakra region. As you do so, feel the circular, pulsing energy of the chakra growing at the center of the region.

There are no negative effects of using binaural beats; however, inappropriate use of beats in conjunction with certain activities can be very dangerous. For example, using binaural beats to create a mind-state that causes sleepiness right before getting behind the wheel of a car endangers both you as the driver and other people on the road. This is why it is important to make sure the beats creating certain mind-states correspond to the activity and intention. In addition, overusing binaural beats can lead a meditator to burn out to the point where the beats are no longer effective. For this reason, meditation experts recommend using binaural beats no longer than one hour a day. The best way to use binaural beats depends on when and how you want to alter consciousness. For someone just starting out, listening 15 minutes a day might produce enough benefits. For advanced meditators looking to increase the length and depth of meditative practice, 60 minutes a day might work better. Binaural beats are available on Youtube channels courtesy of uploaders who also use them. If you want to download binaural beats as an MP3 file or buy as CDs, several online stores include:

1. The Unexplainable Store® **www.unexplainablestore.com**
2. MindSync **www.worldofalternatives.com**
3. Meditation Power **www.meditation-power.com**
4. HoloThink **http://holothink.com**
5. EquiSync® **http://eocinstitute.org/meditation**
6. BrainSync **www.brainsync.com**
7. Immrama Institute **www.immrama.org/shop**

Beginning Core Meditation with Concentration

As a beginning meditator, you should practice meditating for concentration for at least one week before moving on to other forms of meditation. Getting started is very easy. After you assume the meditative position of your choice (lotus, sitting, kneeling, etc.), close your eyes, relax your face and jaw, and begin the techniques for opening the seven chakras. Since this practice involves focusing on each individual chakra, you have already begun to use a form of Concentration Meditation. Doing so will help slow the mind into mid-stage beta consciousness where you become relaxed and the mind's inner dialogue begins to slow down. Concentration Meditation involves concentration on a thought, sensation, object, or idea. What should be the focus of your attention?

1. **Thought:** You might focus on a mantra that calms the mind. Mantras are affirmations based on energy and create thought waves. Examples of mantras include the sacred word *Om*—the spoken essence of the universe pronounced in three sounds (a), (u), and (m) — or any positive affirmation that resonates with you, such as *I am free from anger,* or *I am happy and safe.*

2. **Sensation:** You might focus on the rising and falling of your chest or abdomen as you breathe in and out. You also can focus on the feeling your breath creates as it passes in and out of your body. For example, simply notice the feeling of your breath as it passes through your nose or brushes your upper lip.

3. **Object:** This may involve open-eye meditation on an object in front of you or visualizing an object in the mind. Your meditation object might be a point on your body, the flame of a candle, a flower, or some other object in your meditative space that you like.

4. **Idea:** You might focus on a particular passage from the Bible or Quran, a poem or other inspirational quote or text. Just be sure to keep the idea or passage short.

Regardless of which you choose, the goal is to direct your entire focus on one thing. The idea of sitting still and thinking about one single thing might seem easy at first, but it can be hard to do in beta consciousness. First, you must get past that part of you that believes "just sitting" means being lazy. Meditation requires giving yourself permission to exercise your mind. You are not wasting time with meditation or taking time away from another "more important" activity.

10-Minute Concentration Exercise No. 1: Using the Mind Quieting Technique as Your First Sitting Meditation

1. **Choose a space that is tidy and free of distractions.** A meditation room is nice but not necessary. You can choose a quiet, tidy corner of any room or even a corner of your yard.

2. **Set a timer for at least 10 minutes. Use an alarm clock, cell phone, or a kitchen timer.** Setting a timer is especially helpful in the beginning when one minute can seem longer than it usually feels. Eliminate the worry about how time is passing by attending to this detail before you sit. If no timer is available, the Insight Meditation Center (**www.insight meditationcenter.org**) offers several meditation timers for online purchase. Sharper Image also sells alarm clocks with earth tones that slowly grow louder in cadence.

3. **Sit comfortably.** Remove or loosen any restrictive clothing, shoes, or jewelry. Give special attention to your posture, eyes, mouth, hands and feet. The following list offers a guide to positioning your body during meditation. Remember that the following only offers a guide, so adjust as needed. Ultimately, what matters is how comfortable you are in your body as you sit

4. **Posture:** Posture is the foundation for effective breathing, which will be the foundation of your meditation practice. As you sit, you should be comfortably erect with the chin tucked in and your spine lined up straight from the base to the crown of your head.

5. **Eyes:** You might choose to meditate with your eyes open or closed. With open eyes, adopt a soft, unfocused gaze. Simply fix your eyes on a point about four to six feet in front of you. If you choose to close your eyes, be aware that this choice often leads to feelings of sleepiness. Posture will be particularly important for supporting alertness if you meditate with your eyes closed.

6. **Mouth:** You can hold your mouth slightly open or closed. What is most important is that your jaw is relaxed. Place your tongue comfortably behind your teeth.

7. **Hands:** If you are sitting in a chair, rest your hands comfortably on your thighs. On the floor, cross your legs and rest your arms and hands on your thighs.

8. **Feet:** If sitting in a chair, place your feet firmly on the floor. Do not cross your legs or ankles. If sitting, consult the illustrations in Chapter 3 to make sure your sitting position is correct.

9. **Breathe normally.** As you sit, begin with one or two deep exhalations to calm and settle yourself into this time. With each breath, you might even want to inhale through the nose and exhale through the mouth. Loud exhales through the mouth affirm feelings of relief and can help you settle into a more relaxed state. After the deep breaths, you have nothing to do but breathe normally; no special breathing is required.

10. **Focus attention on your breath.** Your mind will wander; that is all right. Each time your focus moves beyond your breath, gently bring it back to an awareness of each breath as it moves in and out of your body. Sometimes, it can be helpful to label or count the breaths. For example, as you inhale you might hear the word rising in your head, or you might say inwardly, "exhale," "falling," or "out" as the breath moves out of your body. You might also count each in and out breath cycle to keep your mind focused only on your breathing. It does not matter if you need to do this 200 times. Each time your mind wanders, resist the urge to judge or scold yourself. Instead, simply refocus your attention on your breath. It does not matter if your mind wanders as you begin; expect that it will. It only matters that you start sitting.

Advanced Breathing for Concentration

As you can see from the exercise above, breathing for concentration requires more than just regular breathing. Exercise No. 1, however, is a very basic breathing technique. There are a number of different breathing exercises that can enhance concentration by relaxing the body. By concentrating on breathing, the mind slows down and begins to match the other rhythms of the body. The counting technique is another preliminary exercise that you should use as you spend the first week on Concentration Meditation.

10-Minute Concentration Exercise No. 2: The Counting Technique

1. **Experiment with the meditation positions and try holding them for 10 minutes.** If you can hold one of the lotus positions comfortably, use it for this exercise. If not, sit in a chair or kneel with a seiza bench to support your knees.

2. **Set a timer for at least 10 minutes.**

3. **Close your eyes, take a few deep breaths and exhale slowly.** Do not try to control your breath; it is better to let your breath find its own rhythm.

4. **Once your breathing has found its natural rhythm, begin counting each inhale and exhale.** Count each breath until you reach 10. You can do this in two ways. The first way, count "1" on the inhale, "2" on the exhale, "3" on the inhale, "4" on the exhale, and so forth. The second way, disregard counting the exhales and count "1" on the first inhale, "2" on the second inhale, "3" on the third inhale, and so forth.

5. **Extend the numbers as you whisper them in your mind.** Obviously, it is impossible to whisper numbers aloud while breathing, and if you tried, it would become distracting. By mentally counting the numbers and extending them for the length of the inhale and exhale, you can synchronize the counting with the breath. For example, as you begin the inhale, you would think "onnnnne." On the exhale, you would think "twoooooo," and on the next inhale, "threeeeee..."

6. **If you lose track while counting, simply start again.** It does not matter how many times you lose track; each time you lose track the mind is learning about concentration.

During these two breathing exercises, thoughts occasionally will arise. When a pleasing thought arises, the temptation is to stay with it because the beginning meditator assumes that this is the point of meditation. Good feelings are important, but they are not the main goal of Concentration Meditation. Any thought, emotion, or sensation that arises during meditation will inevitably fade and give way to a new thought, emotion, or sensation. The point is not to hold on to them, but to notice them, and let them pass. Meditators who dwell in pleasing thoughts, emotions, or sensation during beta consciousness try hard to hold on to them. What ultimately occurs is frustration when they eventually pass, which gives way to anger if the next thought, emotion, or sensation is troubling. Do not examine any of these things while in beta consciousness. If you do, the inner dialogue will grow louder to the point where it gains your attention and it becomes harder to return to focus. Simply let these thoughts, emotions, or sensations go without judging or examining them, and return to the in-and-out breath.

10-Minute Concentration Exercise No. 3: The Breath Wave

1. **Set a timer for at least 10 minutes.**

2. **Lie down in a corpse pose.** You cannot perform this exercise in a sitting position because it requires expansion of the belly, which sitting can limit or impair. To execute the corpse pose, lay down a tatami matt or lie in bed.

3. **Close your eyes, take a deep breath by breathing through the nose and expanding the stomach like a balloon on the inhale.** The emphasis of the inhale should be breathing into and oxygenating the pelvic area.

4. **Let the chest rise slightly just before the end of the inhale.** Do not let the chest rise too much at the end of the inhale. Keep the movement of breath in the high chest shallow, remembering that most of the movement should be in the stomach, not the diaphragm. In many ways, your focus is the lower half your body, in connection with your breath.

5. **Exhale through the nose.** Keep the respiratory and stomach muscles relaxed on the exhale. Do not worry about expelling all the air out of the lungs. Before you lie down in corpse pose, try this breathing technique standing up or sitting and watch how the front of your body creates an undulating "wave" that rises and falls.

The breath wave is more than just a technique for concentrating. It opens the respiratory system which allows the body to deliver oxygen to areas that normally receive little amounts due to restricted breathing patterns. Yoga uses a variation of this technique whereby the meditator expands the stomach like a balloon on one inhale, and then, without exhaling, contracts the stomach muscles inward to force oxygen up the spinal column and into the chest. Expanding oxygen into the pelvic area and sending it up to the diaphragm in this manner cleanses the body from the root chakra to the crown chakra. This is why a yoga instructor might instruct you to use the respiratory muscles to "send the breath" into an area of the body that may feel tension during a long-held yogic pose. Oxygen has a healing quality that gets rid of pain.

If you wish to cleanse the body further, exhale through the mouth instead of the nose at the end of each breath. Continue exhaling through the mouth, contracting the diaphragm as much as you can, thus pushing the air forcefully out of the lungs. When there appears to be no more air left to exhale, push a little harder until you achieve a wheezing sound. Take a moment to inhale regularly to recover, and then repeat this process again. This exercise is cleanses the lungs of any stale air that has accumulated from limited breathing and oxygen distribution over long periods. To determine if your lungs have stale air, or if your body needs more oxygen distribution, start monitoring the trends in how you normally breathe. If your breathing is too short or shallow, then you are not distributing or expelling enough oxygen throughout your body. In this case, consider adding the breath wave to your 10-minute meditation.

10-Minute Concentration Exercise No. 4: Breath Motion Synchronization

1. **Set a timer for at least 10 minutes.**

2. **Stand upright, feet together, hands at your side and close your eyes.** You will remain standing throughout the duration of this exercise.

3. **Begin the breathing technique in exercise 1, this time standing instead of sitting.** Begin with a deep exhalation through the nose, but as you do so, slowly raise both arms up in a sun salutation. A sun salutation is the motion you make with both arms whereby the arms extend away from your hips as you raise them, similar to a flapping motion. As you slowly raise both arms to the sky, gently lift your chin so your head is tilting upward by the time your hands meet above your head.

4. **Exhale through the mouth.** As you exhale, begin to bring your hands and chin downward in the same motion you brought them up. When both hands reach the side, begin the next inhale and repeat the process.

5. **Keep the focus of attention on the synchronicity between the movement of your body and your breath.** When your mind wanders, gently bring it back to an awareness of this synchronicity. Once you have tried this exercise a few times, consider incorporating the counting technique where by you inwardly synchronize the words "inhale" and "exhale" with the movement of the sun salutation. You could also inwardly use the counting technique instead of thinking words.

Beginning meditators usually find this exercise to be one of the more powerful antidotes to mind chatter because of the results often felt within a single practice. Breath motion synchronization is about incorporating any type of motion with breathing techniques. The sun salutation is just one type of motion for this exercise. It can be something as simple as moving one hand back and forth. In breath motion synchronization, the object of attention does not even have to be the breath. For example, you might start paying attention to the breath, and then focus on your pulse rate, the sound of your breathing, or a sensation that naturally arises from the practice. As an alternative, try closing both eyes and visualizing bodily motion as you breathe if this sounds like too many things to do at once.

Auditory Meditation

Most beginning meditators find themselves in a serious struggle with distractions when they first begin to meditate. One technique for reducing the impact of distractions is to name the distraction. The first wave of distractions for beginning meditators typically comes in the form of external distractions. This may be something as faint as a voice on the street, the general hum of traffic, or a bird chirping outside. One method for getting rid of these distractions is to make external stimuli the object of focus. This is the practice of auditory meditation. The beauty of this meditation is that it requires no specific position or space, and is a good way of turning any environment (such as a bus ride) to your benefit. Sit down, lie down, or stand. Close both eyes or keep them open, just find a spot to rest your gaze. Follow your breath for a few minutes using any of the breathing techniques that suit your situation. After focusing on the breath, turn your attention to the sounds around you. Some sounds may be close while others may be distant. You do not need to respond to these sounds, just let them continue or fade as they please. Passively hearing sounds eventually settles the mind and moves it through beta consciousness.

Naming Your Distractions

As you settle into meditation and move through beta consciousness, the external distractions are more likely to fade because you have begun the process of turning inward. Turning inward means opening up to the internal distractions that might have been just background noise in your consciousness. The sound of that bird chirping is no longer distracting, but the sound of your inner voice is louder than before. You cannot continually focus on distractions, but you cannot continue to ignore them either, especially if inner distractions carry important messages. Being able to name your distractions can reduce their power in your mind, so you can limit the time they take away from your focus. For example, if you hear the bird chirping outside, tell yourself (in your mind), "bird chirping." If an inner voice starts replaying an argument with your parents, say (in your mind),

"argument with parents." If the naming technique does not quiet the distractions, try naming the emotions. For example, if an argument becomes a distraction, ask yourself how this argument made you feel while you were having it. In your mind, name the feeling associated with the memory of this argument. Whether the feeling is anger, despair, frustration, or some other emotion, naming it satisfies the subconscious emotions trying to reach the surface. In other cases, you may feel a distraction related to a bodily sensation. If a painful sensation related to your position becomes too great stop meditating. To see if it passes, try naming the sensation repeatedly in the mind for at ten or 15 seconds before deciding to stop.

10-Minute Concentration Exercise No. 5: Releasing Thoughts Meditation

1. **Set a timer for at least 10 minutes.**

2. **Lie down in corpse pose and leave your eyes open or let them close.** If you leave them open, find a spot ceiling to rest your gaze.

3. **Begin breathing in a normal way, feeling the inhale and exhale.** Center your attention on breathing through the nose. Feel the sensation and (in your mind) say the word "breath" for each inhale and exhale.

4. **When a thought arises, say (in your mind) the words "not breath."** Even if the thought is pleasing, saying the words trains the mind to resist even good distractions. No matter how many positive or negative thoughts arise, the entire purpose of this exercise is to learn detachment by acknowledging thoughts as not belonging to focus.

5. **At the end of 10 minutes, get up and continue your day.**

Inner Quieting with Big Mind Meditation

As we have learned, quieting the mind means going into a deeper state of consciousness. We have also learned that distractions cannot be ignored forever and, at some point, have to be dealt with. This is what makes auditory meditation an effective means of confronting and quieting external distractions. If you can directly confront the external distractions using auditory

meditation, how do you confront inner voice? If you need an alternative to naming distractions as a means of quieting the inner voice, the answer is big mind meditation. Big mind meditation involves the process allowing your thoughts to express whatever they please. This form of meditation requires some degree of visualization, so imagine that a central brain (or big mind) controls all the conscious and subconscious voices running through your head. The trick here is to remain respectful of the big mind and talk to it like an equal. Your goal is to convince the big mind that while you may disagree on things, you both have shared interests. Whatever benefits you also benefits the big mind. Whatever hurts you also hurts the big mind. Once you have gained the big mind's trust, ask the big mind for permission to control the conscious and subconscious thoughts it currently controls. What you are asking the big mind is to have control over yourself. At this point, visualize the big mind giving you control. Using that control, you begin talking to the voices. They listen because you now control them. You visualize changing negative thoughts, habitual behaviors, and other undesirable things about yourself. Since you now have access to the central brain, you have access to files you can now erase. If two voices arise that present two sides of an argument, listen to them and work to reach a conclusion that both sides can live with. Working through problems this way can sometimes quiet inner voices that will not go away until you have satisfied them with a solution.

Keeping a Journal

A journal is important for several reasons. It also allows you to reflect on your previous meditation and set an intention for the next one. When reflecting on previous sessions, it is important to remember that self-judgment is not part of meditative progress. At the beginning of your meditative journal, it may be helpful to record inner dialogue that comes up during meditation. When a thought comes and goes, it probably does not need much attention. However, any thoughts that continue to arise during meditation will need special attention, and it is a good idea to write

them down to see if a theme exists. The best time to write in a journal is when your mind feels most alert, analytical, and open to observations. In other words, the best time to write in a journal is in beta consciousness. Exploring inner dialogue through a journal is a good way to figure out the intention you want to set for the next session. After devoting one week of practice to each of the three core meditations, use a journal to customize your own 10-minute meditation. Based on your intentions, customize each session by mixing-and-matching the techniques learned in this chapter as well as the chapters to come.

CASE STUDY: FOCUS AND VISUALIZATION WITH TONGLEN

Will Ryken
St. Petersburg Shambhala Center
willryken@gmail.com
http://stpetersburg.shambhala.org

Beginning meditators often will find that practicing Concentration Meditation will overlap with Mindfulness Meditation and Lovingkindness Meditation. Tonglen, for example, is a meditative form of lovingkindess that I frequently practice, but it involves concentrating on people and visualizing breath. Tonglen practitioners send and receive the breath by visualizing an exhale as hot, thick darkness, and an inhale as cool, weightless and refreshing breath. Since Tonglen is a form of Lovingkindness Meditation, the meditator will typically practice breathing in peoples' suffering and concentrating on sending fresh, healing air to the objects of the practice. In this practice, we begin with people that we love, continue by concentrating on people that we feel have neutral feelings for and finally to people that we may not like. It is important to begin Tonglen with Concentration Meditation so that we begin with a settled mind.

Whichever meditation you set down to practice, the most important thing is to begin with Concentration Meditation so that you have a settled mind. Sometimes this involves meditating with our eyes open and having a soft gaze. That way, we are practicing to become more awake to our world. We then make a connection with our bodies by simply feeling ourselves being relaxed and present. We bring our attention to the breath by feeling the breath coming in and going out. When a strong thought or emotion breaks concentration, we gently bring ourselves back to our breathing. We are not trying to stop thinking! There are no good or bad thoughts during meditation; we are simply using the practice to strengthen the mind to be in the present moment.

At the beginning of practice, you may notice that your mind is more active and that meditation makes the chatter worse. The more you try to quiet the inner chatter the wilder the mind gets. Watching thoughts with detachment and returning to your breath focus will increase your ability to return to an object of concentration over time. I have found that most beginning meditators come to the meditation with too many immediate expectations. Buddhist master Trungpa Rinpoche once said that more people have reached enlightenment at the sound of the gong ending the sitting session than during the practice itself. The benefits of the practice show up more in our lives outside of sitting because we have strengthened the mind to be more awake to the present moment. Our senses touch us more and we begin to enjoy our lives in the simple things we do, seeing the world with new eyes. It is amazing how the world changes when we are awake at this very moment.

Continuing Core Meditation with Mindfulness

fter you have spent your first week of meditation on developing concentration, your second week will involve developing mindfulness. Mindfulness Meditation, which is the second core practice, involves attention to the present experience. While Concentration Meditation involves the practice of letting go of thoughts, emotions and sensations, mindfulness involves the practice of exploring them. In other words, whatever is happening now, whatever comes mind, should remain the object of attention until it fades from consciousness. When Gautama Buddha first introduced Mindfulness Meditation to his students, he instructed them to develop four types of awareness:

1. Awareness of the body and sensations
2. Awareness of thoughts
3. Awareness of emotions
4. Awareness of the relationship between things

Buddha though that by developing awareness in four ways, the meditator could find out why the mind creates suffering. By directing attention to

difficult emotions, the meditator eventually develops insight, which he or she uses to correct the pattern. Indian culture developed this practice into a form of meditation called *tantra*. Tantra is a meditative practice that uses the sensory experience to gain spiritual realization. In fact, some tantric practices deliberately awaken the *kundalini* as part of this process. Whether you choose to awaken the *kundalini* or not, you will use mindfulness to take an important step in your practice. It is the point in meditation where the mind truly begins to focus inward after quieting down and becoming focused. So the question is, at which point do you stop practicing concentration and begin practicing mindfulness? As the case study in the previous chapter noted, some degree of overlap exists between concentration, mindfulness and Lovingkindness Meditation. To some extent, welcoming thoughts and letting them pass without judgment during periods of concentration is mindfulness. It may not be a full attempt to explore inward, but you are still using awareness to bring your attention back to concentration. In short, the answer really depends on you.

When the mind stops judging and begins concentrating with ease, and when you recognize your descent into deep alpha and theta consciousness, you can begin Mindfulness Meditation. At that point, be ready to begin exploring the inner experience by shifting your focus from concentration to awareness. Remember that meditation is not about ignoring negative feelings that build up inside. Until you face buried emotions, nothing is going to make your problems disappear. Most people who push down painful memories and emotions pay a price mentally, physically and socially over time. Until they learn to release the negative energy accumulated by the chakras and expose the source of their suffering, they continue to move through life without a compass, bumping into one another without understanding why.

How to Explore the Inner Experience

After concentration becomes effortless, the following meditative guidelines will help you turn your attention inward in a way that promotes mindful-

ness. First, it is important to forget about trying to understand the meaning of thoughts and emotions. To do this, consider expanding awareness to bodily sensations. Instead of looking for meaning, simply acknowledge to yourself that this is a thought you are experiencing. If an unpleasant thought comes, and you begin to feel anger or anxiety, shift away from the emotion and notice the bodily sensations created by the anger or anxiety. In other words, instead of asking what the fear or anxiety means, notice the increase in pulse rate, how the stomach tightens, or the way your throat seems to swell up as part of the body's stress response. Second, it is important to shift slowly from concentration to mindfulness rather than all at once.

Third, be aware of how the mind distorts thoughts about the past. Because the mind is always trying to return to a relaxed state, it may try to push down memories or make the past appear rosier in the conscious mind. When this happens, your mind leaves you with distorted memories. Distorted memories are the result of secondhand experience, where the mind aims to escape the present and live in a distorted memory of a more comforting past. Different from secondhand experience is direct experience. Direct experience is the experience of the present moment.

This is why experts recommend expanding to sensations during Mindfulness Meditation. Sensations are part of direct experience, while thoughts and emotions tend to be rooted in secondhand experiences. If you find yourself slipping into the distorted memories and emotions generated by secondhand experience, shift away and expand to the bodily sensations of direct experience. The final guideline of exploring the inner experience is to remember that the most important part of this exploration is being rather than doing. When we talk about shifting from one mind-state to another, what we are really talking about is shifting from a state of doing to a state of being. When you are in a state of simply being, you are meditating.

Expanding to Sensations

After you have used the concentration exercises in the previous chapter to stabilize breathing, expand your awareness to any of the five senses: taste, feel, sight, smell and hearing. If you meditate with your eyes closed, you can still focus on what you see (floaters, pinpricks of light, etc.). Do not actively look for sensations; just sit and practice being until a sensation arises. Pain is the most likely sensation to arise first. Sitting in the same position for 10 minutes is bound to bother beginning meditators, especially meditators with weak core muscles. During Concentration Meditation, try to ride out a painful sensation by redirecting attention back to the breath. If the sensation continues to break your concentration or it has not dissipated after a minute or so, consider stopping and try to meditate in a different position. If a painful sensation arises after you have shifted to Mindfulness Meditation, turn your attention to the pain instead of redirecting attention back to breath. By exploring the painful sensation during Mindfulness Meditation, you may find that the pain eventually subsides until it no longer holds your awareness.

Awareness develops in stages as the mind enters deeper states of consciousness. If you are still trying to turn secondhand experience (*i.e.* past thoughts and emotions) into direct experience (*i.e.* sensations), trying a concentration technique such as naming your distractions can help you get there. You can mix-and-match techniques from different core practices in order to meet meditative challenges and achieve balance. Expanding to sensations is a perfect way to go into a deeper state of consciousness. However, as you edge closer to delta consciousness, the challenge is creating a balance between maintaining awareness and not falling asleep.

One way to balance this challenge is by alternating between sensations rather than focusing on just one. Focusing on one sensation can become boring and cause the mind to relax until you fall asleep. For example, if a sensation arises in your toes, put your focus there for a bit, and then shift

to another sensation, such as the hum of an air conditioner or your heartbeat. By expanding awareness to sensations, thoughts and sensations are no longer distractions, and you are ready to examine your conscious and subconscious mind. At this point, your receptivity grows to the point where you see everything in more detail and from a new point of view. This is the point at which you can take awareness a step further; you pick something out of your thoughts and emotions and begin to explore it in full. This is why Mindfulness Meditation typically begins with exploring sensations.

10-Minute Mindfulness Exercise No. 1: Body Scan Meditation

1. **Set a timer for at least 10 minutes.**

2. **Lie down in corpse pose and stretch.** Relax every muscle for a few moments. Once settled, raise your arms all the way over your head, lift your feet and point your toes away from your body. To get a full body stretch, clasp your hands and reach above you as if being pulled in the opposite direction of your toes. Pointing your toes, use them to push in the opposite direction of your head.

3. **Continue stretching for 20 seconds, then bring both arms to your side, feet down, and relax the entire body, including the toes.** Take a minute to sense your body as a whole. Feel the effect of the stretch. Let go of any tension.

4. **Start a body scan.** Begin by bringing awareness to individual parts of your body and imagine each muscle group softening as you bring awareness. Start with the toes, then to the lower legs and hips, and continue to the abdomen, the chest, the neck, the throat, the shoulders, the arms, the hands, the head, the face and finish with the eyes.

5. **Think of your body as a whole again, and imagine a red line acting as a bio-scanner.** After bringing awareness to individual parts of the body, the red line moves up and down your body, detecting any remaining areas of tension.

6. **Stop scanning and remain motionless in corpse pose until the timer sounds.** During this time, keep the awareness on your entire body as a whole and allow it to settle into deep relaxation.

7. **At the end of 10 minutes, either get up and continue your day, or start Mindfulness Meditation.** If you want to include Mindfulness Meditation into the 10-minute practice, simply shorten the body scan technique down to a couple of minutes and begin Mindfulness Meditation using the remaining minutes on the timer.

Body scan meditation is a way of training the body to become more aware of sensations. It is especially important to stay with direct experience when pain arises. If the mind falls into the trap of thinking on the past or future, the meditator may begin to compare the current experience of pain with pain from the past or future. If this happens, the present moment may dissolve into a distorted memory or the anticipation of pain in the future. For example, if a sudden physical pain arises, the mind starts to wonder how many minutes the pain is going to last. Anxiety sets in, the inner dialogue begins and the overwhelmed mind distorts the immediate future by making the pain seem unbearable. Being stuck in a pattern of habitual responses to pain clouds us from understanding the difference between actual experience and distorted experiences that we add. Not reacting to physical pain teaches us not to react to emotional pain. In her book, "Real Happiness," meditation expert Sharon Salzberg writes, "Meditation helps us see what we're adding to our experiences, not only during meditation sessions, but elsewhere. These add-ons may take the form of projecting into the future (*my neck hurts, so I'll be miserable forever*), forgone conclusions (*there's no point in asking for a raise*), rigid concepts (*you're either with me or against me*), unexamined habits (eating comfort food), and associative thinking (yelling at your daughter and revisiting your own childhood problems)." Seeing what we are adding to our experience allows us to realize that pain is not permanent, and there is no need to feel overwhelmed by it.

Muscle Relaxing Techniques

A version of the body scan is the muscle tensing technique, which is a very relaxing way to expand to sensations. To use this technique, sit in corpse

pose (as you would to prepare for a body scan). Lying down, the muscle tensing technique starts the same way; you begin to focus on each muscle group in anatomical order. The difference here is that instead of starting with a full body stretch, you tense and relax each muscle group as you move through them. Starting with the toes, tighten the muscles as hard as possible by curling them. Hold the tension for about 15 seconds and release. Enjoy the sensation of releasing stress for a few moments, then move focus up toward the calves. Flex the calf muscles as hard as possible, hold for 15 seconds, release and enjoy the sensation for a few moments and move further up toward the thigh muscles. Repeat the tension/release/relax method for the stomach muscles, chest muscles, shoulder blades, biceps and triceps, hands, larynx, and facial muscles. To flex your neck muscles, press the chin down to the collarbone and apply pressure. To flex the hands, curl them into fists and squeeze as hard as possible. To flex the larynx, contract the muscles used to swallow.

Some yoga instructors use the muscle tensing technique at the beginning of yoga practice to release muscle tension. These sessions typically end with meditators laying in corpse pose while meditating on the relaxing physical sensations produced by tension release. If you only have 10 minutes to spare, try this exercise at the beginning of practice. It is a great way to release not only physical stress, but also mental and emotional stress. The technique works best in the morning because it increases blood flow and produces a feeling of relaxed alertness.

Visualization exercises also work well as muscle relaxing techniques. The purpose of visualization, as defined by Buddhist monks, is to use the imagination to transform negative energy into spiritual realization. When you lie down in corpse pose, visualize taking a warm shower and the feeling of warmth that slowly rolls down your body as the water drips to your feet. Imagine the warmth of the water taking the muscle tension with it as the water flows down your body and into the drain. To create your own visual-

ization exercise, find a physical sensation that you find deeply relaxing and create a scene in your head where the physical sensation heals the tension.

10-Minute Mindfulness Exercise No. 2: Body Sensation Meditation

1. **Set a timer for at least 10 minutes.**

2. **Sit down in one of the lotus positions, eyes open or closed.** Take a few deep breaths to calm the mind, and then begin to focus on sound. Let any sound that enters your awareness come and go as it pleases.

3. **Shift attention to the sound of breathing.** Focus on how the air sounds going in and out through your nose, then your mouth and then your chest. Continue listening to the sound of the breath until another physical sensation becomes a distraction.

4. **Shift focus to distracting physical sensation and name the distraction.** For example, if you develop an itch, think the word, "itch." If you experience a chill, think the word "chill."

5. **Continue to welcome and sit with physical sensations until 10 minutes are over.** The important part here is to practice present moment awareness so that the mind does not begin to wonder how much time is left.

6. **At the end of 10 minutes, sit up and either go about your day or extend your practice with more Mindfulness Meditation.**

Slowing Down Daily Activities to Encourage Mindfulness

While you may not feel improvements in your meditative practice during the first few weeks, you may begin to notice improvements in your everyday life. Improvements may take the form of feeling centered or having a greater sense of awareness and appreciation of things that you never noticed. This type of awareness is what colors life and makes it more interesting. Even so, the busy schedules that come with having a busy lifestyle have a way of jolting people out of present moment awareness and back into constant anxiety and anticipation of the future. If you begin losing the

centeredness created from daily meditative practice, several mindfulness techniques can help return the mind to this desired state. The goal of each practice is to slow things down to the point where you are back to experiencing things directly (i.e. sensations) rather than experiencing things indirectly (i.e. distorted memories/future dread). The best way to do this is to apply this concept to everyday activities that are part of your normal routine. Normal activities where you can apply Mindfulness Meditation to might include:

1. Eating a meal
2. Exercising
3. Walking
4. Cleaning your room
5. Watching television

Slowing down time in normal activities with Mindfulness Meditation is about slowing down the actual activity itself. Rather than rushing through something, you want to take time to notice the smaller details of the experience. For example, if you apply Mindfulness Meditation to an activity such as washing the dishes, the point is not to think about cleaning the dishes. The point is to experience everything that involves such a seemingly simple routine that you would ordinarily rush through without thinking about. In this case, set the faucet to medium, begin making slow, circular motions with the sponge, and notice how the lukewarm water feels against your skin as you clean each dish. Expand your awareness to multiple sensations (the sponge, the sound of the water, the smell of the food, etc.) until your mind has returned itself to the type of awareness that made everyday experience more interesting after meditative practice. The keys to maintaining that centered feeling with you into high stress situations (such as school) are to set the tone for the day by meditating, stay mindful as you go through the day and notice how your mind unnecessarily adds indirect experiences to direct experiences, and practice breathing exercises and mini-meditations throughout the day. Practicing everyday meditations is a great way to deep-

en the enjoyment of simple pleasures. When choosing an everyday activity to transform into a meditative practice, the best choice is an activity you have performed a thousand times on autopilot.

10-Minute Mindfulness Exercise No. 3: Walking Meditation

1. **Find a time during the weekend to visit a park or nature preserve.** You may think a walking meditation depends on the weather and time of year since the ideal time for a walk in nature is during warm months. The natural habitat may provide more sensations during warmer months, but even winter months in cold regions offer sights and smells that can cultivate mindfulness. This may include fresher air, seeing breath, or the feeling of snow and cold.

2. **Use your cellphone as a 10-minute timer and pick a starting point along a walking path.** Very slowly, place one foot in front of the other and feel the distribution of weight as you take the first step.

3. **Begin walking at normal speed. Instead of starting with focus on breath, shift attention to the legs and the sensation of your feet as you lift them and bring them down.** To keep the focus at your feet, visualize seeing things from the perspective of your feet. Continue this way for at least a few minutes.

4. **Shift your focus to the sensations caused by the constant redistribution in weight.** To do so, slow your pace and see if it is possible to feel the full range of sensations as the heel lifts, then the foot, then the leg, and the foot again as it comes back down. Here is where you can implement a walking version of the counting technique. Instead of counting each breath, or mentally thinking "inhale/exhale," try thinking, "lift/land" or "up/down" every time your foot comes up and down off the ground.

5. **Expand your awareness.** This can be the way leaves or snow crunch underneath your feet. It also can be sensations outside the feet, such as birds chirping or the feeling of sunlight through the trees.

6. **Consider walking for longer than 10 minutes if time provides.** In this exercise, longer walks mean more opportunities to expand the sensory experience. Being in the quietude of nature for longer periods also offers a peaceful way of reconnecting to spirituality.

If you want to meditate in nature, but are not sure how what is a good place for this activity, think about the following. First, avoid a public park or nature preserve that has too many people. Finding a place where people are constantly jogging back and forth is a potential distraction for the mind. Second, if you go into the wilderness, make sure the area is safe and free of wild animals. Third, for this type of meditation, the time of day does matter. Any place too dark may not bring enough visual sensations to focus on, and you do not want to run the risk of getting hurt if you cannot see where you are walking. You do not want to be alone at night in an empty public place or park either, since these can be opportunities for crimes to occur. At the same time, any place in broad daylight or with too much light can hurt the eyes and make the mind too active. If you live in a city, public parks can be surprisingly quiet breaks from the sounds of traffic.

If you cannot make time to walk in nature, consider a drinking tea meditation. Drinking tea meditation is a popular practice that originated in Japanese teahouses as a form of Zen. Tea became an important part of Japanese culture and meditation in the eighth century when two Japanese monks named Kukai and Saicho returned from China after spending years studying Buddhism in China. When they returned to Japan, they introduced tea seeds to the home country. After tea became part of everyday life, tea master Murata Juko built the first teahouse in a secluded area with the intention of using it as a place where one could drink tea and engage in spiritual contemplation. In Japan today, teahouses are as common as Buddhist temples. In Western life, it is a perfect everyday meditation for anyone who enjoys tea in the morning or uses rituals to get the day going. Drinking coffee is not part of this meditation due to the nature of caffeine and its acidic effect on the body. When it comes to tea, choose green over black, as black tea contains too much acidity. Morning is an ideal time to double up on Mindfulness Meditation because of the habitual routines most often practiced while getting ready for school or starting each day. For example, instead of visualizing a shower as an everyday meditation, mindfulness might start with the actual act of talking a shower and slowing

it down to experience deeper sensations. Drinking tea meditation might follow, or perhaps using breakfast as a form of meditation, feeling the sensations of taste and texture in your mouth as you slowly chew the food.

10-Minute Mindfulness Exercise No. 4: Drinking Tea Meditation

1. **Brew a pot of tea.** Slow down all the actions involved. Feel the weight of the pot as you place it on the stove; smell the tea packet before you dip it into the water.

2. **Stand in front of the stove.** Note the changes in water as the temperature in the pot rises and watch the bubbles form and gain movement. Close your eyes and listen to the sound of the steam. Inhale the fragrance of the vapor.

3. **Pour a cup of tea.** Listen to the sound of the tea is it pours into the glass. Cup the glass with both hands and focus on the heat coming from the tea.

4. **Lift the tea to your mouth and place the cup to your lips.** Feel the vapor in your nostrils. Drink slowly, noting the first taste of the tea as it hits your tongue. Let the tea linger in your mouth for a moment before swallowing.

5. **Explore the different flavors as you drink the rest of the cup.** You do not have to be right about which flavors exist. Simply contemplate what the flavors could be. Slow down the entire process of drinking the cup. Do not focus on how much tea is left. Instead, focus on each individual sip.

Working with Difficult Emotions during Mindfulness Meditation

It is almost certain that meditation will stir up buried emotions that may be difficult to confront. The further you explore the inner experience the more likely this becomes. For this reason, mindfulness is a process of recognizing difficult emotions, accepting them as part of what cannot change, understanding that they do not define you, and then investigating their true meaning. This process cannot be undermined. Any attempt to avoid negative thoughts will only serve to keep the chakras blocked and keep the positive energy from flowing.

Instead, welcome the difficult emotions that arise during Mindfulness Meditation and develop an understanding about their existence. In Tibetan tradition, the story of a master named Milarepa follows one man's meditative retreat into the Himalayas where he encountered demons that attempted to take him from his path. First, he tried to subdue them. When that failed, he decided to give them love and compassion. The fear controlling the demons could not understand the concept of love and compassion, and so they fled. Your interaction with difficult emotions is much the same. They are demons governed by fear, and the solution is acceptance, love, and understanding. It is also the point at which Mindfulness Meditation and Lovingkindness Meditation may overlap. The same is true for people. When you combine mindfulness with lovingkindness, particularly disagreeable individuals no longer seem like trolls, but rather lost souls in need of healing. To heal an emotion, that emotion first needs your understanding and patience.

Difficult Emotion #1: Anger

Due to expectations about what is considered civil behavior, anger is one of the most suppressed emotions in modern society. When children learn that anger is not an appropriate reaction in any situation, feelings that cause anger become internalized and emotions stay buried deep in the subconscious. Over time, suppressing anger becomes a pattern that children carry with them throughout their lives. By the time they get older, years of suppressed emotions have created an individual with an unexamined inner life. People who live unexamined inner lives do not know themselves well enough to understand why they do what they do, which in turn leads to more suppressed anger and confusion. When the expectation of life does not match the result, people feel wronged. The tragic fact of life is that bad things happen to good people, and people who deserve better may not always get what they want. However, if you open your eyes to true wisdom, if you see that the things others convinced you to want are not what you really need, you will see that you already have everything you need. There

is no shame in falling; what matters is whether you continue to get back up, as many times as required.

The key to dealing with anger during Mindfulness Meditation is to first unblock the emotions with chakra healing or allow them to rise and flow without suppressing them. At that point, expand to sensations by focusing on how the stress response triggers physical reactions within the body. For example, the stress response may come in the form of stomach butterflies or a rise in blood pressure. Focusing on sensations caused by anger allows the meditator to observe with detachment. Being able to observe through detachment enables the process of recognizing difficult emotions, accepting them as part of what cannot change, understanding that they do not define you, and being able to investigate their true meaning. Most people who explore their anger eventually discover that the true suppressed emotion behind the anger is hurt or fear.

Difficult Emotion #2: Anxiety and Fear

Self-image is one of the most closely guarded aspects of individualism in modern society because for most people, it directly affects self-esteem. Self-image can appear through one's own opinion or through the opinions of others. However, the opinions of others should not matter. "Know thyself," as the ancient Greek saying goes. Think about how many people make "fitting in" an important goal. If you are like most teens, you probably worry about how your teachers, parents, or friends see you, and this causes you anxi-

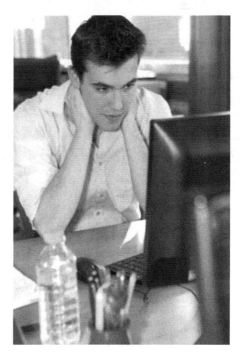

ety. Many people deny their true self because they fear others may find it unacceptable.

If you have ever joined a club you hated, been in a bad relationship, or formed bad habits, meditation may reveal that fear and anxiety was part of the problem. It is no surprise that the struggle to belong causes these emotions when you consider the Buddhists belief that an individual's false sense of separateness is the source of all suffering. When you feel like you do not belong because some group or clique has not welcomed you, you feel like an outsider. Suddenly the opinion of others matters more than your own. Often the emotions of anxiety and fear are what cause repressed anger.

The key to dealing with fear and anxiety during Mindfulness Meditation is the same for dealing with anger. After unblocking the chakras, use mindfulness to recognize an emotion as anxiety or fear using the naming technique. After that, focus on the physical sensations created by the fear or anxiety. This will allow you to explore and observe the true causes of fear and anxiety. As new insights come, any fear and anxiety generated by a false sense of separateness will decrease.

Difficult Emotion #3: Sadness and Depression

Sadness and depression are two of the most paralyzing emotions because the underlying causes may attribute themselves to feelings of emptiness and despair. Depression can be the result of unresolved conflicts and repressed emotions. People who are depressed often experience lack of focus, lack of interest, lack of confidence, and lack of energy. At the same time, the person relives negative memories and emotions that eat away at the spirit and completely remove them from the present. More than any other emotion, the destructive effects of depression are far reaching. The key to dealing with sadness and depression during Mindfulness Meditation is to begin by focusing on any tightness in the heart (commonly known as a heavy heart). After that, focus on opening the heart chakra (explored further in Chapter 7), and begin to meditate on the thoughts and emo-

tions that cause the sadness or depression. To begin a thinking meditation, assume any meditative position, close both eyes and feel the support coming from the ground beneath you. Next, settle down the mind with any choice of breathing technique. As thoughts arise, pleasant or otherwise, to take you away from the breath, use a version of the naming technique by naming the thoughts as "thinking." As you progress, name thoughts more specifically, such as "planning" or "remembering." When difficult emotions arise, name them accordingly as "hating," "worrying," "stressing," and so forth. The point of thinking meditation is to recognize what arises as nothing more than a thought that does not have anything to do with the self. Practicing thinking meditation during mindfulness can clear the way to unraveling habitual patterns until they no longer control the mental and behavioral aspects of self-image.

Working with habitual patterns is also a point where Mindfulness Meditation overlaps Lovingkindness Meditation. In order to unravel habitual patterns, it is necessary to confront difficult emotions by respecting them, or as the Milarepa story demonstrated, to heal your demons by loving them. The more these patterns unravel, the more we begin to release long-held negative energy. Infusing positive energy into thoughts promotes the karmic law of cause and effect—whatever you express into the universe comes back to you.

10-Minute Mindfulness Exercise No. 5: Positive Thinking Meditation

1. **Set a timer for at least 10 minutes.**

2. **Sit, stand, or lie down in one of the meditative positions.** Close both eyes or keep them open.

3. **Think of a positive memory or recent experience.** This memory or experience should be something that evokes a positive emotion whenever you have previously thought about it, such as happiness, contentment, gratitude, joy and so forth.

4. **Capture one image from this memory or experience in your mind as a video recording.** Explore what it feels like to sit with this memory in a state of deep meditation and mental stillness. Allow yourself to smile if the impulse arises, and focus on the sensation of the smile (e.g. the pulsing sensation at the lips, the crease of the mouth, etc.).

5. **Maintain mindful awareness of body sensations created by the recollection of this memory.** For example, if you feel a sudden rush of excitement, notice how it manifests as a sensation, but allow the sensation and the image to pass. Trying to hold on to a pleasurable sensation or thought may invite anxiety or a sense of loss; both are negative thoughts and emotions.

6. **Notice what thoughts arise when you evoke positive memories.** Do you start thinking about how wonderful it feels to be free, to feel part of something? Do you start thinking about how you wish it could always be like this? Does that thought begin to spiral into worries or negative thoughts about being stuck? If you start to have negative thoughts, practice mindfulness by reminding yourself that the negative thoughts are add-ons from the distorted mindset created by your ego. If the negative thought continues, bring your attention back to breath. When the thought disperses, go back to dwelling in the positive memory and experience.

7. **End the meditation by taking a few moments to focus back on breathing.**

Mindfulness-Based Stress Reduction (MBSR)

If you feel more comfortable working with people in the medical profession than people in the new age movement, Dr. Jon Kabat-Zinn created Mindfulness Based Stress Reduction (otherwise known as MBSR), which combines medical research with traditional forms of meditation. MSBR is a behavioral medicine offered in more than 200 integrated medical centers, hospitals and clinics around the world. The majority of students who enroll in the MSBR program suffer from either severe stress or chronic diseases. Studies on MBSR show the program improves conditions such as rheumatoid arthritis, lower back pain, and side effects from HIV and cancer treatment. MBSR is essentially meditation without the spiritual aspects. To learn more about Mindful Based Stress Reduction, go to **https://goamra.org**. If you have a smartphone, consider downloading the Mindfulness Meditation™ app available at **www.mentalworkout.com**.

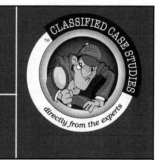

CASE STUDY:
BECOMING MORE
CONSCIOUSLY AWARE

Djuna Roberts
Asheville NC 28805
droberts0001@live.com

I started using positive visualization exercises when I was a kid participating in high school sports. During these exercises, I would visualize how I wanted to play and would often experience a mental state called "being in the zone." Getting into the zone is about finding an inner peacefulness. As my practice evolved, I decided to attend the NC School for Natural Healing where I discovered a practice called "energy healing." This practice helped me learn more techniques for meditating and "getting into the zone."

My favorite technique involves the simple but profound use of various breathing techniques, as well as emotional cleansing, which involves breathing to go into deeper states of consciousness and relaxation in order to clear repressed emotions. I have found that following the breath is the best form of connecting with inner quietness.

Meditation has helped me become more consciously aware of my emotions, thoughts, and general energy during my normal daily activities. It has also helped me become present with the emotional energy, not from a "thinking" mind, but from a place of feeling the currents of various emotions. Emotions during regular meditation do not feel as turbulent when I am looking at them from the inner/higher self and being an observer. In this detached, observing state, I can allow the energy of emotions to exist as energy that moves through me. I practice Mindfulness Meditation each day to stay aware of tension that I need to address. It also helps me stay in a meditative state while walking about in my daily activities. It always will be my challenge to remember to check in with my breath at various times during in day. If my breath feels too shallow, I just take a moment to breathe deep. This expands my awareness immediately and helps me return to centeredness.

I also think Mindfulness Meditation has helped me become more aware of certain emotional patterns. It is only when I become aware of certain patterns of thoughts or behaviors that I am able to make a more conscious choice to try to change the pattern. Meditation helps people become an observer of mental thoughts from a detached place of loving kindness and acceptance. Many patterns are contained in the subconscious, and I feel meditation helps bring that material to conscious awareness. When the mind becomes conscious of a problem, the meditator becomes more equipped to deal with and eventually break any pattern that might be harmful to everyday living and wellness.

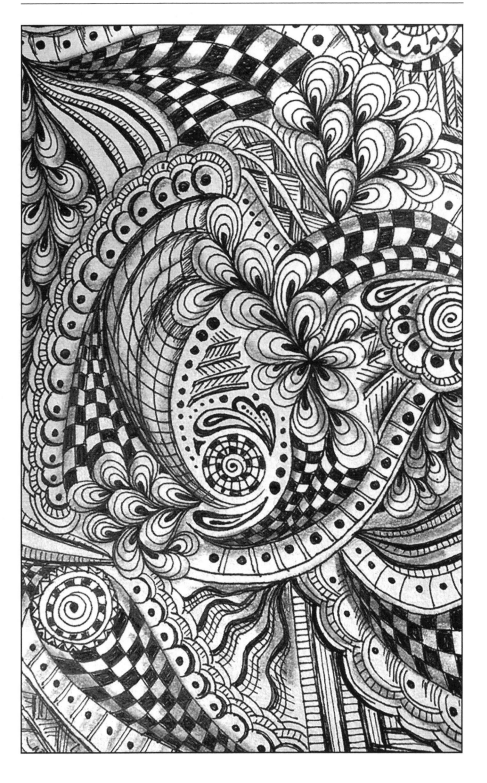

Finishing Core Meditation with Lovingkindness

After you have spent your second week of meditation on developing mindfulness, your third week of meditation will involve developing lovingkindness. Lovingkindness Meditation, which is the third core practice, focuses on bringing love, compassion, sympathy and joy into your life. To review, Concentration Meditation involves the practice of quieting the mind and letting go of thoughts and emotions, and mindfulness involves the practice of exploring them once the mind becomes quiet. Lovingkindess meditation is the meditative practice where you extend caring to yourself and others to bring universal harmony. Once you have quieted the mind and explored the meaning of thoughts and emotions, you will use Lovingkindness Meditation.

The Benefits of Practicing Lovingkindness Meditation

Learning how to love yourself and others sounds simple, yet so many people behave in unloving ways toward themselves and others on a daily basis.

If we apply the ancient Greek saying, "know thyself," to the practice of lovingkindess, we begin to realize that part of knowing oneself means loving oneself. To truly love oneself means never needing to search for love anywhere else. Many people look for the approval of others as a form of love to makeup for what feels lacking within. For this reason, we can identify several benefits of practicing lovingkindness. When we practice lovingkindness, we experience peace and well-being without having to depend on any particular reason to make us feel this way. Life itself becomes joyful. We feel freed from the ego drive when we feel happy. When the ego drive does not define our happiness (*e.g.* getting what we want in order to be happy), the mind lives in the beautiful moment, unconcerned by what may or may not come to us in the future. Likewise, the past does not hold us in fear of repeating old hurts, and we live forward with courage and optimism.

Love energy is Tao energy that gives us vitality. This vitality heals us physically. We feel more awake and renewed when before we may have felt tired and worn down. The love energy we draw from lovingkindness keeps us in good health, nourishes our body and extends our lifespan. Dr. Dean Ornish, author of "Program for Reversing Heart Disease", conducted a well-known series of lovingkindess meditation studies that linked physical healing to patients that made changes in their psychological, emotional and spiritual lifestyle. Notable improvements in patients included discontinuation of medications, less chest pain, higher energy levels, increased calmness, significant weight loss and reduced blockages in arteries. From these studies, Dr. Ornish developed the Opening Your Heart Program which includes meditation, breathing exercises, and guided imagery to treat addictions, lower cholesterol and reduce stress. When we practice lovingkindness, we expand our sense of connection to others; life feels more meaningful. It is this sense of meaning and connection that leads to a greater spiritual awakening.

Directing the Flow of Love Energy

When you begin to extend love to yourself and others, you enter an expanded state of awareness and begin to experience energy flow. During

Lovingkindness Meditation, the individual encounters pure Tao consciousness by drawing in the universal energy of eternal love. Tao is a concept in Buddhism that represents the energy of the universe. By directing this energy flow to yourself and others, you begin to build a connection to all things. The single greatest source of all suffering is the false sense of separation. Lovingkindness removes this sense so that the meditator can feel peace, love and joy. The heart chakra is the energetic opening that assists in this process. In its most fully realized form, lovingkindness is the expression of unconditional love. No matter what others do, no matter what you do to others or to yourself, this love never diminishes.

It is worth noting, however, that using lovingkindness to direct the flow of positive energy as a means of fulfilling ambitions and desires only strengthens the ego drive. For example, you set an intention to love someone hoping that good things will happen for you in life. While the universe may respond to this lower intention, it may keep you from reaching higher states of divine consciousness (explored further in chapter 8). Directing love toward yourself or others on the belief that the universe will give you a material reward is not an expression of true unconditional love. Giving love when motivated by the ego drive is a purely conditional intention and therefore is not a higher intention. Since the true purpose of your spiritual journey is to break free of the ego, you are encouraged to use lovingkindness for higher intentions rather than lower ones. In addition, when we talk about lovingkindness as a practice of extending love to others, we are not talking about liking people or accepting bad behaviors. We are talking about extending love to understand that our lives are spiritually connected. It is an expression of understanding that our own flaws (and the flaws of others) are the result of the ego drive, a disconnection from spirit, and a lack of true understanding.

Deepening the practice of lovingkindess also means using it to achieve compassion for others. Compassion takes love a step further. When you feel compassion for others, you not only love them but also feel their pain

and suffering as you would your own. Developing compassion for others strengthens your bond with everything. The individual begins to lose his or her sense of feeling separate from others. However, compassion does not mean that the individual expressing it feels the same level of sadness as another person. Instead the individual simply understands it. Sympathy is the result of compassion. When lovingkindess meditation reaches its fullest expression of love and compassion, the meditator experiences genuine joy and happiness for another's good fortune. No longer is the individual filled with jealousy.

The best way to practice lovingkindness is to look for the good in people, to want the best for them, and to understand that some people need more love and understanding than others. To prepare for Lovingkindness Meditation, begin to think about how you see other people. Some thoughts of others may be positive while others may be more negative. Either way, the important thing to realize is that, despite your differences with other people, everyone wants the same things. It's just that some have different ways of expressing or trying to get these things, right or wrong. All people, no matter who they are, want love, admiration, respect and so forth. Try putting yourself in that person's place, and ask yourself how you would feel in those shoes. You also might think about the suffering of someone you do not know and imagine that person's problems belonging to a loved one. When we feel separate, we only feel suffering when it touches us. When we feel connected, everyone's suffering matters.

10-Minute Lovingkindness Exercise No. 1: Extending Love to Yourself and Others

1. **Set a timer for at least 10 minutes.**

2. **Sit, stand, or lie down in one of the meditative positions.** Close both eyes or keep them open.

3. **Offer lovingkindness to yourself.** To do this, silently say the words: *"May I be happy. May I be safe. May I be healthy. May I live with ease."*

4. **Keep repeating the words in your mind.** As you continue, it is important keep an even pace between each declaration so that the mind can focus on each one. Breath is not important in this exercise. The main focus is the words.

5. **After a couple of minutes, or when you feel a loving sensation, choose a person you like or has been kind to you, and extend lovingkindness to that person.** If thoughts and memories associated with this person arise, just let them pass. To extend this person lovingkindness, silently say the words, *"May you be happy. May you be safe. May you be healthy. May you live with ease."* To deepen this practice, choose someone who you know may be hurting or sad, and extend the words of lovingkindness.

6. **After a couple of minutes, choose a person you feel neutral about, and extend the words of lovingkindness to that person.** This person might be someone you do not know well or a person you encountered for a brief moment in public, such as an unhappy looking grocery clerk, a nervous child, or a lonely looking woman at the bus stop.

7. **After a couple of minutes, choose a person you have negative feelings toward, and extend the words of lovingkindness to that person.** This might be a difficult person you encountered for a brief moment on the road or someone you see on a regular basis who may be making your life difficult. If you find it difficult to extend lovingkindness to someone you feel wronged you, extend the words of lovingkindness to yourself since that is an indication of suffering. Your inability to express unconditional love may also mean you still hold negative energy due to a blockage in the energetic opening of the heart chakra.

Opening the Heart Chakra

Opening the heart chakra allows the meditator to release energetic blockages in the chest created by negative energy. If the heart chakra is closed, the individual cannot radiate love, compassion, joy, or peace. Freeing these openings and releasing blockages allows the meditator to receive and direct the flow of energy in lovingkindess meditation. The practice of opening this chakra works well at the beginning of a meditation or at the end. If you open the heart chakra before you begin a meditation, follow the instructions outlined at the end of Chapter 3. If you open the heart chakra at the end of your meditation, consider using it as a dedication to someone. For example, after practicing lovingkindness, feel the sensation of peace, joy and love in the body, and offer the energy to someone else. With both eyes closed, bring yourself into a sitting position (if you are not sitting already), and picture this person in your mind. When in sitting position, bring both hands together, and say in your mind, "May my practice be dedicated to your well-being." Having dedicated the practice, offer the energy by slowly parting your hands into a V shape as you raise them over your head. Keep in mind that to direct the flow of love energy, the heart chakra needs to be open, so before you extend love to someone else, it makes sense to extend love to yourself first. However, this is not a strict rule because meditation is not about following rules. No one is going to tell you that you cannot extend lovingkindness to others as a means of opening the heart chakra. Try different methods. Whichever methods work best for you are the ones you should follow.

Another way to open the heart chakra and direct the flow of love energy is through visualization exercises. For example, instead of extending love individually to people who have been kind to you, visualize them in a group, and in your mind merge them together. As they begin to merge, imagine seeing the love and kindness of each person as bright light. As each individual merges, the light becomes even brighter. When each individual has merged, imagine them shaping into a ball of light. With both eyes remaining closed, extend your chest as if pushing your heart chakra forward, and visualize this ball of light descending into the heart chakra. You might also

consider using the Tonglen exercise discussed in the Chapter 5 case study. In this exercise, you imagine a person who may be suffering from negativity or a sense of separation and breathe in the negative energy they radiate. On the exhale, concentrate on sending positive, healing energy to them.

The same exercise works for sending love to where people live. For example, you might visualize a poor neighborhood or a war zone. First, use a technique to open the heart chakra and imagine a white ball of light in the middle of your chest. Next, visualize a place, perhaps one you have seen on television or in person, and breathe in any negative energy, depression, or spiritual darkness you feel in the environment. As you draw in the negative energy, visualize it moving down into the chest area, absorbing into the ball of light, and transforming into love energy. On the exhale, breathe out the love energy and direct the flow toward the environment. You can apply this technique to yourself when you are suffering, to others who may be suffering, and to situations that create suffering.

The important thing to remember is that a healthy heart chakra is the gateway to experiencing love, compassion, sympathy and joy. Visualization techniques have a transformative power over undesired emotions, especially if you find it difficult to extend love to someone who has caused you problems. To transform any difficult emotions you may have toward others, join each index finger with the thumb on the same hand, and put the right hand to your chest. Close your eyes, concentrate on the heart chakra. After a few breaths, visualize the white glow in the center again, and begin chanting the sound "YAM." As you chant, imagine the sphere increasing in size until it surrounds your entire body. Bring this difficult person and the feelings of anger or anxiety they caused to mind. See them filled with the same white light and let your energy body merge with theirs to create a sphere twice as big. Continuing to chant "YAM," let all of your emotions absorb into this light and listen for the hidden message in them.

10-Minute Lovingkindness Exercise No. 2: Seeing the Good in Everyone

1. **Set a timer for at least 10 minutes.**

2. **Sit, stand, or lie down in one of the meditative positions.** Close both eyes or keep them open.

3. **Think of one good thing you did yesterday.** Nothing is too inconsequential. It can be something as minor as a smile you gave someone on the street or something as meaningful to you as accomplishing a goal you set for yourself.

4. **Meditate on the good thing you did.** Just sit and be with the memory for a couple of minutes Do not examine it; simply meditate.

5. **Think of someone who has helped you.** Think about the center of good within that person and the qualities you admire about them.

6. **Think of someone you feel neutral about and recall something that may reflect their center of good.** For example, if you witnessed an act of kindness by a stranger in public, think about how they helped someone when they did not have to. Imagine the center of good in them as being similar to the person who helped you.

7. **Think of someone you may dislike and try to recall a time when this person demonstrated an admirable quality.** It may be difficult to view someone you don't like in a positive light. When this happens, the mind is resisting an established pattern, so think about a choice this person made or some good thing this person accomplished. Meditate on this good thing and imagine the center of good in this person as being similar to the people you like.

Mantra Meditation

In Sanskrit, the word mantra refers to a sacred sound that caries the energy of the universe. The word *man*-tra means "mind-tool" or "magical spell." In the ancient tradition of Buddhism, monks used mantras to connect to higher levels of consciousness. By chanting a sacred sound, the meditator joins a higher level of consciousness. It is like hearing a tune being played by a band and whistling along with the music. It is made up of three

Sanskrit letters, "aa," "au," and "ma"…it is believed to be the basic sound which contains all other sounds." Other common mantras include:

1. HAMSA
2. OM MANI PEME HUNG
3. OM AH HUNG

There are many ways to chant a mantra. Some people chant aloud (on the exhale); others chant in their own minds. The basic key to chanting is to do it slowly, avoid thinking about meaning, and to blend the chant with the breath. The more the meditator repeats the mantra, the louder the chant grows in the mind. Different mantra sounds have different vibrations that trigger different effects in our bodies. For example, the mantra "HUNG" resonates in the chest and holds the energy there. When you try a new mantra, feel where the vibration appears in your body and use it to open a corresponding chakra. Third eye meditation involves mantra chanting the sound "AUM." Therefore, you might also consider visualizing the white sphere of light between the eyes for this chant.

Using the HAMSA chant, you might visualize the breath as a wave rolling back and forth from head to toe. This chant is useful for healing physical pains. Mantra meditation requires longer mantras chanted faster and spoken as a three-beat (for example, OM-*MA*/NI-*PE*/ME-*HUNG*). In the case of OM MANI PEME HUNG, the accent would fall on the second, fourth and sixth syllables. Accenting these syllables, the sound would come out as "om-MA/ni-PE/me-HUNG." OM MANI PEME HUNG is a mantra that Tibetans use to extend friendliness to all living things. For this reason, OM MANI PEME HUNG is a heart opening mantra appropriate for Lovingkindness Meditation. If you do not feel comfortable chanting mantras that involve Sanskrit, consider using affirmations. In this case, an affirmation would be a phrase repeated in English, such as "peace," "joy to all," or "quiet mind." To choose an affirmation, think about your intention. If you want to change a negative behavior, choose a phrase that counters this behavior and repeat it aloud or in your mind as an affirmation.

**10-Minute Lovingkindness Exercise No. 3:
Lovingkindness in Nature Meditation**

1. **Find a time during the weekend to visit a park or nature preserve.** The time of year matters less for this walking meditation, because it does not involve focusing on sensations (i.e. sights, sounds, smells, etc.).

2. **Use your cellphone as a 10-minute timer and pick a starting point along a walking path.** Instead of concentrating on movement, talk a few deep breaths and begin to walk.

3. **Choose an affirmation or chant and begin repeating it.** The chant is the object of your focus. If repeating a chant or affirmation aloud makes you feel self-conscious, repeat it in your mind. Since this is a Lovingkindness Meditation, choose a chant that extends love to yourself, to others, or to all living beings.

4. **Focus on the repetition.** It is all right to rest some attention on the environment, as long as you keep returning focus to the chant.

5. **Extend lovingkindness to the environment.** If someone walks by you on a nature trail, or you hear a dog bark in the distance, acknowledge their presence by extending the chant to include them. For example, if you are chanting, "May I be happy, may I be safe," etc., then include the passersby and chant, "May you be happy, may you be safe," etc. After a few moments, come back to extending the chant to yourself.

6. **If a person you have negative feelings about enters your thoughts, extend them lovingkindness.** After thoughts of this person dissipate, come back to extending the chant to yourself.

Causes of Energetic Blockages in the Heart Chakra

No matter how balanced meditation makes you, life will always throw curveballs your way. The pressures that come with going to school, being an athlete or living up to your parents' expectations begin to build if you do not meditate. When this happens, the chakras begin to close

and the body stores negative energy that causes blockages in the chakra system. If you begin to feel angry or hurt, this energy will clog the heart chakra. This is why opening the chakras should be a routine practice in Lovingkindness Meditation. The key to finding a blockage is to locate an area of the body feeling physical pain and determine its chakra region. For example, a closed heart chakra may take the physical form of chest or shoulder tightness.

Evidence of an energetic blockage in the heart chakra caused by patterns of behavior may take a less noticeable form. To determine whether patterns of behavior have caused a blockage in the heart chakra, look for any recent behaviors rooted in fear, resentment, grief, jealousy or ego drive. Fear, for example, closes the heart when the ego fears criticism from others. When fear blocks the heart chakra, a person's behavior turns confrontational. The fearful mind sees everything as an attack, causing the person to express outrage and become judgmental. If you find yourself constantly criticizing others, including yourself, look to open the heart chakra and release the negative energy causing you to act in these ways. By unblocking the heart chakra, you give yourself an opportunity to unravel the pattern of dwelling in the past. Jealousy is a form of resentment directed inward. People express jealousy when they feel something in themselves is lacking. In this instance, the object of your anger is you. In this instance, you would unblock the heart chakra by extending love to the person who is really suffering. When the heart releases jealousy, it releases you from the blame you lay at your own feet for not measuring up to some type of standard. If jealousy continues to block the heart chakra, resentment eventually becomes grief. Much like resentment, grief can hold people in the past. Grief is an emotion often felt after regret. Regret comes with a sense of loss for something that used to be. The realization that we cannot recover what is lost causes grief. Grief keeps the heart chakra blocked when we turn away from the pain caused by our grief.

When grief lingers, the pain it causes creates an ego-constructed wall in the heart that refuses to let emotions enter or leave. Over time, we come

to believe that this wall keeps us from feeling pain when it really keeps us from feeling love and moving on. At this point, emotional experiences stop and the heart becomes dead inside. If you find yourself trapped in one of these patterns, do something selfless for someone. The mere act of doing something selfless can open the heart chakra. The more you selflessly do for others without any expectation of reward, the more you keep the heart chakra open. The more you keep the heart chakra open, the more life rewards you with its love.

10-Minute Lovingkindness Exercise No. 4: Cultivating Optimism

1. Set a timer for 10 minutes.

2. Choose a meditative position, close your eyes and start a breathing exercise.

3. After a few deep breaths, imagine being the person you aspire to be. When the image of your ideal future self comes, imagine having the life you always hoped to have. This might include anything to do with your relationships, social life, or hobbies.

4. After spending 10 minutes visualizing this future self, open your eyes and spend a few minutes writing anything about this future self.

5. Go about your day and notice if you feel more positive toward life than before. If so, consider doing this activity on a daily basis and see if your optimism builds exponentially over time.

Additional Tips for Deepening Lovingkindness

The positive effects of lovingkindess meditation usually become more noticeable outside of practice. People who continue to meditate over time begin to feel the deepening of love, joy, compassion and sympathy. Outside of practice, there are ways to deepen the effects of lovingkindness even further through reflection. Reflecting on meditative practice might mean taking a few moments to write down observations of the past week in a journal, or it might mean thinking about them. Reflection is a way of noticing

positive changes and any changes about your practice, your behavior, or your thoughts that you would still like to make. To deepen lovingkindness, take an active role in extending love outside your practice. This may mean agreeing to becoming more flexible to change, learning to forgive people, finding the beauty in even the smallest things, or feeling thankful for what you have. Being more flexible to change involves accepting the fact that change is unavoidable. Life moves in forward motion, and you must move with it the way like a tree swaying without resistance in the direction of the wind. If you keep a journal, note when change happens and the thoughts you had as you learned about this change. Ask yourself if you approached this change with less resistance or the same as usual. If nothing in this area of your life has changed, take this to your practice and make developing flexibility to change part of your intention in meditation.

It is the same for learning forgiveness. Instead of thinking about when someone hurt you or betrayed your trust, think about a time when you hurt s omeone or betrayed someone's trust. Follow this person in your mind and see the effect your behavior had on them. Practicing lovingkindness is about understanding that people are the same and need the same things. If you feel their pain, dwell on it for a few moments, and think about how much you would like this person's forgiveness. When the memory of this person passes, relate your desire for their forgiveness to someone who has hurt you and forgive that person. Afterward, reflect on what you learned about that person you hurt and how you have grown since then.

Another way to deepen lovingkindness outside of your practice is to find the beauty in things. Finding the beauty in things can happen through reflection or in present moment awareness. Find the beauty in objects and living creatures. Look at a piece of steel and think about the heating process that created it. Watch a butterfly crawl along a flower and think about the transformation process of the butterfly from a caterpillar or a seed to a colorful flower. When you have time to reflect or write in a journal, think about all the good things that happened over the previous two days. If at

first you have trouble finding anything, remember that beauty exists in even the smallest things, a gesture, an offering, an experience, and so forth. Think about your positive contributions to the world in that time. Perhaps you opened a door for someone, got an essay finished on time, tutored a struggling student or cooked someone dinner. In your thoughts, express gratitude toward life for giving you the opportunity to make the world better in some way. When you have done this, think back further in time and look for the beauty in your memory or positive contributions to the world. If time provides, reflect further back in time — a month, a year, a decade, and so forth. In your reflection, realize there is enough happiness to go around. It is not in limited supply. Joy, peace, beauty, etc., are limitless. There is enough for everyone, and it is open to you at any time.

10-Minute Lovingkindness Exercise No. 5: Altar Meditation

1. **Set a timer for t10 minutes.**

2. **Create a meditation altar of a spiritual leader.** The altar should comprise a compilation of anything that reminds you of this spiritual leader (for example, a Bible, a picture, a cross, etc.) This this spiritual leader can be a historical figure such as Jesus, Mohammed, or Buddha. It also can be a personal figure, your own teacher or someone you feel expresses unconditional love.

3. **Sit in a meditative position, focus on the altar and start a breathing exercise.**

4. **After a few deep breaths, imagine this leader's loving energy radiating outward and in your direction.** Imagine the radiating energy continuing to expand until it surrounds you. Imagine receiving and absorbing this energy for yourself.

5. **Repeat a lovingkindness mantra.** You might start by extending lovingkindness to yourself by saying or thinking, "May I be happy, may I be safe, may I be at peace, may I be free of suffering." After a few minutes, imagine holding this love energy from your spiritual leader and extending it through mantra to someone you care about, someone you feel neutral about and someone you feel negatively about.

---

6. **End the meditation.** Go about your day and notice if you feel more positive toward life than before. If so, consider doing this activity on a daily basis and see if your love energy builds exponentially over time.

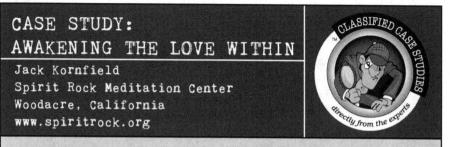

CASE STUDY:
AWAKENING THE LOVE WITHIN

Jack Kornfield
Spirit Rock Meditation Center
Woodacre, California
www.spiritrock.org

Excerpt Taken From: **http://www.kripalu.org**

Article Title: **Balancing Act**

What transformations can people have when they practice meditation?

There is a glow people have, a "meditation facelift" that leaves people profoundly refreshed, their eyes open and skin clear. You do not have to become a card-carrying Buddhist. You can tend to the awakened inner beauty from meditation practice in moments, by skillful use of intention, and the practice of loving-kindness. You can do this anywhere—in the airport, supermarket, or workplace. In any circumstance, even tending young children, having the skills of wise intention is invaluable and makes that circumstance more alive.

Body-based practices, such as being aware of the breath, can help you embody the power of mindfulness and live fully in the present, whether you are jogging or cooking. The result is the ability to live your life in the reality of the present, rather than in the worries of the future and regrets of the past. And you have the flexibility and ability to respond to your circumstances with a tremendous sense of inner power.

How can someone use mindfulness and loving-kindness every day?

You can sit on a subway in New York City and begin, without looking weird at all, to direct the force of loving-kindness to those around you. You might imagine people in their original beauty as children. In a minute, your relationship to them transforms and they connect with your heart. Look into your heart, and it will show you that you are looking for ways to connect and create bridges.

What mantras do you like to use, if any?

I use a loving-kindness meditation at times, for inner recitation. When I encounter people, I use, "May you be well, may you be safe."

Sometimes, I use one from the Beatles: "Let it be." I really take it to heart in a deep way when I recite that. There is a way I'm letting the world be as it is, I know how to respond, and I don't have to be worried or rushed. I feel what response comes from silence.

What are your goals as a teacher?

My goal is for people to awaken to their fundamental dignity, nobility, and freedom of the heart regardless of their circumstances. My goal is for them to remember how to love and bring compassion to all parts of their lives. Also, to give people ancient practices and tools they can use when they return to their everyday lives so they can quiet the mind, open the heart, and develop a spirit of compassion no matter where they are. People can heal and transform themselves and learn to be their own enlightened master. My goal is for them to trust their innate wisdom

Divine Meditation

Once you have finished three weeks of core meditation practice, you have the option to either customize your own 10-minute practice using the techniques that work best for you or go further into divine meditation. While lovingkindess lifts the meditator into pure Tao consciousness (love, joy, peace), divine meditation aspires to the highest point of consciousness: divine (or ultimate) consciousness and enlightenment. Divine meditation is any meditation that seeks to contemplate, communicate and become one with God. Divine meditation helps the meditator to become more spiritual.

Entering Deeper Realms of Spirituality

To achieve cosmic consciousness, we first have to recognize the levels of spiritual transcendence. In the first stage of spiritual transcendence, the meditator comes to believe in spirituality. Practicing divine meditation may begin to trigger glimpses of spiritual dimensions and cause the spirit within you to awaken. Once the spirit within you awakens, you feel transformed and have a sense that something is communicating directly to you.

As your divine meditation progresses the spirit within not only awakens; it also joins with your consciousness, and you have no doubt of your transcendence.

Those who reach this transcendent stage still have a distinction between the physical body and the spirit. As you progress through divine meditation, the ego drive that connects you to your sense of self begins to dissolve and you become one with spirit, meaning that everything you do in life is for the spirit communicating to you. In the final transcendent stage of spirituality, every moment, person, action, or thought contains some form of divine expression, without the slightest trace of separation. No longer does anything appear as a random coincidence devoid of meaning. At this stage, it becomes possible to attempt to foresee future events or understand everyday situations with greater clarity.

Common Experiences in Divine Meditation

Because we typically experience three dimensions, the concept of the spiritual dimension is difficult for us to understand. Where does the spiritual dimension exist? The answer is, anywhere you look. Some encounters are internal, and others occur in the external environment. The separation does not exist literally. We just need to change how we look at reality. As the Dalai Lama said, "This is my simple religion. There is no need for temples; no need for complicated philosophy. Our own brain, our own heart is our temple; the philosophy is kindness."

Meditators who experience spiritual transcendence often report understanding deep truths that others might not be able to understand. Deeper levels of transcendence create a deeper sense of peace. Meditators on this spiritual level also report a continual revelation of truth.

Through divine meditation, consciousness expands from the physical body into your self-image and ego. Expansion into these areas acts as a type of cleansing and rebirth. From there, consciousness expansion continues be-

yond the mind into your energy body. Your energy body is your surrounding energy known as the *aura*, which expands and contracts depending on the emotions and thoughts you give off. Meditators who achieve the higher levels of divine meditation may experience communication with otherworldly beings. Spiritual gurus at this level often experience astral projection and report contact with divine historical figures such as Christ, Mohammed, and others. Because divine meditation requires a lengthy session to achieve an intense level of stillness and concentration, you are not likely to achieve astral projection within 10 minutes. If you attempt astral projection, make sure you are breathing regularly, paying attention to the sounds around you and noting all sensations. Try to visualize yourself sitting in place as though being an observer to your body. As an observer, watch your body's movements as you breathe. Visualize your astral body rising up like a mist out of your physical self. As an observer, study your astral body the same way you studied your physical body. Next, visualize you the observer moving toward your astral body and merging with it. After merging with your astral body, look down at your physical body, and then begin to move across the room, visualizing yourself passing through the walls, floating outside, away from your community, into different parts of the world, and into the universe. The deeper you fall into the practice of astral projection, the more intense images may become. In a sense, astral projection is both a search for God and another method to cultivate spirituality. Other ways to cultivate spirituality include:

1. Developing and living life by virtues that adhere to natural law
2. Cultivating unconditional love
3. Transcending duality

Developing and living life by the virtues that adhere to natural law requires you to know and understand the seven laws of nature. To read and put into practice the seven laws of nature, go to Appendix B. Likewise, cultivating unconditional love requires you always extend lovingkindness to people who have wronged you.

10-Minute Divine Meditation Exercise 1:
Experimenting with Aura

1. **Close your eyes and take a few deep breaths.** Feel yourself relax further upon each exhale.

2. **Visualize yourself with someone or some place that you love.** Imagine your aura experiencing an energetic expansion with the positive feelings this person or place brings. As it reaches its fullest expansion, study its appearance (color, brightness, thickness, etc.).

3. **Visualize yourself in a taxing situation, one that has caused you distress in the past.** Imagine your aura experiencing an energetic contraction with the negative feelings this situation brings. Study the contraction. Note how the physical characteristics you noted earlier seem diminished.

4. **Open your eyes, stand up and move to the center of the room.** Note the boundaries of the room, close your eyes and visualize filling the entire room with your energy body.

5. **Retract your energy body until it forms a sphere around you.** Expand and contract it a few more times, then relax, open your eyes and notice how you feel.

Third Eye Activation and Meditation

The third eye is the sixth chakra, the energetic opening where the stream of prana feeds into human form. Located between the eyes, mystics call this chakra "the seat of intuition" because it connects us to higher dimensional consciousness, namely the fourth dimension. Every chakra is involved in some form of extrasensory perception, but the extrasensory perceptions of the sixth chakra include:

1. Intuition
2. Clairvoyance
3. Precognition
4. Astral projection
5. Seeing people's aura

10-Minute Divine Meditation Exercise 2:
Third Eye Activation

1. **Limit your physical vision.** Darkness is an important factor in third eye activation/meditation because it stimulates the pineal gland to produce melatonin. Melatonin plays an important role in getting the brain to higher states of consciousness. This is why people produce melatonin when they dream. Dream sleep is a form of astral projection.

2. **Sit in lotus position and begin breathing.** On the inhale, breathe through the nose. On the exhale, breathe through the mouth. As thoughts occur, let them pass without judgment and allow them to pass. After a few breaths, focus on facial tension. Facial tension reduces your ability to open the third eye, so focus on tense areas and relax them.

3. **Take a deep breath and hold it for as long as you feel comfortable.** Part your jaw slightly, and on the exhale, and create the sound, "Thohhhhh-hhhhhh" and extend it for as long as is comfortable. Specific sounds such as this will cause a vibration in the midbrain that stimulates the pineal gland. Repeat this breathing process six times in a row.

4. **Breathe deep and hold the inhale for six seconds.** On the exhale, create the sound "Maaaaaaaaaaaaaaay," and repeat this breathing process six times. You can experiment with different tones to see which tone best causes a vibration in the midbrain. For example, Step 6 in Chapter 4 stretches out the tone "OM." Use whichever tone works best to make the area between your eyes vibrate. Eventually, you should feel a vibration from the crown chakra. This vibration is the seventh chakra bringing extra-sensory information to your third eye.

5. **Eyelids remaining shut, rotate your eyes upward as if looking toward the center of your head.** This may feel like a strain, but it helps activate the third eye. Some meditators can open their third eye without looking toward the center of the eyes, so try this step if you are having trouble activating the third eye.

6. **Looking toward the center, imagine your third eye opening slowly..** At this point, you may start to see patterns or colors. Observe what you see or feel without judgment. You will eventually begin to see extra-dimensionally.

7. **To end the session, shift your focus back to the breath for several moments and open your eyes.**

riences, go back to the four types of extrasensory perceptions and see which one, if any, matches your experiences.

Third eye mediation requires some physical preparation. While an acid-alkaline diet can be an important step toward adopting healthier lifestyle, some recipes may contain meats or other foods that in prevent third eye activation. To avoid such ingredients, consider adopting a vegan diet. Veganism is a type of vegetarian diet that completely excludes meat, eggs, refined sugar, dairy products, processed foods, and all other animal-derived ingredients. To reiterate, a vegan diet essentially includes the same foods found in an acid-alkaline diet, but some acid-alkaline diets may allow for foods, such as chicken, that are not vegan. Meats such as chicken are spiritually grounding. Vegan foods such as oatmeal, vegetables, cereal, whole wheat bread, frozen fruit desserts, lentil soup and chickpeas may not have the optimal acid-alkaline balance, but they are spiritually elevating. If you plan to activate your third eye, choose a vegan diet or an acid-alkaline diet that does not include meat. For more information about veganism, go to **www.vrg. org**. To activate the third eye, go back to Chapter 4 and follow the instructions from step 6 under section that covers opening the seven chakras or practice the exercise on the following page.

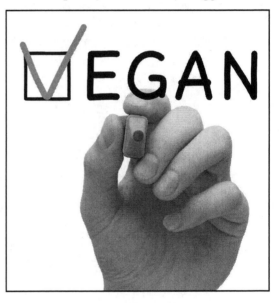

tion, it is especially important to open the sacral chakra, which controls fear and releases negative energy. You need to be aware that certain dangers exist if you implement incorrect procedures for third eye activation, which mainly involves activating and opening the third eye without opening the prior chakras. For example, activating the third eye requires that you open the root chakra beforehand to release excess energies that might overwhelm you during third eye meditation. If you fail to open the sacral chakra, and you encounter frightful images during third eye meditation, you may not be able to distinguish your projections from what is real.

If you continue your practice over a lengthy period, the third eye will eventually stay activated and you can constantly channel for extra-dimensional information in between meditative sessions. Some of the symptoms you might experience include the extrasensory perceptions listed above. Additional symptoms might also include food and noise sensitivities, increased creativity, changing perception of time, experiencing life changing events, random encounters with spiritual teachers, and so forth. Everyone who practices third eye meditation receives extrasensory information in different ways. The four main ways are physical, emotional, spiritual and mental. For example, mental psychics have clairvoyance, emotional psychics feel intense empathy for other beings, spiritual psychics know things without being able to provide an explanation, and physical psychics feel extrasensory information. Most people possess at least one psychic sense that is stronger than the rest. However, as you continue your practice in third eye meditation, your strongest psychic sense will expand to the point of exhaustion and begin to increase the strength of your other psychic senses. A mental psychic who practices third eye meditation may then begin to experience increased physical, emotional, or mental extrasensory perceptions. Before you activate your third eye, consider using your core meditation to explore which psychic sense you believe is your primary strength. For example, you might quiet your mind and meditate on how you often hear sounds that no one else seems to hear. Based on your expe-

6. Lucid dreaming

Everything we see with our physical eyes narrows our perception to three-dimensional reality. We are born into this world with enhanced third eye perceptions that gradually close the more we see with the physical eye. By activating the third eye, you can reverse this process and experience higher, multidimensional aspects of consciousness. Quantum physics tells us that reality has 10 different dimensions. In his book, "Hyperspace: A Scientific Odyssey Through Parallel Universes, Time Warps, and the Tenth Dimension," renowned quantum physicist Michio Kaku states that the 10th dimension is the dimension at which all the laws of the universe become unified. Since we experience life in the third dimension, much of what exists remains hidden from us.

You might be asking yourself, what might third eye meditation in a higher dimension look like? The answer is not limited to one thing. For example, you might use an affirmation that tells fourth dimensional reality to organize itself in a way that is understandable to you. Remember that you are interacting with fourth dimensional reality, where time does not exist linearly, so you only need to think something in order for it to happen. In the fourth dimension, you can get creative in your exploration, and you do not necessarily have to experience things through sight alone. You might ask the universe a question and have it explained to you. To gain insight, you might ask for an experience from a different perspective. As Teal Scott elaborates, "Let's take a given event. Let's say you wanted to go back and experience Hiroshima. You could experience what it was like to be a small boy being bombed, or what it was like to be a soldier dropping bombs. You could experience the universal conscious mind and experience its perspective about that event. There is no perspective that is off limits to you."

Before you activate your third eye, it is important to have already explored your inner self through your core meditation. This helps you understand your fears, which have the potential to cloud your perceptions, interpretations, and projections during third eye meditation. For third eye medita-

6. Lucid dreaming

Everything we see with our physical eyes narrows our perception to three-dimensional reality. We are born into this world with enhanced third eye perceptions that gradually close the more we see with the physical eye. By activating the third eye, you can reverse this process and experience higher, multidimensional aspects of consciousness. Quantum physics tells us that reality has 10 different dimensions. In his book, "Hyperspace: A Scientific Odyssey Through Parallel Universes, Time Warps, and the Tenth Dimension," renowned quantum physicist Michio Kaku states that the 10th dimension is the dimension at which all the laws of the universe become unified. Since we experience life in the third dimension, much of what exists remains hidden from us.

You might be asking yourself, what might third eye meditation in a higher dimension look like? The answer is not limited to one thing. For example, you might use an affirmation that tells fourth dimensional reality to organize itself in a way that is understandable to you. Remember that you are interacting with fourth dimensional reality, where time does not exist linearly, so you only need to think something in order for it to happen. In the fourth dimension, you can get creative in your exploration, and you do not necessarily have to experience things through sight alone. You might ask the universe a question and have it explained to you. To gain insight, you might ask for an experience from a different perspective. As Teal Scott elaborates, "Let's take a given event. Let's say you wanted to go back and experience Hiroshima. You could experience what it was like to be a small boy being bombed, or what it was like to be a soldier dropping bombs. You could experience the universal conscious mind and experience its perspective about that event. There is no perspective that is off limits to you."

Before you activate your third eye, it is important to have already explored your inner self through your core meditation. This helps you understand your fears, which have the potential to cloud your perceptions, interpretations, and projections during third eye meditation. For third eye medita-

10-Minute Divine Meditation Exercise 2: Third Eye Activation

1. **Limit your physical vision.** Darkness is an important factor in third eye activation/meditation because it stimulates the pineal gland to produce melatonin. Melatonin plays an important role in getting the brain to higher states of consciousness. This is why people produce melatonin when they dream. Dream sleep is a form of astral projection.

2. **Sit in lotus position and begin breathing.** On the inhale, breathe through the nose. On the exhale, breathe through the mouth. As thoughts occur, let them pass without judgment and allow them to pass. After a few breaths, focus on facial tension. Facial tension reduces your ability to open the third eye, so focus on tense areas and relax them.

3. **Take a deep breath and hold it for as long as you feel comfortable.** Part your jaw slightly, and on the exhale, and create the sound, "Thohhhhh-hhhhhh" and extend it for as long as is comfortable. Specific sounds such as this will cause a vibration in the midbrain that stimulates the pineal gland. Repeat this breathing process six times in a row.

4. **Breathe deep and hold the inhale for six seconds.** On the exhale, create the sound "Maaaaaaaaaaaaaaay," and repeat this breathing process six times. You can experiment with different tones to see which tone best causes a vibration in the midbrain. For example, Step 6 in Chapter 4 stretches out the tone "OM." Use whichever tone works best to make the area between your eyes vibrate. Eventually, you should feel a vibration from the crown chakra. This vibration is the seventh chakra bringing extra-sensory information to your third eye.

5. **Eyelids remaining shut, rotate your eyes upward as if looking toward the center of your head.** This may feel like a strain, but it helps activate the third eye. Some meditators can open their third eye without looking toward the center of the eyes, so try this step if you are having trouble activating the third eye.

6. **Looking toward the center, imagine your third eye opening slowly..** At this point, you may start to see patterns or colors. Observe what you see or feel without judgment. You will eventually begin to see extra-dimensionally.

7. **To end the session, shift your focus back to the breath for several moments and open your eyes.**

Using Binaural Beats for Third Eye Meditation

Using binaural beats is another way to activate your third eye. You do not necessarily have to be in delta consciousness to open the third eye, but this state is usually optimal for divine meditation. Therefore, if your initial goal is to activate the third eye with a binaural beat, you might choose a 13 Hz low beta frequency, which contains enough stimulation to vibrate the pineal gland. For example, a binaural beat set at 13 Hz for third eye opening might utilize 70 Hz tone for the left ear, and an 83 Hz tone for the right ear. The 70 Hz frequency would stimulate mental and astral projection while the 83 Hz frequency would stimulate third eye opening. In addition to binaural beats, some meditators use (and even prefer) isochronic tones for meditation. Isochronic tones are the most powerful and differ from binaural beats in that they combine two equal intensity pulses with intervals of silence while gradually increasing pulse speeds. Headphones are necessary for binaural beats, and optional (though still recommended) for isochronic tones. To get an idea about which audio may be more suitable for your personal use, consider the following pros and cons.

Binaural Beats (Pros)

1. Greater variety of audio options
2. More effective for deep trance delta consciousness
3. Research well established

Binaural Beats (Cons)

1. Less effective than isochronic tones outside the delta frequency range
2. Headphones more necessary than for isochronic tones, which may be less convenient

Isochronic Tones (Pros)

1. More effective than binaural beats in beta, alpha and theta frequency ranges

2. Headphones not necessary which is more convenient

Isochronic Tones (Cons)

1. Smaller variety of audio options
2. Less effective for delta consciousness
3. Research less established

10-Minute Divine Meditation Exercise 3: Using Binaural Beats or Isochronic Tones

1. **Find a dark room and assume a meditative position.** You can use any comfortable position, or the step 6 position from Chapter 4.

2. **Put on your headphones.** Begin playing the binaural beat or isochronic tone, and close your eyes.

3. **Use any breathing technique and focus the breath into and out of your third eye chakra.** On the inhale, feel the oxygen entering your third eye. On the exhale, feel the chakra pulsate as it receives the air.

4. **Repeat step 3 for the length of the audio.** The audio for a binaural beat or an isochronic tone is usually between 30 and 60 minutes.

5. **When the audio ends, stay with the meditation or come back to the breath to end the session.** Take a few deep breaths, and slowly open your eyes. Continue this practice daily for at least three weeks. The more you do it, the more fourth dimensional sight your third eye will gain.

After each session, rub your hands quickly together to heat them up, and bring them to your face to absorb the energy. This helps integrate your brain to the new experience. Third eye meditation can be the most interesting practice when it comes to keeping a journal. After you come out of a session, write down what you experience. Continue this meditative process for at least three weeks and examine what has changed. It is common for some third eye mediators to experience symptoms such as headaches, migraines, or dizziness after activating this part of the brain. Understand that this is normal, that you are still in control, and that it is not easy to awaken and open up to what the universe wants to show you.

Chanting Meditation to Evoke the Divine

If you have trouble opening the third eye, try mixing a chanting meditation into your practice. Chanting meditations are not for everyone, but those who practice devotion to a religion such as Christianity or Islam may be more inclined to use them. Again, this is where different forms of meditation intersect with devotional religions. Singing gospel is a form of devotional chanting much the same way that the prayers used by various religions are a form of meditation. Chanting also serves as a preparation for meditation when combined with some of the other methods described in Chapter 4.

Insight vs. Devotion

Ultimately, the point of practicing divine meditation is discovering who you are in relation to everything else. Divine meditation offers two paths, insight and devotion. Devotional meditation, typically practiced in religions such as Christianity or Islam, uses representations of divinity as the focus. In devotional meditation, you work to achieve spiritual union with ultimate consciousness. You allow the universal creative source to work through you and affect every aspect of your life. Insight meditation uses present moment awareness and spiritual connectivity to investigate further into the nature of things. Doing so reveals the deeper reality, achieving a divine meditation in its essence, but without the characteristics of devotional practice.

If you have an interest in gaining insight into your existence but do not have an interest in cultivating spiritual devotion, it is best to choose divine meditative practices that cultivate insight rather than devotion. Buddhism, for example, practices insight rather than devotion, and some religions, while devotional in nature, offer insight practices as an alternative. The Judeo practice of Kabbalah is one such practice that focuses on this path. Insight meditation teaches that reality has two levels, relative and absolute. The relative world is the physical reality and everything it encom-

passes such as classes, the homework you have to do, the job you may have, etc. While these things contain meaning for people, they do not contain true cosmic meaning. Absolute reality is true cosmic meaning, the divine presence that gives everything its reason for being. Accessing the points at which *relative* and *absolute* reality intersect to create enlightenment is what insight meditation aspires to achieve. Therefore, consider any meditative exercise designed to expand boundaries a path to insight.

CASE STUDY: MEDITATIVE DRAWING

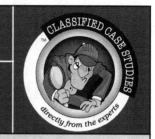

Meg Buchner
Meditative Drawing Instructor
Ferryville, WI

Meg Buchner is an art teacher in Wisconsin who teaches students of all ages to reach a state of relaxation and meditation through drawing. Often referred to as "directed doodling" meditative drawing focuses on creating repetitive lines, shapes or patterns. Drawings are typically done in black and white.

Buchner says, "The key to meditative doodling is to clear your mind and focus on the lines and shapes. When you are drawing, you should not have any idea of what the "finished" drawing will look like. There is no right or wrong or any exact way the drawing should look."

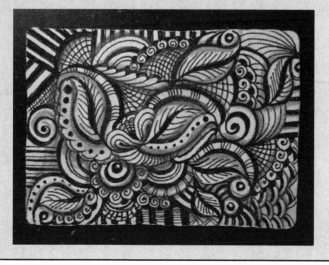

Here are some general steps to creating a meditative doodle.

1. Start with a small, blank piece of paper or card stock. Many people prefer square or circular titles about 3" x 3", so the finished drawing is symmetrical.

2. Use a black pen. Any pen will do, including a regular ballpoint. People who practice meditative doodling on a frequent basis usually prefer pens with varying widths.

3. To begin, divide your paper into random sections with wavy lines and fill each section with a different pattern.

4. Start in any section. Draw a simple shape or line and repeat. Squares, spirals, circles are often used.

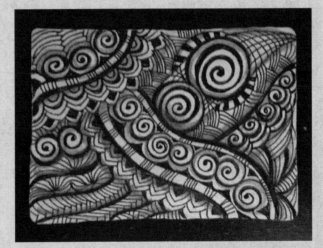

Buchner adds that there are many examples online of finished drawings as well as sample shapes you can use for inspiration. You can also look for sample patterns and step-by-step explanations of how to create them. Pinterest has many boards devoted to meditative doodling and YouTube has a multitude of instructional videos. A few examples are:

- www.pinterest.com/megadesn/zen-tangles-and-doodles
- www.pinterest.com/sharieob/zentangles-patterns
- www.pinterest.com/steensd/zentangle-and-meditative-drawing
- https://youtu.be/uAYcB9pOWos
- https://youtu.be/m3y-9XVnjTo

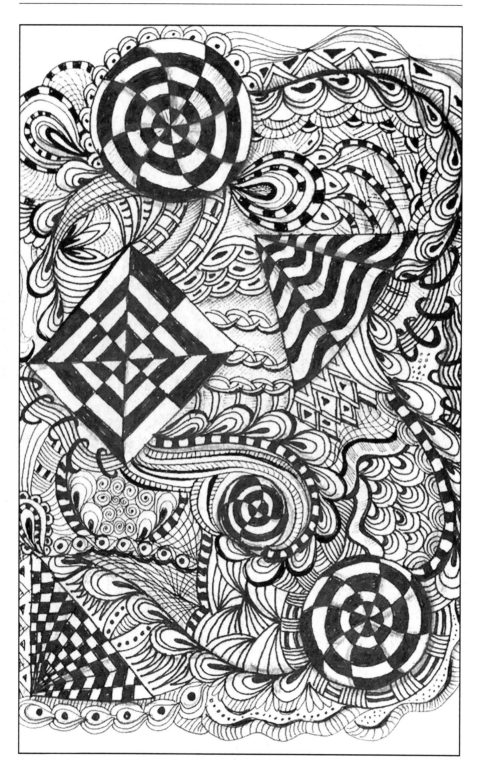

Meditation in Everyday Life

ooks on meditation attract different people for different reasons, but one thing most people want is to see its results extended into everyday life. Meditation yields the kind of mental and physical results most people in modern life need to run their everyday lives. In addition to being a devotional and insightful art, it also prepares the body for physical activity. No better example of meditation as a performance art exists than in the martial arts. When people think about martial arts (tai-kwan-do, judo, jujitsu, and so forth), meditation is not the first thing that comes to mind. However, meditation plays a large part because it involves achieving a connection between the body and mind. Meditation not only helps martial artists but also a wide variety of people in competitive sports and performing arts because it causes what athletes call "being in the zone." If you suffer from anger, anxiety, or depression and you try to learn a martial art, play a competitive sport, or pursue a performing art, negative mind-states are likely to affect your training and level of performance without some form of meditation.

Meditation as a Performance Booster in Martial Arts

Why do people learn martial arts, and what are its benefits? Some people practice martial arts to get fit, while others use it to reduce stress. Martial arts are an action form of meditation which develops the mind and what the Chinese call the semi-sleeping state. The semi-sleeping state is the meditative component of marital arts that focuses on concentration; it awakens the subconscious mind and tells the conscious mind to release control. Practicing meditation to develop the semi-sleeping state allows the martial artist to achieve a level of focus where outside distractions do not register. To reach full potential as a martial artist, training begins with calming the mind so that it will focus and allow your body to work with it. Without meditation, the martial artist can tense up with fear. When this occurs, the mind doesn't let the body flow with what the Chinese call *Qi* energy. The two different parts of the body that regulate Qi energy are the brain and the abdomen region, otherwise known as the yin and yang. The brain (or yin) regulates the quality of energy. The abdomen (or yang) stores and supplies the body's energy quantity.

As Bruce Lee attested in a 1971 interview with Pierre Berton, "Martial arts have a very deep meaning in my life because everything I have learned as an actor, as a martial artist, and as a human being I have learned from martial arts. It is a combination of natural instinct and control, and you have to combine the two in harmony. In either extreme, you become unscientific or mechanical, no longer a human being. Therefore, martial art is the art of expressing the human body." Through martial arts, the yin and yang communicate through the spinal cord, which enables the two Qi energies to act as one. Martial artists also use meditation as a way to mentally review techniques in their mind. During meditation, a martial artist will replay moves with precise changes, focusing on footwork, balance, state of mind, timing, power, and so forth. They might also use it as a form of self-reflection with respect to training. For example, if performance train-

ing becomes difficult, meditation is a place where you can examine your motives, contemplate your weaknesses, and refocus your approach. Those who sustain injuries in combat also use meditation as a way to heal faster. As a way of gaining a competitive advantage, martial artists may also use meditation to understand the opponent. In the seminal book, "The Art of War," Sun Tzu writes, "If you only know yourself, but not your opponent, you may win or you may lose."

Meditation as a Performance Booster in Competitive Sports

Athletes who play at peak performance often describe an experience they call being "in flow" or "in the zone." Athletes describe this experience as a state in which extremely difficult tasks come easier than normal, and the brain flows smoothly from one activity to the next. Hall of Fame basketball player Michael Jordan once described an experience where his shooting accuracy was near perfect because the basketball net seemed much bigger than normal, and it felt as if he could not miss. Joe Greene, Hall of Fame defensive end for the Pittsburgh Steelers once said, "A lot of players talk about being in the zone, but for me, it only happened one time in my career. In fact, the one time it happened, it felt like the whole team was in the zone and we were playing as one unit. We could anticipate exactly what our opponent was going to do and we executed to perfection."

Many professional athletes have trouble figuring out how or why they get into the zone, but those who meditate to enhance their performance are likely to find the zone more often than those who do not. When athletes do poorly in the big moments, it is because anxiety and the fear of failure overwhelms them. However, athletes who meditate are calmer in these situations and more likely to succeed. Many athletes meditate before a game to reduce stress and increase their focus. Other athletes meditate during resting periods in between to develop the energy and endurance necessary for later use. According to sports meditation consultant George Mumford,

who was hired during Phil Jackson's tenure with the Chicago Bulls, "Meditation offers opportunity to be in the moment. In sports, what gets people's attention is this idea of being in the zone or playing in the zone. When they are playing their best, they can do no wrong, and no matter what happens they are always a step quicker, a step ahead. That happens when we are in the moment, when we are mindful of what is going on. There is a lack of self-consciousness, there is a relaxed concentration, and there is this sense of effortlessness, of being in the flow." In his book, "Flow: The Psychology of the Optimal Experience," Mihalyi Csikszentmihalyi identifies several characteristics of athletes who surpass the dimension of human experience, which include:

1. Deep concentration
2. The transformation of time
3. Letting go of control
4. Loss of self-consciousness

Although some athletes are naturally faster and stronger, the athlete that masters meditation and being in flow is far more likely to outperform the physically superior athlete that does not. Bruce Lee was by no means a physically imposing person, but to this day many consider him the greatest martial artist of all time. What being in flow demonstrates is that consciousness plays an essential role in athletic training. Csikszentmihalyi writes, "Because optimal experience depends on the ability to control what happens in moment-by-moment consciousness, each person has to achieve it on the basis of his or her own individual efforts and creativity. This happens when psychic energy is invested in realistic goals, and when skills match the opportunities for action."

Csikszentmihalyi teaches athletes that having the right skills to perform requires that the activity be stimulating and enjoyable when trying to perform it. When beating the opponent is more important than performing as well as possible, enjoyment tends to disappear and flow goes with it. This is what some mean when they say that sports and competition cause you to

become spiritually disconnected. Out of fear, anger, or anxiety comes the fear of being controlled, out of which comes the desire to control others. Having real control means allowing one's self to let go of control. As Csikszentmihalyi notes, "The flow experience is typically described as involving a sense of control or, more precisely, as lacking the sense of worry about losing control that is typical in many situations of normal life. What people enjoy is not the sense of *being* in control, but the sense of *exercising* control in difficult situations. However, when a person becomes dependent on the ability to control an enjoyable activity, he or she then loses the ultimate control: the freedom to determine the content of consciousness." Whether the miracle underdog comes out of nowhere and surprises everyone, or the dominating favorite runs through the competition with ease, what we often witness is what coaches call "team concept." While competition does drive some to develop unhealthy egoistic tendencies, the most unforgettable moments in sports do serve to remind us of our own inner potential.

Meditation as a Performance Booster in the Creative Arts

What is inspiration and where does it come from? Whether you are someone pursuing an education as a creative artist or just enjoy hobbies like painting or writing as a creative outlet, people have sought the answer since the first great works of art appeared in human history. Inspiration implies the idea that some external source must create an internal spark. The truth about inspiration is that it is nothing more than the act of gaining insight by accessing a creative source that exists within each person at any given moment. One of the most common questions asked by creative artists is where ideas for great works come from. According to renowned Hollywood screenwriting teacher Robert McKee, "Stories unearth themselves inside the mind of the writer. They are not buried somewhere in the ground of life trying to come up and tell themselves. The stories worth telling already exist within you. You are responding to your own inner life, whether

Csikszentmihalyi also presented a Flow Chart diagram (illustrated below) which measures the point at which the skill of the individual and the challenge of the task begin to create flow.

As the diagram shows, anxiety, worry, and apathy are typical emotions of individuals who have negative perceptions toward the task and therefore low skill level. However, these negative emotions differ when it comes to the individual's *perception* of the task. Those who demonstrate apathy may not care about completing the challenge and therefore have less skill to complete it. Since these individuals do not worry about completing the task, it makes no difference whether they succeed or fail. Those with an interest in completing the task demonstrate worry and anxiety about their ability to do so. Since these individuals have little experience or skill, they focus on their own fear of failure rather than on the task itself. Individuals with mid-level skill experience apathy more often than boredom. For these individuals, the goal is to simply complete the task rather than excel at it. Once able to complete the minimum requirements, they quickly become bored. However, those with mid-level skills who demonstrate extreme interest in the task have an aroused desire to excel further. This is the point at which optimal conditions for flow state exist.

To get to flow. the perception of the task as enjoyable, interesting, and challenging must combine with having attained at least a mid-level skill. Even without these conditions, meditation can still allow the skilled individual to relax while completing the challenge. However, if the task does not create enough enjoyment at this stage, flow is not possible. As a mild interest, the skilled individual may use meditation to exhibit greater control but still not flow. As the individual's perception of the challenge as interesting and enjoyable begins to rise in concert with skill level, meditation can take the individual into higher levels of consciousness that create flow. Use the Csikszentmihalyi Flow Chart to find out where your true passion lies. The greater the match between your skills and interests, the greater the chance of choosing a path that allows your flow. The conditions necessary to use

meditation as a means of inducing your flow state before you meditate include:

1. Finding a challenge, something you enjoy doing
2. Developing enough skill to meet the minimum requirements of the challenge
3. Having set clear goals that make the task challenging enough
4. Eliminating other distractions before attempting the challenge
5. Making sure there is enough time set aside time to get in flow state (roughly 10-15 minutes) and to complete the challenge
6. Developing mindfulness of what emotions typically arise when attempting this challenge

Using Guided Visual Imagery

The Buddhist practice of using visual imagery in meditation incorporates the use of the imagination to invoke spiritual forces that fuel spiritual realization. Any meditation that requires you to visualize or imagine something is a guided visual meditation. This includes some of the previous mediations discussed earlier, such as Big Mind meditation or experimenting with aura. Instead of invoking spirituality, some meditations using guided visual imagery can work specifically for getting in flow. According to Belleruth Naparstek, author of "Staying Well with Guided Imagery," visualized meditation consists of three basic principles.

Principle #1: The body and mind cannot tell the difference between a current sensory experience and a past sensory experience. In other words, once you immerse the mind and body with a visualization of a past or imaginary experience, the body interprets the experience as real and happening now. If you have ever recalled an embarrassing experience, you probably noticed that your body reacted as if the experience was happening all over again.

Exercise: To employ this principle to a meditation, take 10 minutes to close your eyes and visualize yourself immersed in your task or challenge as if it is happening right now. Note the physical or emotional sensations and become mindful of how your body reacts.

Principle #2: Altered states induced by meditation have a healing effect that can cause the individual to grow and change. Altered states allow you to explore new behaviors and change existing ones. When dealing with performance boosting techniques, the best way to excel is to learn how to do something better. Meditation allows you to think about mistakes and see what you can improve for next time.

Exercise: To employ this principle to a meditation, take 10 minutes to close your eyes and visualize a time in the past when you attempted your task or challenge. Become mindful of the mistakes you made and meditate on what you need to change about your approach.

Principle #3: Imagery makes mastering a challenge seem more possible. Some guided meditations call for visualizing a near impossible task, so that when you take on the actual task, it seems that much easier. For example, some guided meditations ask professional swimmers to visualize swimming through molasses so that when they prepare to swim through water, it seems much easier than what they mentally prepared for.

Exercise: To employ this principle to a meditation, take 10 minutes to close your eyes and visualize a similar but much harder version of your task or challenge. Notice how your body and mind reacts to this near impossible task. When you come out of the meditation, notice how much easier the task feels compared to your visualization. This exercise is one of the most common meditations used among martial artists, athletes and creative artists. However, this exercise, like most others, is more useful when the conditions for flow are right. A more skilled individual using this guided meditation may enter relaxation, control, or flow, whereas a less skilled individual may evoke apathy or boredom.

10-Minute Performance Meditation:
Guided Visuals for Enhanced Creativity

1. **Close your eyes, take 10 deep breaths – through the nose on the inhale, through the mouth on the exhale.** Say the world "Relax" on each out breath.

2. **Imagine standing at the top of 10 steps. Imagine seeing a door at the bottom of these steps.** Imagine taking a step and feeling more relaxed, then another and feeling even more relaxed.

3. **Imagine reaching the bottom of the steps.** Imagine opening the door and seeing your ideal place of relaxation (for example, a beach, a home, a garden).

4. **Imagine stepping through the door, into your ideal place of relaxation.** Use your senses and begin to explore this place. What does it look like, sound like, smell like, and feel like?

5. **Visualize an imaginary lake appearing in the middle of this ideal relaxation place.** Visualize a stone on the ground, then pick it up and throw the stone into the lake. Watch the ripples in the water created by the stone.

6. **As you watch the ripples, imagine that creative thoughts are beginning to flow to you.** Do not try to force anything. Just enjoy this place and stay relaxed while waiting for the creative mind to activate.

7. **When you feel sufficiently relaxed, open your eyes and take on your creative task.**

Will Power Concentration

Will Power Meditation is similar to the Big Mind Meditation in that you use visualization to gain cooperation with larger parts of your brain. The difference is that this meditation works well for performance enhancement. Using Will Power Concentration requires keeping a journal. Write down a list of objectives and goals for tomorrow's daily activities or meditative practice. Writing these goals the night before gives you some time to think about them and "sleep on it." As you lay down in bed, close your eyes and practice a breathing technique. If nothing about the challenge causes

negative emotions that may inhibit your performance, visualize the stages of each task and begin to visualize completing each with ease. It may also help to visualize challenges that arise, and overcoming these challenges. If something about the challenge causes fear or anxiety, say the task aloud and ask yourself what about this task causes fear or anxiety. As discussed earlier, sometimes naming a fear serves to lessen its power in the mind. The purpose of will power concentration is to command the unconscious mind into an understanding of what you are asking it to do and gaining its compliance.

Healing Meditations

In Chapter 1, we explored how meditation correlates with mental, physical and emotional well-being. When we meditate, the nervous system activates *the relaxation response* which lowers the body's adrenaline levels, softens the muscles, and decreases blood pressure. The same concept applies to healing meditations. Healing meditations work to eliminate injuries caused by the stress response. Since healing meditation works to maintain the body's wellness, it can also be seen as a way to boost performance. Light is a common visual image that meditators use for healing. To experiment with light as a healing practice, assume any meditative posture, begin breathing to quiet the mind, and after a few minutes, imagine a sphere of light suspended a foot above your head. Imagine this sphere full of positive, healing energy. If you are religious, this sphere may represent your spiritual leader. Next, imagine the sphere of light growing more luminous as it draws in all the benevolent forces of the universe until the light radiates everything around you. As the light radiates, imagine it streaming its energy down into your body, replacing pain and stress with vitality and health. Feel the light energy soaking into your muscles and cells, leaving you energized and strong. Imagine the sphere itself descending into your heart, creating harmony and peace until you begin to radiate this energy to every other being in the world. For aches and pains, also consider using the meditative practice below.

10-Minute Healing Meditation: The 4-4-8 Procedure

1. Assume a meditative posture, close your eyes, and inhale deeply for four seconds.

2. At the end of four seconds, hold your breath for another four seconds.

3. At the end of four seconds, release your breath and exhale for another eight seconds.

4. **At the end of eight seconds, inhale for four seconds and visualize that you are breathing in a cool, bluish, healthy air.** Visualize the air flowing like water into your nose, feeling it cleanse your body, and feeling its coolness soothe your lungs.

5. **At the end of four seconds, hold the healthy air on your lungs for four seconds.** As you hold the breath, envision the tension and stress gathering in your lungs, ready to expunge on the exhale.

6. At the end of four seconds, exhale for eight seconds, and release the tension gathered in your lungs.

7. Repeat as many times as you want, and adjust the length of the inhale and exhale according to your needs.

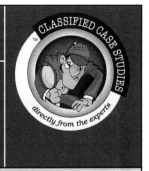

CASE STUDY: PERFORMANCE ENHANCEMENT

Brian Sheen
Florida Institute for Complementary
and Alternative Medicine
Boynton Beach, FL
drbriansheen@yahoo.com
www.BrianSheen.com

Meditation is a developmental process of learning how to create attention and inner focus while expanding your awareness of the bigger picture of Life. Feeling grounded and connected to existence provides an opportunity to tune in to the deeper powers of the body and mind when you feel aligned to the flow of life energy. Instead of struggling to fulfill your desires, you learn to move with the currents and ride the waves of existence. Being in tune with the life energies can enhance the result of *any* action, as the action becomes an expression of life and existence. You become the vehicle for extending this action in whatever action that involves you.

For the last 40 years, I have practiced and taught thousands of individuals to develop their attention to enhance their task performance objectives. I have worked with presidents of Fortune 500 companies, major hospitals, politicians, actors, writers, football players, golfers, doctors, nurses, teachers, accountants, waiters, secretaries, and students. Using meditative practices, my students have developed improvements in their ability to get results in their personal and professional actions. As a part of a core practice, I have developed a Seven Keys for Attention Development Program, which has helped individuals become calmer and more focused.

Most of my students attend my classes to improve upon a number of different personal or professional tasks, such as wanting to focus better at work, wanting to improve sleep patterns, wanting to increase their creativity, wanting to improve communication with co-workers or loved ones, or wanting to reduce blood pressure medications. To achieve performance results, I have found that the clear mind--open heart meditation is one of the most effective techniques. In addition to enhanced task performance, my students report drastic improvements in their emotional state of being. When the mind is calm, only then can the body function at optimal levels. This is so important to being happier, healthier, and more empowered in every area of life.

Conclusion

Our hope in writing this book is that you have come away with a better understanding of what it takes to reduce stress and anxiety through effective meditation. An experienced meditator uses many methods to quiet the mind and reduce stress. As you continue to practice the techniques described in this book, you will gain experience and become the kind of person with inner and outer balance. When the outside world becomes stressful that is where your practice comes in. You will be a master of the balanced mind. The way the world creates stress may change over time, but its changes will always create new opportunities for you to balance your life. Make it your mission in life to remain awake *and be the change you want to see in the world.* The road ahead is both challenging and rewarding. We wish you luck.

Before closing this book and heading off to use these techniques, examine the questions at the end of this conclusion as they will help you determine just how ready you are to achieve effective meditation within 10 minutes. As you set out in life, remember that true knowledge is knowledge of self, and true happiness means releasing yourself from ego-driven attachments,

desires and beliefs. As Bruce Lee once said, "Empty your mind. Be formless, shapeless…like water. If you put water into a cup, it becomes the cup. If you put water into a bottle, it becomes the bottle. If you put water in a teapot, it becomes the teapot. Water can flow, or it can crash. Be water, my friend."

Questions to ask after reading this book

1. Do I have a better understanding of meditation?
2. Do I feel comfortable using the strategies and protocols outlined in this book?
3. Do I feel it is feasible to support my meditative practice in the manners described?
4. Do I feel these strategies will reduce stress, eliminate anxiety, eliminate misunderstanding, reduce conflicts and enrich my life?
5. Is there any information I am unsure about?
6. Where can I find information (in this book or otherwise) that will lead me to my answer?

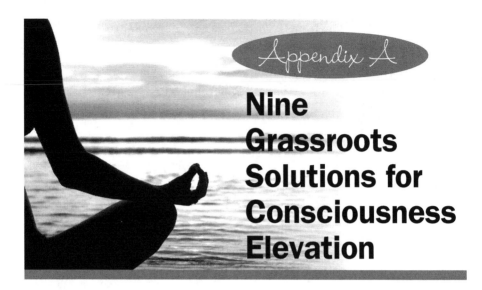

Nine Grassroots Solutions for Consciousness Elevation

1. **Heal your individual worldview.** Help ease the suffering of others instead of seeking personal comfort.

2. **Change the quality of info you give your attention to.** Information that creates depression puts you into a negative trance state of mind. You are the product of the information you take in.

3. **Develop true present moment awareness.** Do not focus on regret over the past or anxiety of the future. Avoid focusing on the tiny details of everyday living. Be in the moment but see the bigger picture around you from a global perspective.

4. **Change diet; eat healthy whole foods.** Avoid unnecessary drugs and detach from poisonous foods. Focus on organic local food production. Start an alkaline diet. Lower your intake of carbohydrates and sugars. Eating right will help you focus your mind. You are what you eat.

5. **Practice non-support of the ego-based dominator culture.** This culture continues to unbalance people more and more. Participants of this culture are people we know, even those we love. Try to bring the information to people to the extent that they are capable of under-

standing it. We think of them as contributors to the negative, but they are the most in need of spiritual healing because their consciousness may be the most devastated. When enough people come to a level of consciousness that prevents manipulation by external influences, then local and global conflicts will end.

6. **Develop mindfulness by quieting the mind.** Empty your thoughts for a time to experience pure conscious awareness. But do not allow it to shut down critical thinking permanently. Different meditations — sitting walking, stretching, binaural beat music, and scented candles — are helpful. Relinquishing control is the message you hear if you turn down the volume. The illusion of control is what brings suffering upon you. Live in harmony with that which is. You are only in control of the way you think, feel, and act. Watch your actions.

7. **Learn to generate the divine within and use it for the correct reasons.** Recognize and develop consciousness. Meditative techniques can open up vistas of creativity because they open up consciousness and allow deeper connection with right brain consciousness.

8. **Practice positive thinking.** Keep a sense of humor even if your life is difficult. It is important to see the glass as half-full and recognize small steps in the right direction.

9. **Help others awaken.** So many people have a poisoned worldview and need your understanding, not your hatred, contempt or resentment. They remain attached to egoism and want to stay in that state of disconnection. It is hard because you want to be angry that they do not understand. Work with them, and if they do not want to listen then you have to allow them to stay in that state. Eventually, they will discover the true nature of existence. It is a lesson that no one escapes, only delayed. Always examine yourself before you examine others. Remember that you have fallen from your higher self and acted in ways you are not proud to admit. A true teacher always remembers

to enable the proper operation of the mind. Responsibility is "response ability," the ability to respond in a balanced way to the circumstances and the situation that you find yourself in. Understand that everything is connected. Every beings' suffering is our own suffering; we are all connected.

List presented by Mark Passio, 2012 Free Your Mind Conference.

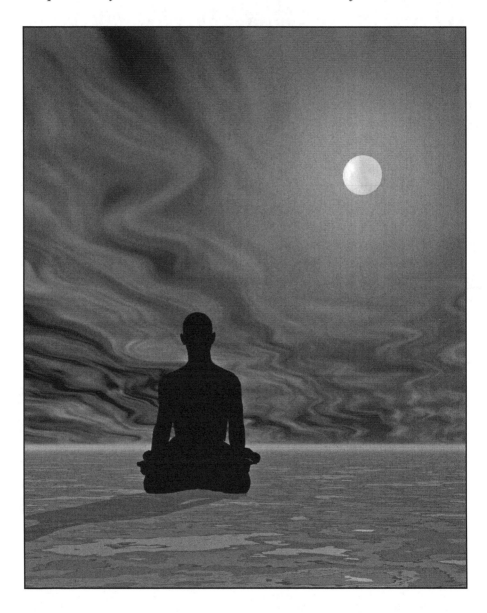

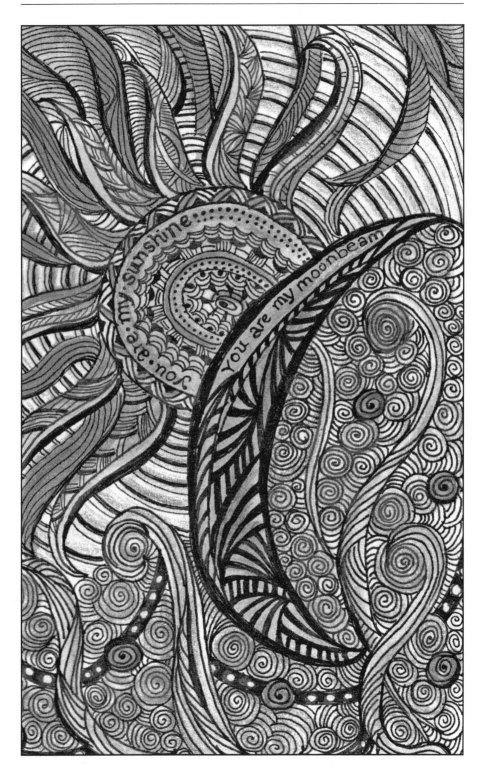

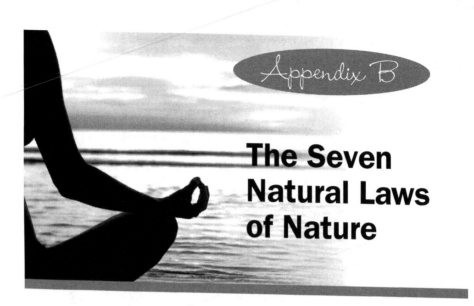

The Seven Natural Laws of Nature

The law of perpetual transmutation — Directed energy always manifests into physical form. Ideas that we hold in our mind and give attention will manifest in reality.

The law of relativity — Nothing is good or bad, nice or ugly, smart or stupid. We have to relate all of it to something. If you think something is bad, relate your situation to something much worse, and it will become good. (Ex: saying, "This situation is bad, but I don't have cancer.")

The law of vibration and attraction — Nothing rests, everything vibrates. Feeling is conscious awareness. Vibrations in our mind dictate what we attract, so think positive to attract positive situations.

The law of polarity — Everything has an opposite: smart/stupid, good/bad, left/right.... You must look for the good in people and situations, and you will attract more good things in your life.

The law of rhythm — Good and bad things in life happen in rhythms and cycles. When you encounter a bad stretch in life, do not feel bad. The rhythm of life will not stay that way forever. Things will get better, so think of good times that are coming.

The law of cause and effect — Whatever we think and feel will manifest in some way in the future. Action creates reaction. Think good thoughts and treat every situation and everyone with respect; it will come back to you.

The law of gestation —Your goals and ideas are spiritual seeds that need time to incubate. They will manifest when the time is right.

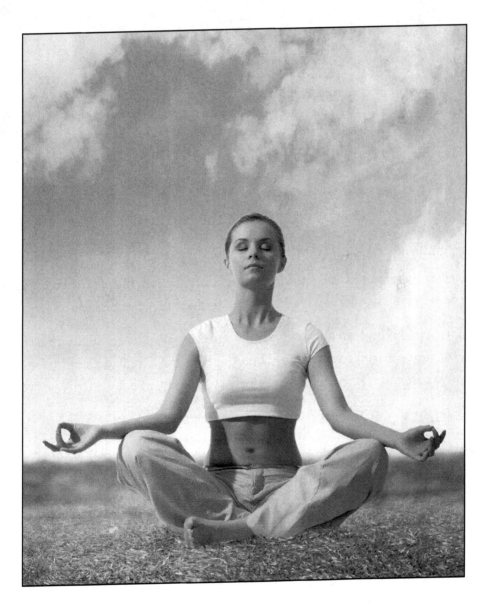

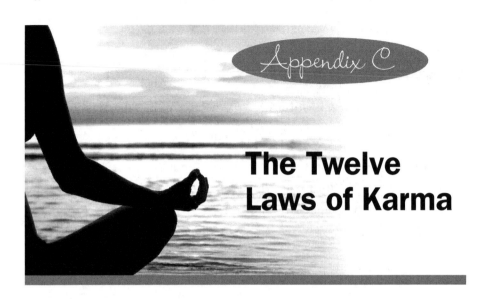

The Twelve Laws of Karma

The law of cause and effect — Whatever we put out in the universe comes back to us.

The law of creation — Life does not just happen; it requires our participation. What we want to have in our life requires action.

The law of humility — If we refuse to see the good in people, but instead see them as enemies or possessing negative traits, we are not tuned into a higher level of existence.

The law of growth — Wherever we go, there we are. To grow in spirit, we must change ourselves, not the people, places or things around us. When we change our heart our life changes, too.

The law of responsibility — Nothing is ever wrong except what we need to change in ourselves. We mirror our environment and our environment mirrors us. We must take responsibility for what we create in our lives.

The law of connection — No task, thought, gesture, behavior or intention is inconsequential because everything in the universe is connected. Past, present and future are connected.

The law of focus — We cannot think of two things at the same time. When our focus is on spiritual values, it is impossible for us to have lower thoughts such as greed or anger.

The law of giving and hospitality — When we learn valuable life lessons, we must put into practice what we have learned.

The law of here and now — Dwelling in the past prevents us from being present. Hanging on to old thoughts, patterns, behaviors, and dreams prevents us from having new ones.

The law of change — History repeats itself until we learn the lessons that we need to change our path.

The law of patience and reward — All rewards require an honest effort. True joy is the process of doing rather than achieving.

The law of significance and inspiration — Whatever we put into life is what we get back. Weak efforts have no impact. Loving efforts lift up and inspire the whole.

Source: 12 Little Known Laws of Karma (That Will Change Your Life)
http://www.in5d.com/12-little-known-laws-of-karma.html

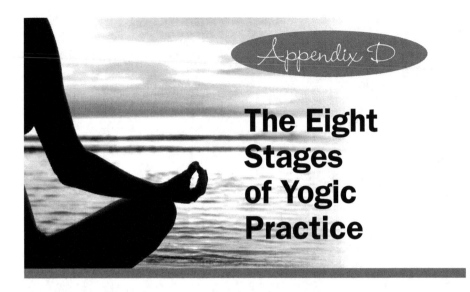

The Eight Stages of Yogic Practice

Sanskrit	English
1. *Yama*	Moral codes (what you should not do)
2. *Niyama*	Self-purification (what you should do)
3. *Asana*	Posture
4. *Pranayama*	Energy control
5. *Pratyahara*	Withdrawal from the senses
6. *Dharana*	Concentration
7. *Dhyana*	Deep meditation
8. *Samadhi*	Union with God

Source: "10 Minute Meditation for Deep Relaxation," by Dr. Alka Khurana

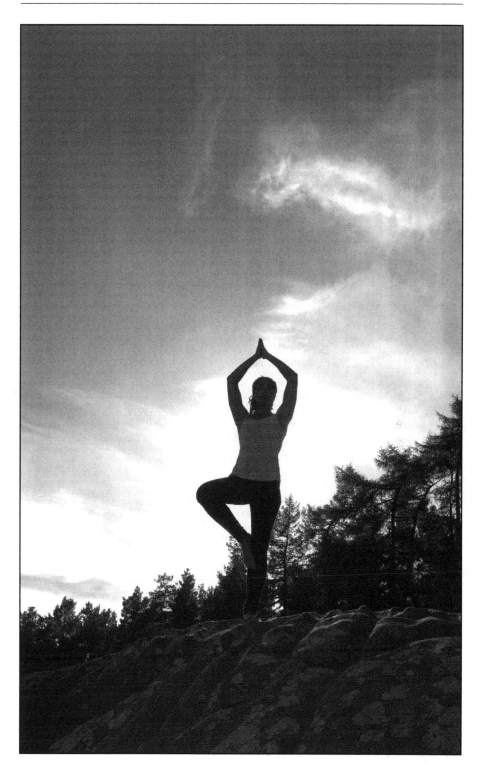

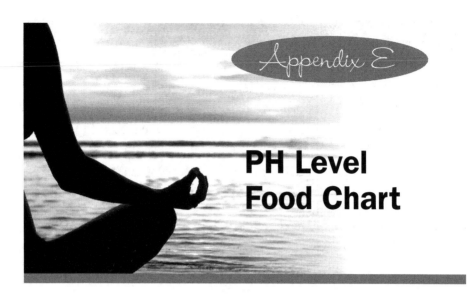

PH Level Food Chart

Your targeted acid/alkaline balance should be 7.2 (or slightly alkaline).

The body needs 20-30 percent of acid-forming foods and 70-80 percent of alkaline forming foods to maintain an acid-alkaline balance.

Acid ratio should come from the acid-forming foods of grains, legumes and nuts, not the other acid forming foods.

Healthy Alkaline Foods (Eat lots of them!)	Foods For Moderate Consumption	Acidic Foods (Eat less of them!)
Vegetables	**Fruits**	**Meat, Poultry, And Fish**
Alfalfa Grass +29.3	**(In Season, For Cleansing Only Or With Moderation)**	Beef -34.5
Asparagus +1.3	Apples -8,5	Chicken (to -22) -18.0
Barley Grass +28.1	Apricot -9.5	Eggs (to -22)
Broccoli +14.4	Banana, Ripe -10.1	Liver -3.0
Brussels Sprouts +0.5	Banana, Unripe +4.8	Ocean Fish -20.0
Cabbage Lettuce, Fresh +14.1	Black Currant -6.1	Organ Meats -3.0
Cauliflower +3.1	Blueberry -5.3	Oysters -5.0
Cayenne Pepper +18.8	Cantaloupe -2.5	Pork -38.0
Celery +13.3	Cherry, Sour +3.5	Veal -35.0
Chives +8.3	Cherry, Sweet -3.6	

Healthy Alkaline Foods (Eat lots of them!)	Foods For Moderate Consumption	Acidic Foods (Eat less of them!)
Comfrey +1.5	Coconut, Fresh +0.5	**Milk And Milk Products**
Cucumber, Fresh +31.5	Cranberry -7.0	Buttermilk +1.3
Dandelion +22.7	Currant -8.2	Cream -3.9
Dog Grass +22.6	Date -4.7	Hard Cheese -18.1
Endive, Fresh +14.5	Fig Juice Powder -2.4	Homogenized Milk -1.0
French Cut Green Beans +11.2	Gooseberry, Ripe -7.7	Quark -17.3
Garlic +13.2	Grape, Ripe -7.6	**Bread, Biscuits (Stored Grains/Risen Dough)**
Green Cabbage December Harvest +4.0	Grapefruit -1.7	Rye Bread -2.5
Green Cabbage, March Harvest +2.0	Italian Plum -4.9	White Biscuit -6.5
	Mandarin Orange -11.5	White Bread -10.0
Kamut Grass +27.6	Mango -8.7	Whole-Grain Bread -4.5
Lamb's Lettuce +4.8	Orange -9.2	Whole-Meal Bread -6.5
Leeks (Bulbs) +7.2	Papaya -9.4	
Lettuce +2.2	Peach -9.7	**Nuts**
Onion +3.0	Pear -9.9	Cashews -9.3
Peas, Fresh +5.1	Pineapple -12.6	Peanuts -12.8
Peas, Ripe +0.5	Raspberry -5.1	Pistachios -16.6
Red Cabbage +6.3	Red Currant -2.4	
Rhubarb Stalks +6.3	Rose Hips -15.5	**Fats**
Savoy Cabbage +4.5	Strawberry -5.4	Butter -3.9
Shave Grass +21.7	Tangerine -8.5	Corn Oil -6.5
Sorrel +11.5	Watermelon -1.0	Margarine -7.5
Soy Sprouts +29.5	Yellow Plum -4.9	
Spinach (Other Than March) +13.1	**Non-Stored Grains**	**Sweets**
Spinach, March Harvest +8.0	Brown Rice -12.5	Artificial Sweeteners -26.5
	Wheat -10.1	Barley Malt Syrup -9.3
Sprouted Chia Seeds +28.5		Beet Sugar -15.1
Sprouted Radish Seeds +28.4	**Nuts**	Brown Rice Syrup -8.7
	Hazelnuts -2.0	Chocolate -24.6
Straw Grass +21.4	Macadamia Nuts -3.2	Dr. Bronner's Barley
Watercress +7.7	Walnuts -8.0	Dried Sugar Cane Juice -18.0
		Fructose -9.5

Healthy Alkaline Foods (Eat lots of them!)	Foods For Moderate Consumption	Acidic Foods (Eat less of them!)
Wheat Grass +33.8	**Fish**	Honey -7.6
White Cabbage +3.3	Fresh Water Fish -11.8	Malt Sweetener -9.8
Zucchini +5.7		Milk Sugar -9.4
	Fats	Molasses -14.6
Root Vegetables	Coconut Milk -1.5	Turbinado Sugar -9.5
Beet +11.3	Sunflower Oil -6.7	White Sugar -17.6
Carrot +9.5		
Horseradish +6.8		**Condiments**
Kohlrabi +5.1		Ketchup -12.4
Potatoes +2.0		Mayonnaise -12.5
Red Radish +16.7		Mustard -19.2
Rutabaga +3.1		Soy Sauce -36.2
Summer Black Radish +39.4		Vinegar -39.4
Turnip +8.0		
White Radish (Spring) +3.1		**Beverages**
		Beer -26.8
Fruits		Coffee -25.1
Avocado (Protein) +15.6		Fruit Juice Sweetened
Fresh Lemon +9.9		Fruit Juice, Packaged, Natural -8.7
Limes +8.2		Liquor -38.7
Tomato +13.6		Tea (Black) -27.1
		Wine -16.4
Non-Stored Organic Grains And Legumes		
Buckwheat Groats +0.5		**Miscellaneous**
Granulated Soy (Cooked Ground Soy Beans) +12.8		Canned Foods
Lentils +0.6		Microwaved Foods
Lima Beans +12.0		Processed Foods
Quinoa +		
Soy Flour +2.5		
Soy Lecithin (Pure) +38.0		
Soy Nuts (soaked Soy Beans, Then Air Dried) +26.5		

Healthy Alkaline Foods (Eat lots of them!)	Foods For Moderate Consumption	Acidic Foods (Eat less of them!)
Soybeans, Fresh +12.0		
Spelt +0.5		
Tofu +3.2		
White Beans (Navy Beans) +12.1		
Nuts		
Almonds +3.6		
Brazil Nuts +0.5		
Seeds		
Caraway Seeds +2.3		
Cumin Seeds +1.1		
Fennel Seeds +1.3		
Flax Seeds +1.3		
Pumpkin Seeds +5.6		
Sesame Seeds +0.5		
Sunflower Seeds +5.4		
Wheat Kernel +11.4		
Fats (Fresh, Cold-Pressed Oils)		
Borage Oil +3.2		
Evening Primrose Oil +4.1		
Flax Seed Oil +3.5		
Marine Lipids +4.7		
Olive Oil +1.0		

Table: pH scale of alkaline and acid forming foods

*Table Reprinted with Permission from **www.balance-ph-diet.com**.*

Hip Opening Postures

ip Openers powerfully stimulate and balance the muladhara (root) and svadisthana (sacral) chakras.

Hip openers work the epicenter of your body, where many old emotions can get stuck. Through creating balance in these chakras, we can become grounded, comfortable within our own identity and inherently creative.

Reclining Butterfly

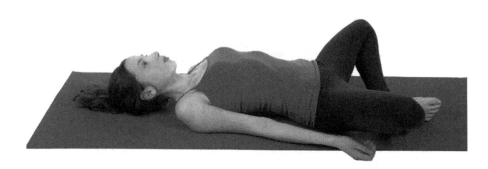

Wide-legged Forward Bend

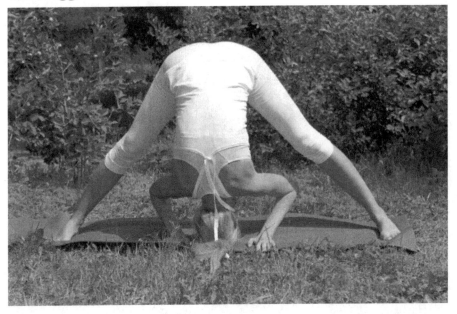

Warrior II

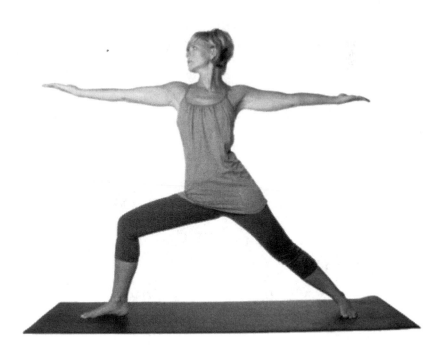

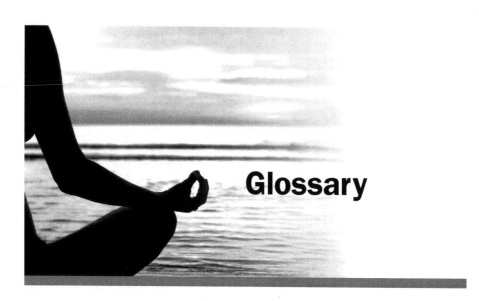

Glossary

acid — Any watery solution with a pH of less than 7, and thus a higher concentration of hydrogen ions.

alkaline — Any watery solution with a pH of more than 7, and thus a lower concentration of hydrogen ions.

alpha — The frequency range of brain wave activity that falls between 8 and 12 Hertz, or cycles per second.

ambient — A type of music that emphasizes tone and atmosphere.

asanas — The third path of Yoga. Postures for internal discipline.

ashtanga vinyasa Yoga — Form of Yoga focusing on strength building through the alignment of movement and breath. Also known as Power Yoga.

astral projection — An out-of-body experience that assumes the essence of spirit, which separates from the physical self during meditation to explore time and space.

aura — Vibratory energy that expands and contracts depending on the emotions and thoughts you emit.

beta — The frequency range of brain wave activity that falls between 12.5 and 30 Hertz, or cycles per second.

bikram Yoga — Form of Yoga that focuses on breathing techniques in a room set to 105 degrees Fahrenheit.

binaural beats — A sound with specific amplitude and frequency created by combining two different tones. Used for the purpose of altering brain waves and consciousness.

bodhicitta — Buddhist term for an awaked heart and mind.

bodhisattva — Buddhist term for person who seeks enlightenment with the goal of benefiting others.

cardiovascular system — The body's organ system responsible for transporting nutrients and removing gaseous waste from the body.

chakras — Energetic openings located at seven points along the body.

citta — Buddhist term for emotional and mental states, or mind and heart.

corpse pose — Yogic pose that requires lying down on your back with both arms and legs slightly spread apart, letting all the body's muscles relax.

delta — The frequency range of brain wave activity that falls between 0.1 and 3 Hertz, or cycles per second.

dharma — Hindu term for behaviors considered to be in accord with life and the universe.

dhyana — The seventh path of Yoga. Meditation.

diksha — Sanskrit word for the preparation of a religious ceremony in Hindu and Buddhist religions.

dharana — The sixth path of Yoga. Concentration.

ego — Latin or Greek term referring to the psychic apparatus that sees itself as "I."

ego drive — The impulse derived from the ego to protect and satisfy itself.

empty stance — A common standing meditation used in Qigong to relieve back pain whereby the meditator shifts weight off one leg and raises both arms.

energetic openings — Synonym for charkas.

energy body — Your surrounding vibratory energy known as the aura.

electroencephalogram (EEG) — A test that measures and records electrical brain wave activity by using sensors called electrodes.

esoteric — Knowledge known only by few people.

exoteric — Knowledge known by many people.

feng shui — The Chinese tradition of using colors to promote harmonization with the surrounding environment.

flow — An egoless state of consciousness characterized by effortless concentration and skilled execution of a task or challenge; also known as "being in the zone."

gamma — The fastest frequency range of brain wave activity, falls between 40 - 70 Hertz, or cycles per second.

gastrointestinal system — The body's organ system responsible for digestion.

gomden — A square meditation cushion.

hatha Yoga — Form of Yoga focusing on relaxation and stress reduction through exercises and postures.

hertz — The unit of frequency in the International System of Units.

horse stance — A common standing meditation used in Tai Chi whereby the arms raise while the knees and hips bend as if the meditator is about to sit down.

hot Yoga — Form of Yoga practice in a room temperature of 105 degrees for the purpose of sweating toxins out through the pores.

hypnotherapy — Therapy practiced by psychologists to create unconscious changes in patients' thoughts, attitudes, behaviors or emotions.

immune system — Biological structures and processes within the body that protects against disease.

isochronic tones — A form of audio brainwave entrainment that combines two equal intensity pulses with intervals of silence while gradually increasing pulse speeds.

kundalini — The divine feminine "Shakti" or spiritual body energy released during in a state of deep meditation, which purifies the body and mind.

kundalini Yoga — Form of Yoga that focuses on raising the kundalini

energy through the spine to produce a feeling of ecstasy.

lymphatic system — The part of the circulatory system that serves an important function for the immune system.

mantra — A acred utterance that caries the vibratory energy of the cosmos. Used in Buddhism as a "mind tool."

mindful-based stress reduction (MBSR) — A secular form of meditation that combines medical research with traditional forms of meditation to improve chronic disorders and diseases.

metta — Buddhist term for lovingkindness or unconditional friendliness, especially toward the self.

musculature system — The body's organ system consisting of skeletal, smooth and cardiac muscles.

nervous system — Part of the body that coordinates the voluntary and involuntary actions and transmits signals.

niyamas — The second path of Yoga. Keeping the body and mind free of impurities, being austere, and studying the sacred texts.

orgonite — A solid material cured mold that combines fiberglass resin, metal shavings, and quartz crystal. Used by meditators for protection against negative energy.

pineal gland — Gland located in the midbrain which stimulates third eye perception.

pH — The abbreviation for "power of hydrogen, " which measures is the level of hydrogen ion concentration in the human body.

prana — Sanskit term for breath.

pranayama — The fourth path of Yoga. Regulation and control of the breath.

pratyahara — The fifth path of Yoga. Withdrawl of the senses in order to still the mind.

qi — Referred to in Chinese culture as the energy regulated by the yin and yang.

relaxation response — A physical state of deep rest that the body strives to achieve.

samadhi — The eighth and final path of Yoga. Achieving unity of self with all things.

samsāra — Buddhist term for the continuous flow or repeating cycle of birth, life and death in reincarnation.

shamatha — Sanskrit term for peacefully abiding.

seiza bench — Specially designed Japanese support for sitting in proper meditative position.

shakti — Sanskrit term for energy.

stress response — the body's transition from a resting state into a state of increased biological activity.

sun salutation — Yogic pose whereby the meditator raises both arms from each side of the body until both hands touch overhead.

sushuma — Sanskrit term for the meditator's body.

systolic — The rate of blood pressure when the heart is contracting.

tantra — The meditative practice of channeling energy directly from the Universe.

tao — A metaphysical concept in Buddhism that signifies the formless and nameless energy of the universe.

theta — The frequency range of brain wave activity that falls between 4–7 Hertz, or cycles per second.

third eye — The brow chakra, or invisible eye which provides perception beyond ordinary sight.

vinyasa — Sanskrit term for practicing a series of poses.

yamas — The first path of Yoga. Non-violence, truthfulness, moderation in all things, and non-covetousness.

yang — Referred to in martial arts as the part of the body (abdomen) which stores and supplies the body's energy quantity.

yin — Referred to in martial arts as the part of the body (brain) which regulates the quality of energy collected, stored, and released by a martial artist.

zabuton — Japanese cushion for sitting.

zafu — A round meditation cushion.

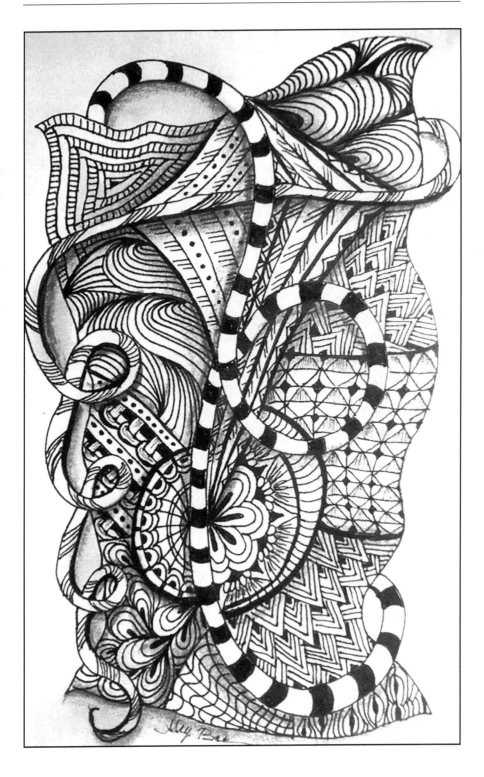

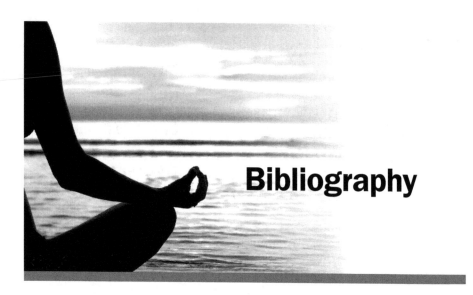

Bibliography

Allaboutspirituality.org. "Meditation and Contemplation." 2014. **www.allaboutspirituality.org/meditation.htm**.

Allen, Marc. *How to Quiet Your Mind: Relax and Silence the Voice of Your Mind, Today!* Empowerment Nation, 2011.

Amazing-green-tea.com. "Japanese Tea History: A Thousand Year Journey From China, Chanoyu to Sencha." 2014. **www.amazing-green-tea.com/japanese-tea-history.html**.

Askteal.com. How to Activate and Open Your Third Eye. 2013. **www.askteal.com/videos/how-to-activate-and-open-your-third-eye**.

Askteal.com. "Why are Spiritual Teachers so Contradictory?" 2013. **www.youtube.com/watch?v=uCMBMQjjD7I**.

Balance-ph-diet.com. "Acid Alkaline Food Chart." 2014. **www.balance-ph-diet.com/acid_alkaline_food_chart.html**.

Binauralbeatsonline.com. "Experience Gamma Brain Waves with Gamma Binaural Beats." 2010. **www.binauralbeatsonline.com/experience-gamma-brain-waves-with-gamma-binaural-beats/**.

Bodhiactivity.wordpress.com. "Pitfalls in Meditation." 2013. **http://bodhiactivity.wordpress.com/2011/02/05/potential-pitfalls-in-meditation/**.

Bodian, Stephan. *Meditation for Dummies.* John Wiley & Sons, 2012.

Brainandspinalcord.org. Infections and Organic Brain Injury. 2013. **www.brainandspinalcord.org/brain-injury/infections.html**.

Breathing.com. "The Breathing or Breath Wave and The Speed Bump of Life." 2014. **www.breathing.com/articles/breathwave.htm**.

Buddhism.about.com. "Life of Buddha." 2013. **http://buddhism.about.com/od/lifeofthebuddha/a/buddhalife.htm**.

Daringtolivefully.com. "How to Enter the Flow State." 2014. **http://daringtolivefully.com/how-to-enter-the-flow-state**.

Davich, Victor. *8 Minute Meditation: Quiet Your Mind, Change Your Life.* The Penguin Group, 2004.

Detoxsafely.org. "Herbs Commonly Used in Detox Programs." 2013. **www.detoxsafely.org/herbs_for_detox.html#detoxherbs**.

Eclecticenergies.com. "Opening the Chakras." 2014. **www.eclecticenergies.com/chakras/open.php**.

Energyopening.com. "Energy Medicine." 2013. **http://energyopening.com/index_files/Page483.htm**.

Ezinearticles.com. "Is it Easier to Learn to Meditate in a Group or Alone? The Pros and Cons of Group Meditation." 2009. **http://ezinearticles.com/?Is-it-Easier-to-Learn-to-Meditate-in-a-Group-Or-Alone?--The-Pros-and-Cons-of-Group-Meditation&id=2120516**.

Greatergood.berkeley.edu. "Here's How Mindful You Are." 2011. **http://greatergood.berkeley.edu/article/item/heres_how_mindful_you_are/**.

Harrison, Eric. *Teach Yourself to Meditate in 10 Simple Lessons.* Ulysses Press, 2007.

Healingbeats.com. "Frequently Asked Questions." 2014. **http://healingbeats.com/faq.html**.

Helpguide.org. "How Much Sleep Do You Need?" 2014. **http://www.helpguide.org/life/sleeping.htm**.

Indiaprwire.com. "Avoiding Pitfalls of Yoga and Meditation." 2009. **www.indiaprwire.com/pressrelease/health-care/2009070128604.htm**.

Isochronictone.com. Binaural Beats, Pros and Cons. 2012. **www.isochronictone.com/articles/Isochronic-Tones-Vs-Binaural-Beats-Vs-Monaural-Beats.html**.

Khurana, Alka. *10 Minute Meditation for Deep Relaxation.* Dr. Alka Khurana all rights reserved, 2013.

Livestrong.com. "Core Muscle Stretches." 2013. **www.livestrong.com/article/355186-core-muscle-stretches/**.

Livestrong.com. "Exercises that Strengthen the Diaphragm & Abdominal Muscles to Help in the Breathing Process." 2013. **www.livestrong.com/article/113103-exercises-strengthen-diaphragm-abdominal/**.

Livstrong.com. "How Does Meditation Help Athletes. 2014. **www.livestrong.com/article/458411-how-does-meditation-help-athletes/**.

Massgeneral.org. "Decreased Premature Ventricular Contractions Through Use of the Relaxation Response in Patients with Stable Ischemic Heart Disease." 1975. **www.massgeneral.org/bhi/assets/pdfs/publications/Benson%201975%20Lancet.pdf**.

Martial-art-potential.com. "Meditation in Martial Art." 2013. **www.martial-art-potential.com/meditation.html**.

Mindfullivingprograms.com. "What is Mindfulness-Based Stress Reduction." 2014. **www.mindfullivingprograms.com/whatMBSR.php**.

Ncbi.nlm.nih.gov. "An Update on Mindfulness Meditation as Self-Help Treatment for Anxiety and Depression." 2012. **www.ncbi.nlm.nih.gov/pmc/articles/PMC3500142/**.

Ncbi.nlm.nih.gov. "Brief Meditation Training Induces Smoking Reduction." 2013. **www.ncbi.nlm.nih.gov/pmc/articles/PMC3752264/**.

Ncbi.nlm.nih.gov. "Ultrastructure and X-Ray Microanalytical Study of Human Pineal Concretions." 1995. **www.ncbi.nlm.nih.gov/pubmed/7645736**.

Onlinelibrary.wiley.com. "Acute Treatment with Pulsed Electromagnetic Fields and its Effect on Fast Axonal Transport in Normal and Regenerating Nerve Vibration and Tissue." 2004. **http://onlinelibrary.wiley.com/doi/10.1002/jnr.490420512/abstract**.

Perry, Susan K. *Writing in Flow.* Writer's Digest Books, 1999.

Psy-flow.com. "Flow, the Psychology of the Optimal Experience." 2000. **www.psy-flow.com/sites/psy-flow/files/docs/flow.pdf**.

Ritecare.com. "Implications of Adrenal Insufficiency." 2001. **www.ritecare.com/nutritional/natcell_adrenals.html**.

Salzberg, Sharon. *Real Happiness: The Power of Meditation.* Workman Publishing Company, Inc., 2011.

Sagemeditation.com. "Meditation Cushion." 2014. **www.sagemeditation.com/meditation-cushion/ meditation-cushion.html.**

Scribd.com. "Healing with Water." 2004. **http://www.scribd.com/ doc/47788640/Healing-With-Water-Emoto-2004.**

Storylogue.com "How Do Writer's Unearth the Stories that Want to be Told?" 2010. **www.youtube.com/watch?v=TWxoTpINxxw.**

Swamij.com. "The Four Paths of Yoga." 2013. **www.swamij.com/four-paths-of-yoga.htm.**

Ted.com. "Four Scientific Studies on How Meditation can affect your Heart, Brain, and Creativity." 2013. **http://blog.ted.com/2013/01/11/4-scientific-studies-on-how-meditation-can-affect-your-heart-brain-and-creativity/.**

The-guided-meditation-site.com. "Meditation for Creativity." 2014. **www.the-guided-meditation-site.com/meditation-for-creativity.html.**

Totaltrainer.com. "Discover the Three Special Benefits of Good Body Alignment." 2010. **www.totaltrainer.com/exercises/discover-the-three-special-benefits-of-good-body-alignment/.**

Tripod.com "Physiological Aspects of Meditation." 2000. **http://hanshananigan.tripod.com/meditation.html.**

Wakeup-world.com. "Binaural Beats: A Meditative Gateway to Altered States of Consciousness." 2013. **http://wakeup-world.com/ 2012/07/28/binaural-beats-a-meditative-gateway-to-altered-states-of-consciousness/.**

Ymaa.com. "Why Meditation is Important in Martial Arts." 2011. **http://ymaa.com/articles/why-meditation-is-important-in-martial-arts.**

Young, Robert O., and Shelley Redford-Young. *The PH Miracle: Balance Your Diet, Reclaim Your Health.* Grand Central Life & Style, 2010.

Youtube.com. "Sovereignty, Natural Law, and Grassroots Solutions." 2012. **www.youtube.com/watch?v=pWwPFw7Dk60.**

Youtube.com. "The Healing Begins Now." 2007. **www.youtube.com/ watch?v=GUfk2QnUfQc.**

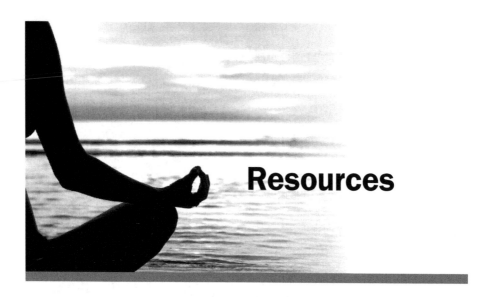

Resources

Meditation-Supporting Dietary Supplements

*The following dietary supplements are available at most health stores. Herbal supplements are listed at the end of Chapter 3.

Liquid chlorophyll or concentrated green powder (wheatgrass, barley grass, kamut grass) — Fiber rich mixture of green grasses that help alkalize the body and remove toxins. Best brands include pHorever, World Organics, Innerlight, and DeSouza's.

Omega-3 and Omega-6 oils — Protection for the heart, lowers triglycerides, cholesterol, and high blood pressure

Alkaline Water — Water that has been ionized, filtered, and contains a high concentration of election energy (Look online for the nearest store that sells alkaline water)

Sodium Bicarbonate — Found in unprocessed mineral salt; reduces bone loss, irritation, and inflammation

Vitamin D — Most common deficiency in the human body, but important to overall health; for people with severe bone density loss, the most potent and effective supplemental form is Vitamin D$_3$

Glutathione — Antioxidant that binds to acids and allows them to excrete from the body; repairs body from damage caused by stress

N-acetyl cysteine — Controls negative microforms that result from toxic hazards such as cigarette smoke

Noni fruit concentrate — Antifungal that renews cells and helps rebuild blood and body tissue

Flavonoids — Supplement for fruits and vegetables; act as acid neutralizers

Rhodium and iridium — Increases cells ability to communicate with each other

List of Companies that Carry Meditation Supplies and Accessories

Source	Purchase	Contact
Wildmind	Music, courses, incense, jewelry, DVDs, meditation timers, and more	http://secure.wildmind.org/store/home.php?cat=
Carolina Morning	Meditation benches, cushions and mats, organic bedding, books, candles, meditation bells, and more	www.zafu.net/benches.html
Dharma Crafts meditation supplies	Clothing, cushions, benches, incense and burners, bells, and gongs	www.dharmacrafts.com/100xMS/DharmaCrafts-Meditation-Supplies.html

Most Popular Ambient Recording Titles

The Orb	*A Huge Evergrowing Pulsating Brain that Rules From the Centre of the Ultraworld*	1990
The Orb	Adventures Beyond the Ultraworld	1991
Global Communication	76:14	1994
Tetsu Inoue	Ambiant Otaku	1994

Monolake	Hongkong	1997
Biosphere	Substrata	1998
Future Sound of London	Lifeforms	1998
Tim Hecker	Radio Amor	2002
Aglaia	Three Organic Experiences	2003
Helios	Eingya	2006

List of Meditation Centers

Organization	Contact Information	About
Insight Meditation Center	Insight Meditation Center of the Mid-Peninsula 108 Birch Street Redwood City, California 94062 (650) 599-3456 **www.insightmeditationcenter.org** **insightmeditationcenter@gmail.com**	Based in Redwood City, California, IMC offers support for Vipassana or Insight Meditation. Practice is guided by Gil Fronsdal and Andrea Fella. The weekly schedule includes dharma talks, Yoga practice, discussions, sitting, and meditation instruction.
Shambala	Shambala 1084 Tower Road Halifax, Nova Scotia B3H 2Y5, Canada (902) 425-4275 **http://shambala.org**	A global community with more than 170 centers around the world, Shambala offers teaching and training. Shambala views every human as fundamentally good. Through meditation, each person's fundamentally good and intelligent nature extends outward to family, society, and community.
Chakrasambara Kadampa Meditation Center	Chakrasambara Kadampa Meditation Center 322 Eighth Ave, Suite 502, New York, NY 10001 (Entrance on 26th Street, between 8th and 7th Ave.) (212) 924-6706 **www.meditationinnewyork.org**	Offers meditation classes, talks, and retreats with guidance from qualified Western teachers. Weekly classes held in Manhattan, Bronx, New Jersey, Brooklyn, Queens, Long Island, and Westchester.

Organization	Contact Information	About
Spirit Rock Meditation Center	Spirit Rock 5000 Sir Francis Drake Boulevard Woodacre, CA 94973 (415) 488-0164 Fax: (415) 488-1025 **www.spiritrock.org**	A Western dharma and retreat center offering classes and programs on Vipassana meditation.
Karuna Meditation Society	**www.karuna.ca**	Based on the teachings of Thich Nhat Hanh and Shunryu Suzuki Roshi, Karuna Meditation Society offers free, six-week meditation and discussion courses five times a year.
Austin Zen Center	Austin Zen Center 3014 Washington Square Austin, TX 78705 512-452-5777 **www.austinzencenter.org**	Based on the teachings of Shunryu Suzuki Roshi, Austin Zen Center offers classes, retreats, talks, seated meditation, and more.
Zen Center of Georgia	**www.zen-georgia.org**	Offering weekly Zazen and Okyo (chanting) meditation classes in the Zen tradition. Classes are offered in Avondale Estates and Alpharetta, Georgia.
Dahn Yoga	**www.dahnYoga.com**	Offering Yoga, meditation, and tai chi classes at centers around the United States. Instruction is also available through books and CDs sold on the website.
Sanatan Society	**www.sanatansociety.org/Yoga_and_ meditation/hatha_Yoga.htm**	Offers education and instruction in Hatha Yoga.

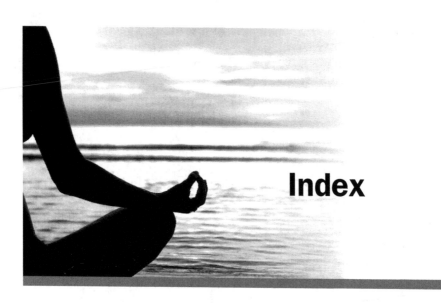

Index